Recent Results in Cancer Research 90

Early Detection of Breast Cancer

Edited by
S. Brünner B. Langfeldt P. E. Andersen

With 94 Figures and 91 Tables

Springer-Verlag
Berlin Heidelberg New York Tokyo 1984

Assoc. Professor Sam Brünner, MD
Department of Diagnostic Radiology
University of Copenhagen, Gentofte Hospital
2900 Hellerup/Copenhagen, Denmark

Assoc. Professor Bent Langfeldt, MD
Department of Diagnostic Radiology
The County Hospital, University of Århus
8000 Århus, C., Denmark

Assoc. Professor Paul E. Andersen, MD
Department of Diagnostic Radiology
University Hospital of Odense
5000 Odense, C., Denmark

Sponsored by the Swiss League against Cancer

ISBN-13: 978-3-642-82033-5 e-ISBN-13: 978-3-642-82031-1

DOI: 10.1007/978-3-642-82031-1

Library of Congress Cataloging in Publication Data. Main entry under title: Early detection of breast cancer. (Recent results in cancer research; v. 90). Based on papers presented at the 2nd International Copenhagen Symposium on Detection of Breast Cancer. Bibliography: p. Includes index. 1. Breast – Cancer – Diagnosis – Congresses. 2. Breast – Radiography – Congresses. I. Brünner, S. (Sam). 1920– . II. Langfeldt, B. (Bent), 1923– . III. Andersen, P. E. (Paul E.), 1917– . IV. International Copenhagen Symposium on Detection of Breast Cancer. V. Series. [DNLM: 1. Breast neoplasms – Diagnosis – Congresses. W1 RE106P v. 90/WP 870 E12 1983] RC 261. R35 vol. 90 616.99'4s [616.99'449075] 83-40292 [RC280.B8]

2125/3140–543210

Preface

The enormous expansion seen over the last decade in the mammographic detection of breast cancer lesions, especially the use of screening procedures for the early detection of clinically unsuspected tumors, has made it necessary to summarize the experience made by various centers in the world. The 2nd International Copenhagen Symposium on Detection of Breast Cancer afforded an opportunity of gathering scientists from all over the world to discuss the various problems of early breast cancer detection with special reference to screening procedures. This book forms a synthesis of the information presented by leading scientists from many of the world's mammographic centers, particularly those in Sweden and the USA. Hence, the reader will have the opportunity to study the outstanding work carried out by various institutes and centers of breast cancer screening. It is our sincere hope that a study of this volume will encourage other scientists to join in the work on screening procedures.

S. Brünner B. Langfeldt P. E. Andersen

Contents

*List of Contributors**

---

* The address of the principal author is given on the first page of each contribution
1 Page, on which contribution commences

Hypothetical Breast Cancer Risk from Mammography

S. A. Feig

Department of Radiology, Thomas Jefferson University Hospital,
Philadelphia, PA 19107, USA

Studies concerning the relationship of radiation and breast cancer are of more than academic value: Their purpose is to determine if there is a health risk from mammography. This chapter will review and analyze these studies in order to quantitate the hypothetical risk. The chapter that follows will compare this risk to the expected benefit from mammography. These analyses are not abstract exercises. The conclusions they draw could influence the way we practice medicine.

Risk from High Doses

An excess incidence of breast cancer has been observed in several groups of women exposed to high doses of radiation when these were compared with similar populations of nonexposed women. These were:

1. Japanese women exposed to gamma and neutron radiation from atomic bombings at Hiroshima and Nagasaki (Jablon and Kato 1972; McGregor et al. 1977; Tokunaga et al. 1979).
2. Nova Scotia sanatoria patients who received multiple chest fluoroscopies during pneumothorax treatment for tuberculosis (MacKenzie 1965; Myrden and Hiltz 1969; Myrden and Quinlan 1974).
3. Massachusetts sanatoria patients monitored by fluoroscopy during artificial pneumothorax treatment (Boice and Monson 1977).
4. Women from Rochester, New York treated with radiotherapy for post partum mastitis (Mettler et al. 1969; Shore et al. 1979).
5. Swedish women who received radiation therapy for a variety of benign breast conditions such as fibroadenomas and mastitis (Baral et al. 1977).
6. Female radium-dial workers who ingested radioactive material from paint brushes which they moistened and pointed with their tongues (Adams and Brues 1980).

Hypothetical Risk from Low Doses

It is not known whether very low doses of radiation such as those from current mammographic techniques can cause breast cancer. The risk, if it does exist, is so small that it has never been observed. Its possible existence has only been inferred from the excess breast cancer incidence seen in women exposed to high doses. Unfortunately, studies on women exposed to high doses provide little or no information regarding the possible effect from low doses.

Recent Results in Cancer Research. Vol. 90

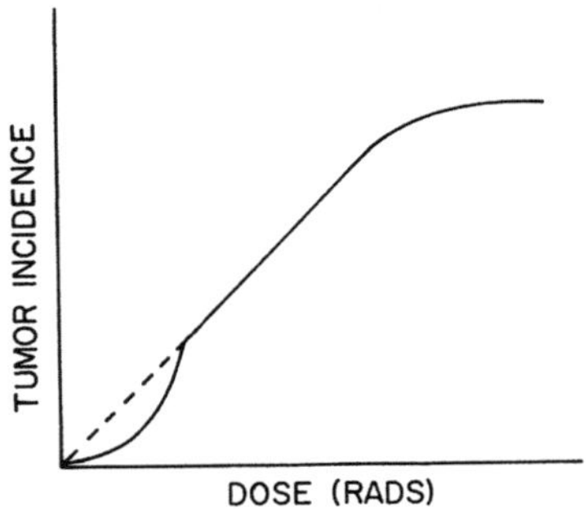

Fig. 1. Dose-response curve for radiation-induced cancers in animals

The effects of low doses of radiation can be postulated from animal experiments involving a variety of radiation-induced tumors. These experiments usually produce dose-response curves consisting of three distinct components (Fig. 1). The midportion of the curve is a rising straight line. It is linear and here the incidence is directly proportional to the first power of the dose. Over this part of the curve, the effect per rad remains constant. At higher doses, the slope decreases due to cell killing and sterilization. The lowest portion of the curve (below 25–50 rads) is concave since the incidence varies as an exponential function of the dose. Here, effect per rad is less than at medium or high doses. Extrapolation downward from the higher doses of the linear portion would result in an exaggeration of the risk (Advisory Committee on the Biological Effects of Ionizing Radiation 1972; United Nations Scientific Committee on the Effects of Atomic Radiation 1972; Casarett 1973).

In several respects, the curves for radiation-induced breast cancers in humans resemble those produced in animal models (Fig. 2). All contain a linear portion that rises with doses above 100 rads. Several studies suggest a lower slope at high doses. Unfortunately, at low doses (below 25–50 rads), the human curves provide little information to choose between a linear or curvilinear response. The lowest dose-group among women in the Rochester mastitis series received 112 rads to both breasts (Fig. 2a). The lowest dose-group in the Nova Scotia fluoroscopy series received 261 rads (Fig. 2b).

No excess incidence of cancer was recorded among Massachusetts sanatoria patients receiving a mean dose of 35 rads (Fig. 2c), among Toronto sanatoria patients exposed to 17 rads (Delarue et al. 1975), or among female radium-dial workers receiving 50 μCi or less. However, the number of women exposed to these low doses was not sufficient to exclude the possibility of the same risk per rad as exists at higher doses.

The Japanese women comprise a larger group, many of whom did receive doses below 100 rads (Fig. 2d). There may have been excess incidences of breast cancer among women receiving an average dose of 70 rads, but not for those over 30 years of age at the time of exposure. Analysis of these data is complicated by uncertainty regarding the dose estimates. Even for women under 30 years of age at the time of exposure, an estimation of risk, if any, from low doses is complicated by uncertainty regarding the dose estimates and choice of a proper baseline incidence for naturally occurring breast cancers. For each of the two cities, Hiroshima and Nagasaki, there are three possible baselines – women exposed to 1–9 rads, residents in the city at the time of the atomic bomb but not exposed to radiation, and residents out of the city at the time of the bombing. The highest possible baseline incidence is approximately 25 cases per 100,000 patient years, a value not very different from the observed incidence at low doses (Fig. 2d).

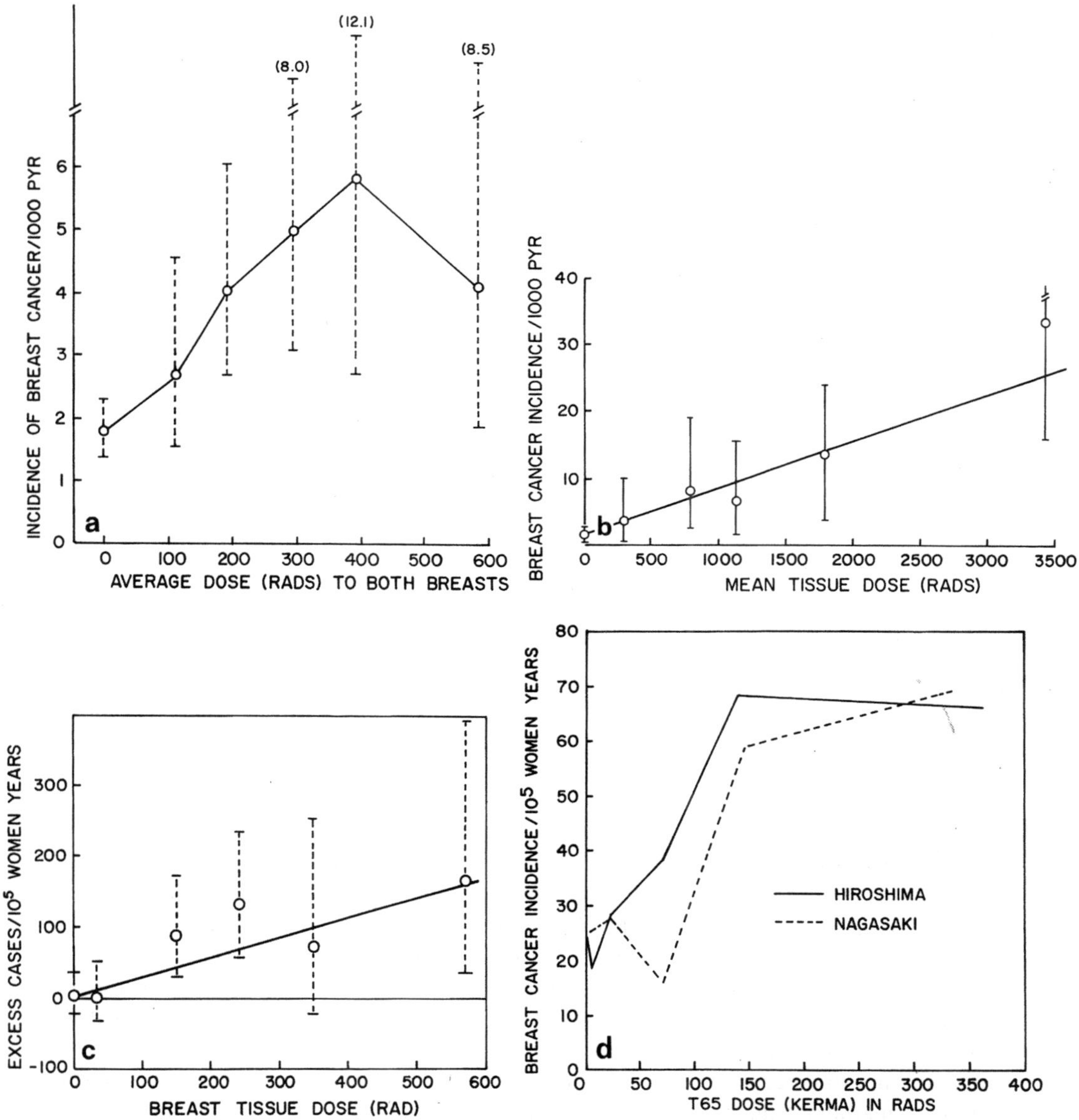

Fig. 2. Dose-response curve for radiation-induced breast cancers among **a** Rochester mastitis patients, **b** Nova Scotia sanatoria patients, **c** Massachusetts sanatoria patients, **d** Japanese A-bomb survivors. (Adapted from Advisory Committee on the Biological Effects of Ionizing Radiation 1972; Mettler et al. 1969; McGregor et al. 1977; Boice and Monson 1977; Shore et al. 1979)

If there is a risk from low doses, its numerical value would depend on the shape one ascribes to the dose-response curve in this region (Fig. 3). In a linear situation, a tenfold reduction in exposure should lead to a tenfold reduction in risk – risk per rad remains constant. In a curvilinear (quadratic) situation, the drop in cancer incidence would be even greater. The risk per rad at low doses would be one-half or one-third that expected from a linear extrapolation.

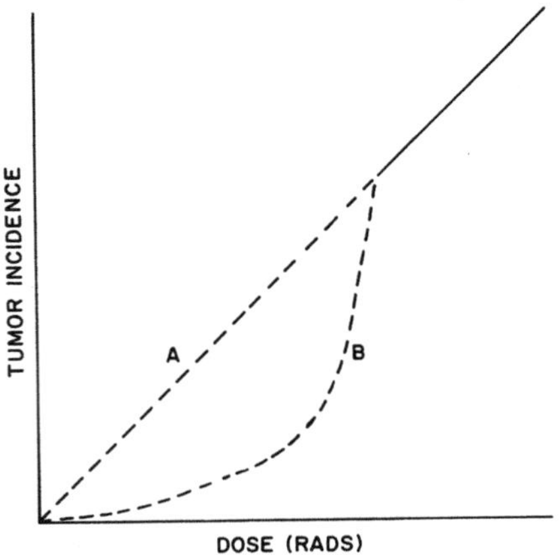

Fig. 3. Possible dose-response curves for low levels of ionizing radiation – linear *(A)* and curvilinear *(B)*

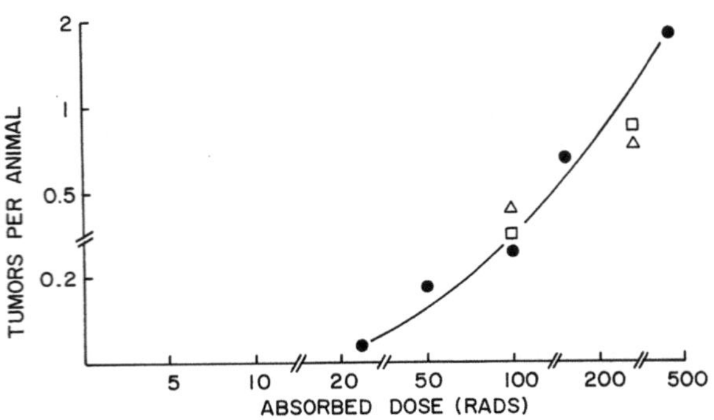

Fig. 4. Breast tumors per rat vs X-ray dose. (Adapted from Rossi and Kellerer 1972)

Most animal experiments involving radiation-induced tumors show a curvilinear response at low doses (Fig. 4). This type of response is also seen for radiation-induced leukemia among Japanese A-bomb survivors. These findings have been explained by the dual radiation action hypothesis of Kellerer and Rossi, in which carcinogenesis results from the nearly simultaneous inactivation of two separate genetic loci. Under conditions of low radiation saturation, one site can repair itself before the second one is hit (Rossi and Kellerer 1972; Kellerer and Rossi 1972).

In an attempt to determine the precise low-dose risk for breast cancer in humans, several elaborate mathematical methods such as curve-fitting and contingency-table analysis have been applied to the human data. These efforts have been basically ineffective because of the small number of women exposed to low doses. There is a strong linear component at moderate to high doses, but below 25 rads it is not certain if a linear or a quadratic component is dominant (Land et al. 1980).

For human cancers in general, the recently issued Committee on the Biological Effects of Ionizing Radiation (BEIR) III report has employed a combined linear-quadratic model, in which risk is intermediate between a linear and a pure quadratic response. In this case, the estimate from the linear model is said to represent the upper limits and the quadratic model the lower limits of risk. It is not known whether the dose-response curve for human breast cancer follows the pattern set by most other human and animal cancers at low-dose levels or whether it represents an exception with a linear response down to 0 rad (Committee on the Biological Effects of Ionizing Radiation 1980).

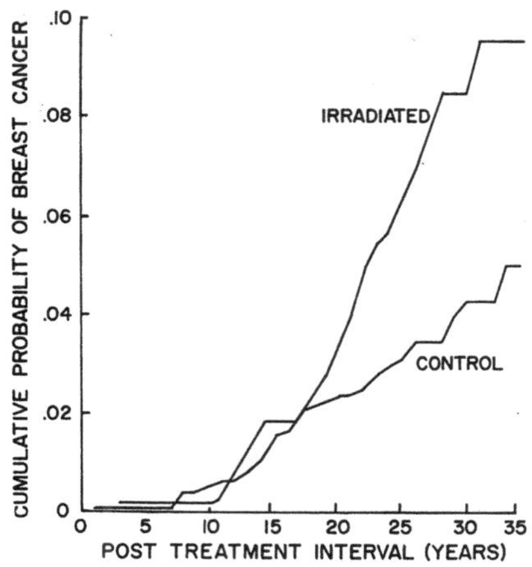

Fig. 5. Determination of latent period for radiation-induced breast cancers in the Rochester mastitis series. (Modified from Shore et al. 1979)

Radiogenic breast cancers in humans do not appear until a minimum of 10 years following exposure. For younger women, such as those in the Rochester mastitis series, the latent period was 15–20 years (Fig. 5). The duration of the carcinogenic effect is unknown, but all studies indicate that it persists for at least another 15 years and a further follow-up is necessary to determine its actual length. For the years following this latent period, a risk estimate of 7.5 excess cancers/million women/year/rad has been made for the three main groups of Western women studied (Committee on the Biological Effects of Ionizing Radiation 1980). This estimate represents a linear extrapolation from high doses and is used in the absence of any significant low-dose human breast cancer data. It probably represents a substantial overestimate, which can be considered the upper limits of risk.

Age-Related Sensitivity

The above estimate is derived from populations consisting largely of individuals under 30 years of age. When these populations are further analyzed, a considerable dependence of radiation sensitivity on the age at the time of exposure is evident. The breasts of women 30 years of age or older at the time of exposure have been found to be considerably less susceptible to radiation than those of younger women (Feig 1977, 1978, 1979a, 1979b, 1980).

For Nova Scotia sanatoria patients, cancer induction in women over 30 years of age was only 20% that seen in younger women when a control incidence of 1% was subtracted from each age interval (Table 1) (United Nations Scientific Committee on the Effects of Atomic Radiation 1972). Among Massachusetts sanatoria patients 30 years of age or older at the time of exposure, no excess breast cancers were evident (Fig. 6). Swedish women, too, showed a decrease in radiation sensitivity with increased age at the time of exposure, although the steep decline (Fig. 7) may be partially due to the higher doses received by older women.

The Japanese data indicate that for women over 35 years of age at the time of exposure, the absolute risk was less than half that seen in younger women (Table 2). In fact, no increased cancer risk was found in Japanese women exposed at 20 years of age or older to doses

Table 1. Breast cancer incidence vs age at exposure for Nova Scotia sanatoria patients (United Nations Scientific Committee on the Effects of Atomic Radiation 1972)

Patients	Age at exposure (years)	Incidence
Monitored by fluoroscopy	0–19	10%
	20–29	13%
	30–60+	3%
Control	0–60+	1%

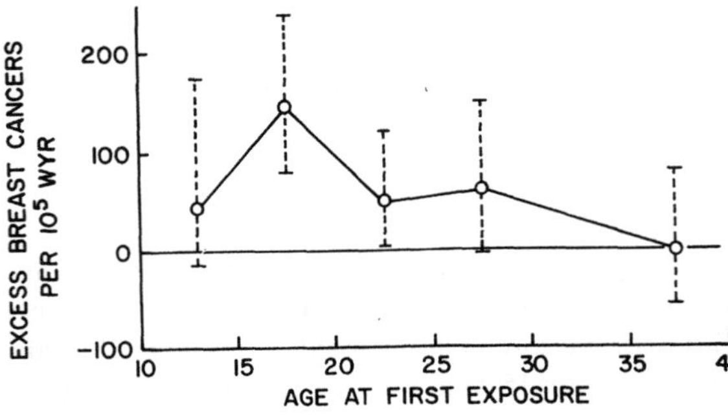

Fig. 6. Excess breast cancer risk vs age at exposure for Massachusetts sanatoria patients. (Modified from Boice and Monson 1977)

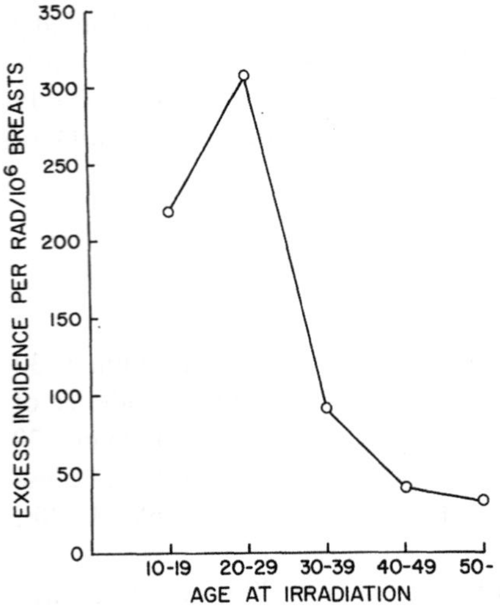

Fig. 7. Excess breast cancer risk vs age at exposure for Swedish radiotherapy patients

below 100 rads. An increased incidence for this dose-range was found only in those exposed between 10 and 19 years of age (Table 3). Since the Japanese population was larger and contained a wider age-range than did the Western groups, the National Cancer Institute used it to obtain a risk adjustment factor of 0.45 for women over 30 years of age. When this factor is multiplied by the risk estimate of 7.5 excess cancers/million women/year/rad seen in Western populations, this estimate is reduced to 3.5 excess cancers/million women/year/rad for Western women over 30 years of age at the time of exposure (Upton et al. 1977).

Table 2. Absolute breast cancer risk vs age at exposure for Japanese A-bomb survivors (McGregor et al. 1977)

Age at exposure (years)	Risk[a]
10–19	4.0
20–34	1.2
35–49	0.9
50+	1.1

[a] Excess cases/10^6 patients/rad/year

Table 3. Relative breast cancer risk vs radiation dose and age at exposure for A-bomb survivory (McGregor et al. 1977)

Age at exposure (years)	Relative risk according to dose[a]	
	10–99 rads	100+ rads
10–19	5.6	8.7
20–34	0.8	3.1
35–49	1.1	1.9
50+	1.0	3.0

[a] Relative risk of 1.0 means no excess risk

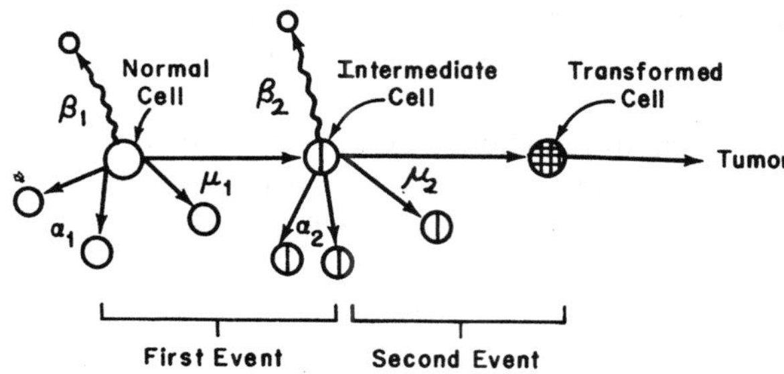

Fig. 8. Two-stage mechanism proposed to explain age-related sensitivity to radiation. (Moolgavkar et al. 1980)

Several theories have been advanced to explain why radiation risk depends on age at the time of exposure. Moolgavkar et al. (1980) postulate that breast cancer evolves in two stages and that the effect of radiation or any other carcinogen is to act on the second step, to transform intermediate cells into tumor cells. Susceptibility to radiation, or any other carcinogen, would depend on the number of cells in this intermediate pool and on the rate of cell division. Parity and older age are believed to reduce both of these factors (Fig. 8).

Korenman (1980) has suggested that the susceptibility to radiation depends on the ratio of estrogen to progesterone in the blood at the time of radiation exposure. This ratio is highest during adolescence, a period of anovulatory cycles, inadequate luteal phases, and unopposed estrogenic stimulation. This so-called estrogen window may be closed by increasing age and/or parity. To a very limited extent, it may reopen during the perimenopausal period.

Hypothetical Risk from Mammography

This risk estimate of 3.5 cancers/million women/year/rad means that if one million women aged 30 years or older each received a mean breast dose of 1 rad, there would, after a minimal latent period of 10 years, be an excess incidence of 3.5 cancers each year in the population. Examination with current low-dose technique (mean breast dose of 0.17 rad for a two-view study) would carry a hypothetical risk of about one excess cancer case/year/2 million women examined. Assuming a 50% breast cancer mortality rate, the hypothetical risk would be one excess death/4 million women examined. This level of risk, one death/4 million women/year, is extremely small and can be equated with the following (Pochin 1978): 100 miles travelled by air, 15 miles travelled by car, smoking one-quarter of one cigarette, $^1/_3$ min of mountain climbing, and 5 min of being a man aged 60 years. Another means of appreciating the very small risk from mammography is by a comparison with the natural breast cancer incidence. A risk of one excess breast cancer per 2 million women examined can be compared with the much larger magnitude of natural breast cancer incidence: 800 cases/million women/year at the age of 40 years, 1,800 cases/million women/year at the age of 50 years, and 2,500 cases/million women/year at the age of 65 years (Seidman 1980).

The pathologic appearance of radiation-induced and naturally occurring breast cancer is indistinguishable when analyzed by such factors as lesion size, lymph node status, histologic type, and grade (Dvoretsky et al. 1980). Radiation-induced and naturally occurring breast cancers can be distinguished only in a statistical sense. For radiogenic cancers in general, the population size required to demonstrate the presence or absence of risk at any given dose level is proportional to the inverse square of the dose. If a population of 1,000 people is needed to demonstrate a risk from 100 rads, then a population of 10 million people is necessary to prove or disprove the risk from 1 rad (National Council on Radiation Protection and Measurements 1980; Land 1980). The necessary sample size would also depend on the natural incidence of the cancer being considered as well as the sensitivity of the organ to radiation. Cancers with a relatively low natural incidence and/or a relatively high organ site sensitivity to radiation would require smaller sample population sizes. For breast cancer, the magnitude of possible risk from 1 rad of radiation is so small that a 20-year follow-up of 25 million exposed and 25 million nonexposed women from the age of 50 years would be required to prove or disprove the existence of risk at this dose level.

Summary

The existence of low-dose risk has neither been proven nor disproven. If there is a risk from the low doses used in current mammographic techniques, it is immeasurably small, especially when compared to the overwhelmingly large incidence of naturally occurring breast cancers, many of which could be detected by mammography at an early curable stage. The risk, if it does exist, would be lowest among women exposed over 30 years of age, a fortunate circumstance since this group would benefit most from mammography.

References

1. Adams EE, Brues AM (1980) Breast cancer in female radium dial workers first employed before 1930. J Occupational Med 22: 583–587
2. Advisory Committee on the Biological Effects of Ionizing Radiation (1972) The effects on populations of exposure to low levels of ionizing radiation. National Academy of Sciences – National Research Council, Washington, DC
3. Baral E, Larrson LE, Mattson B (1977) Breast cancer following irradiation of the breast. Cancer 40: 2905–2910
4. Boice JD, Monson RB (1977) Breast cancer following repeated fluoroscopic examinations of the chest. JNCI 59: 823–832
5. Casarett GW (1973) Possible effects of relatively low levels of radiation. Curr Probl Diagn Radiol 3: 1
6. Committee on the Biological Effects of Ionizing Radiation (1980) The effects on populations of exposure to low levels of ionizing radiation. National Academy of Sciences – National Research Council, Washington, DC
7. Delarue NC, Gale G, Ronald A (1975) Multiple fluoroscopy of the chest: Carcinogenicity for the female breast and implications for breast cancer screening programs. Can Med Assoc J 112: 1405–1411
8. Dvoretsky PM, Woodard E, Bonfiglio TA et al. (1980) The pathology of breast cancer in women irradiated for acute postpartum mastitis. Cancer 46: 2257–2262
9. Feig SA (1977) Can breast cancer be radiation induced? In: Logan WW (ed) Breast carcinoma: the radiologist's expanded role. Wiley, New York, pp 5–14
10. Feig SA (1978) Ionizing radiation and human breast cancer. CRC Crit Rev Diagn Imaging 11: 145–166
11. Feig SA (1979a) Epidemiology of radiation related breast cancer. In: Logan WW, Muntz EP (eds) Reduced dose mammography. Masson, New York, pp 10–20
12. Feig SA (1979b) Anatomic and pathologic basis of radiation related human breast cancers. In: Logan WW, Muntz EP (eds) Reduced dose mammography. Masson, New York, pp 21–34
13. Feig SA (1980) Biological determinants of radiation induced human breast cancer. CRC Crit Rev Diagn Imaging 13: 229–248
14. Jablon S, Kato H (1972) Studies of the mortality of A-bomb survivors. V. Radiation dose and mortality 1950–1970. Radiat Res 50: 649–698
15. Kellerer AM, Rossi HH (1972) The theory of dual radiation action. Curr Top Radiat Res 8: 85–158
16. Korenman SG (1980) The endocrinology of breast cancer. Cancer 46: 874–878
17. Land CE (1980) Estimating cancer risks from low doses of ionizing radiation. Science 209: 1197–1203
18. Land CE, Boice JD, Shore RE et al. (1980) Breast cancer risk from low dose exposure to ionizing radiation: Results of parallel analysis of three exposed populations of women. JNCI 65: 353–376
19. MacKenzie I (1965) Breast cancer following multiple fluoroscopies. Br J Cancer 19: 1–8
20. McGregor DH, Land CE, Choi K et al. (1977) Breast cancer incidence among atomic bomb survivors, Hiroshima and Nagasaki, 1950–1969. JNCI 59: 799–811
21. Mettler FA, Hempelmann LH, Dutton AM et al. (1969) Breast neoplasms in women treated with x-rays for acute postpartum mastitis, a pilot study. JNCI 43: 803–811
22. Moolgavkar SH, Day NE, Stevens RG (1980) Two-stage model for carcinogenesis: Epidemiology of breast cancer in females. JNCI 65: 559–569
23. Myrden JA, Hiltz JE (1969) Breast cancer following multiple fluoroscopies during artificial pneumothorax treatment of pulmonary tuberculosis. Can Med Assoc J 100: 1032–1034
24. Myrden JA, Quinlan JJ (1974) Breast carcinoma following multiple fluoroscopies with pneumothorax treatment of pulmonary tuberculosis. Ann R Coll Physicians Can 7: 45
25. National Council on Radiation Protection and Measurements (1980) NCRP Report No. 66: Mammography. NCRP, Washington DC

26. Pochin EE (1978) Why be quantitative about radiation risk estimates? The Lauriston S Taylor lecture series in radiation protection and measurements, National Council on Radiation Protection and Measurements
27. Rossi H, Kellerer A (1972) Radiation carcinogenesis at low doses. Science 175: 200–202
28. Seidman H (1980) Statistical and epidemiological data on cancer of the breast. American Cancer Society, New York
29. Shore RE, Hempelmann LH, Kowaluk E et al. (1979) Breast neoplasms in women treated with x-rays for acute postpartum mastitis. JNCI 59: 799–811
30. Tokunaga M, Norman JE, Asano M et al. (1979) Malignant breast tumors among atomic bomb survivors, Hiroshima and Nagasaki, 1950–1974. JNCI 62: 1347–1359
31. United Nations Scientific Committee on the Effects of Atomic Radiation (1972) Ionizing radiation: Levels and effects, vol 2. United Nations, New York
32. Upton AC, Beebe GW, Brown JM et al. (1977) Report of the NCI ad hoc working group on the risks associated with mammography in mass screening for the detection of breast cancer. JNCI 59: 481–492

Benefits and Risks of Mammography

S. A. Feig

Department of Radiology, Thomas Jefferson University Hospital,
Philadelphia, PA 19107, USA

In medical practice, mammography may be used as a diagnostic or as a screening procedure. As a diagnostic procedure, it is part of the evaluation of a patient with specific signs and symptoms, such as breast mass, pain, discharge, and abnormalities of the skin and axillary nodes. Because mammography may provide important information regarding these clinical problems, its use for this purpose has never been questioned. In this context, the issue of risk vs benefit does not arise since the value of the answers that mammography furnishes to these diagnostic problems cannot be given a numerical value for insertion into a benefit/risk calculation.

The role of mammography in screening to detect unsuspected breast cancer in women without clinical signs and symptoms is based on its ability to find the disease at a relatively early stage when it is still too small to be clinically palpable. Breast cancer survival depends on two related factors – lesion size and lymph node status. Smaller lesions with no histologic evidence of axillary metastasis at the time of treatment have the best prognosis (Table 1). Current mammographic techniques provide the most effective means of detecting such lesions (Table 2). Thus, it would appear that mammographic screening could greatly diminish the effects of a disease that now afflicts 1 of every 11 American women in her lifetime (Seidman 1983). Its impact on breast cancer could be similar to that

Table 1. Breast cancer survival according to stage of disease and method of cancer detection

Stage of disease	Percent survival after		
	5 years	10 years	20 years
Minimal	98	95	93
Negative nodes	85	74	62
Positive nodes	55	39	23
Distant metastases	10	2	*
Method of detection			
Screening by mammography and physical examination	93	*	*
Clinical detection in absence of screening	64	51	37

* Data not yet available due to insufficient follow-up

Data compiled from National Cancer Institute (1976); Wanebo et al. (1974); Frazier et al. (1977); Letton and Mason (1981)

5- and 10-year survival for minimal breast cancer as defined by Wanebo et al. (1974); 20-year survival for minimal breast cancer as defined Frazier et al. (1977)

Recent Results in Cancer Research. Vol. 90

Table 2. Accuracy of mammography and physical examination in breast cancer screening according to stage of disease (after Beahrs et al. 1979)

Stage of disease	Percent detection	
	Mammography	Physical examination
Minimal carcinoma	97	33
Negative nodes	92	51
Positive nodes	93	77

which the Pap smear had in reducing mortality from cervical carcinoma (Cramer 1978).

Although these data would support mammographic screening for all women in the breast cancer age-group (aged 40 years and older), not all authorities have endorsed this policy (Bailar 1976, 1977, 1978). There has been general agreement that mammographic screening should be performed on women aged 50 years and over, but some investigators have questioned the advisablity of screening younger women between 40 and 50 years of age. The disagreement relates to two major issues. First, concern has been expressed about the potential risk incurred from low doses of radiation. As previously described, this risk now appears to be very slight. Not only has there been a marked reduction in dosage in current mammographic techniques but refined dosimetric calculations have shown the actual dose delivered to the breast tissue per given skin dose to be less than formerly believed. Also, recent epidemiologic investigations, such as the Canadian National Cancer Institute fluoroscopy study, have shown that the risk to women over 35 years of age at the time of exposure is either negligible or nonexistent (Miller and Howe 1981).

It has also been argued that the detection of early lesions and observation of increased survival rates do not necessarily indicate that breast cancer deaths can be diminished (Feinleib and Zelen 1969; Zelen and Feinleib 1969; Zelen 1972, 1976). This line of reasoning may be understood by means of the model shown in Fig. 1 and described below, which show possible relationships of early detection to breast cancer mortality:

1. During its natural history, a malignant tumor will increase in size with time (model 1). Metastasis will begin to occur at some point in its development. When breast cancers are detected clinically in the absence of screening, over 50% show evidence of axillary node metastasis on pathologic examination. The actual incidence of spread beyond the breast must be higher since over 70% of these patients eventually die from breast cancer at time point D (Young et al. 1981; Seidman 1983).
2. Model 2 proposes that the natural course of the disease may be interdicted by mammographic screening if the cancer is detected while still confined to the breast at point A. In this case, breast cancer death is averted by early detection.
3. In model 3, metastases occur prior to detection by mammographic screening at time point A. The patient still dies from the disease at time point D. Actual survival is not prolonged but it may seem to be since it is now measured as D−A rather than D−C. This model is referred to as the lead time bias hypothesis since it postulates that the lead time from screening (C−A) will not alter the predetermined time of the patient's demise.

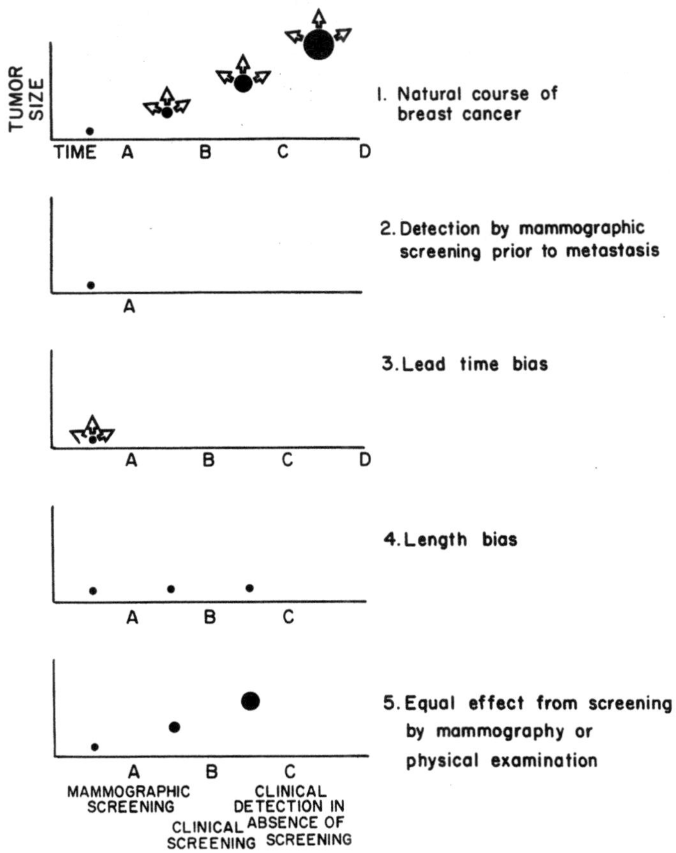

Fig. 1. Models for the possible effects of early detection and treatment on breast cancer mortality

4. The length bias hypothesis postulates the existence of slow growing lesions, which are associated with long duration of the disease. These cancers remain small throughout most of the patient's lifetime and have little or no potential for growth and metastatic spread. These nonaggressive lesions are associated with favorable survival rates even if they remain undetected in the absence of screening.
5. The final model acknowledges that mammographic screening can detect cancers at an earlier stage (A) than possible with clinical screening (B). However, it postulates that similar cure rates may be achieved with either modality since significant metastatic spread does not occur between point A and B.

It can be appreciated that lead time bias, length bias, and decreased mortality through screening are mutually exclusive when applied to a specific cancer. If a lesion metastasizes prior to detection (lead time bias), it cannot be so biologically inert that it would never threaten a patient's life if undetected (length bias). If either of these two hypotheses are true for all cancers, then screening would have no effect on reducing mortality. The effectiveness of screening depends less on which model may apply in a given case than it does on which model is valid for most cases. Are any of these models applicable to a significant proportion of cancers detected in screening? As postulated by the length bias hypothesis, some detected lesions such as lobular neoplasia in situ may not behave as true cancers (McDivitt 1978; Rosen et al. 1978; Haagensen et al. 1978). And, as predicted by the lead time bias theory, some very small minimally invasive ductal carcinomas may already have metastasized at the time of screening (Silverberg and Chitale 1973). But to how many cases are these models applicable? Do they apply to a sufficient proportion of cancers to preclude any true benefit from screening?

This question is best resolved in a randomized clinical trial where breast cancer mortality (breast cancer deaths per number of women screened) rather than survival (percentage of patients alive at a given time post-diagnosis) is measured simultaneously in control and study populations. Both populations are identical in that they are comprised of women volunteering for screening. They differ in that screening is performed only on the study group.

Evidence of Benefit from Screening Projects

Health Insurance Plan of Greater New York (HIP) Study

Such a randomized trial was conducted by the Health Insurance Plan of Greater New York (HIP) (Strax et al. 1973; Venet et al. 1975; Shapiro 1977): 62,000 women, 40–64 years of age, who volunteered for screening, were divided into study and control populations of 31,000 women each. Women in the study group were offered screening by mammography and physical examination for 5 successive years (1963–1968). When compared to the nonscreened control group, a mortality reduction of 33% was found among all screened women. Reduced mortality was still evident in the 12-year follow-up. These results offer incontrovertible proof of benefit from screening. They cannot be negated by the arguments of lead time bias and length bias, which apply only to survival data, not to mortality data in a randomized trial.

The results of the HIP study represent the crux of the mammography controversy in that the entire benefit was confined to women over the age of 50 years at the time of detection (if only these older women are considered, the reduction in mortality was over 40%). No mortality reduction was found among women whose cancers were detected at younger ages.

The results of this study raise questions concerning the efficacy of screening these younger women. First, is breast cancer in younger women a different disease, which is refractory to the benefit of early detection? This seems unlikely since survival rates for breast cancers detected in clinical practice do not vary according to patient age when similar stage lesions are considered (Mausner et al. 1969; Stoll 1976). Secondly, could benefit be existent but unobserved in younger women? This is certainly possible since there may have been a benefit of up to 20%–30%, which was not seen due to the small number of younger women studied. The third and most plausible explanation for the failure to demonstrate decreased mortality in younger women seems to be that mammography as practiced in the HIP project was considerably less effective in detecting cancers among women below the age of 50 years. Among cancers detected on screening women above the age of 50 years, 38% were found from mammography alone. For cancers detected in screening women below the age of 50 years, only 20% were found by mammography alone (Fig. 2). Breast cancers detected by mammography alone in the HIP study did have exceptionally low case fatality rates, i.e., 14% at 8 years following diagnosis vs 35% for cancers detected by clinical examination. Unfortunately, few such lesions were found among women under the age of 50 years.

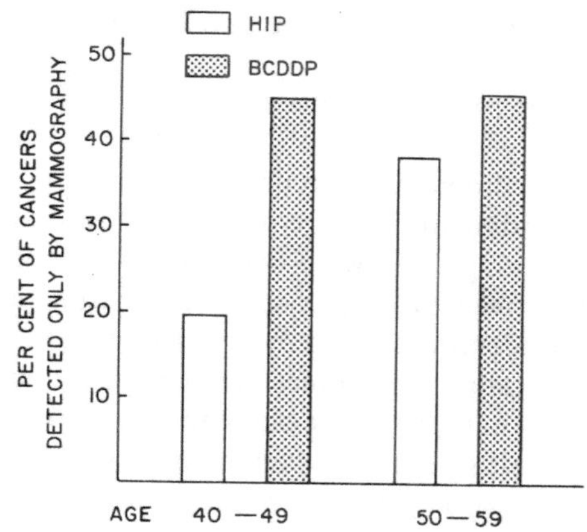

Fig. 2. Detection of nonpalpable cancers according to patient age in HIP and BCDDP Projects. (After Feig et al. 1979)

Breast Cancer Detection Demonstration Projects

The HIP data can be compared to those obtained from the more recent National Cancer Institute – American Cancer Society (NCI-ACS)-sponsored Breast Cancer Detection Demonstration Projects (BCDDP) (1973–1981). Here, due to improvements in mammographic technique and interpretive expertise, the number of nonpalpable cancers detected among younger women rose dramatically. Nearly 50% of cancers in women below the age of 50 years were found by mammography alone compared with 20% in the HIP study (Fig. 2). Cancer detection rates for women of all ages on initial screening at the BCDDP centers were approximately twice as high as those in the HIP – 5.54 vs 2.73 cancers/1,000 women screened, respectively. There was also a remarkable shift in detection toward smaller lesions. Minimal carcinomas (defined here as all invasive carcinomas smaller than 1 cm and all in situ carcinomas) constituted 36% of all cancers in the BCDDP vs only 8% of all cancers at the HIP centers (Beahrs et al. 1979; Beahrs 1983; Beahrs and Smart 1983). This gain was due mainly to mammography. Although the two populations are not strictly comparable, the data do suggest that mammography has become a more accurate modality.

Results from the current BCDDP suggest that the reduction in breast cancer mortality achieved by the HIP study in the mid-1960s for women over 50 years of age at the time of screening can now be extended to women below the age of 50 years by means of current mammographic techniques. It is likely that the 40% mortality reduction seen in HIP women over the age of 50 years at the time of screening can now be equaled or surpassed for all women over 35 years of age.

One unfortunate difference between the two studies is that the BCDDP data do not include comparative mortality rates in control and study populations so that it cannot offer the same degree of proof as would be obtained from a randomized trial. Although final proof must await results from randomized trials now underway, such as those in Sweden (Tabar et al. 1983), there are several lines of evidence indicating that the ability of mammography to detect breast carcinoma at an early stage will be translated into decreased mortality.

Significance of Mammographic Screening

Comparative Effectiveness of Clinical Examination and Mammography

The comparative accuracy of mammography and physical examination in the BCDDP according to the stage of cancer detection is shown in Fig. 3. Among the cancers found by screening, 93% were detected by mammography and 54% by physical examination. The effectiveness of physical examination is seen to decline as earlier stage lesions are considered. It was only able to find 50% of cancers with negative axillary nodes, 39% of infiltrating carcinomas smaller than 1 cm, and 30% of in situ carcinomas.

Although physical examination is considerably less sensitive in detecting cancers at the earliest stage now possible, one could speculate that it might still be able to detect cancers at a sufficiently early stage to achieve cure rates similar to those expected with mammography. However, the study by Feig et al. (1979) based on data from the Breast Diagnostic Center at Jefferson University Hospital in Philadelphia indicates that if mammography had not been performed and patients were screened by physical examination alone, most cancers would have metastasized before they had reached sufficient size to be palpable (Table 3). Among cancers smaller than 2 cm, only 13% had

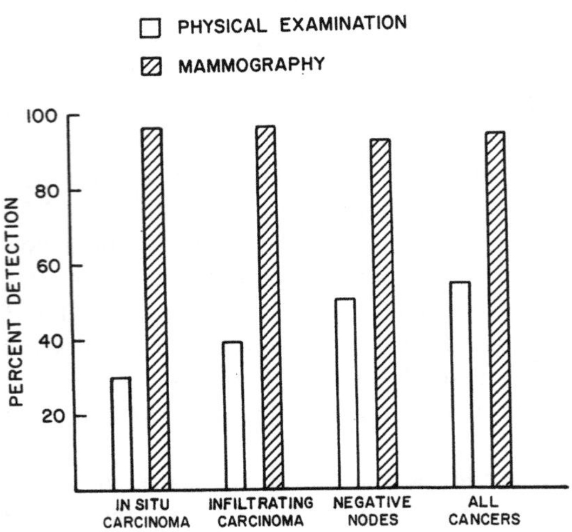

Fig. 3. Comparative accuracy of mammography and physical examination in breast cancer screening at the BCDDP Center. (Adapted from Beahrs et al. 1979; Beahrs 1983; Beahrs and Smart 1983)

Table 3. Relationship of cancer size to detection by physical examination and presence of lymph node metastases (after Feig et al. 1979)

Cancer size (cm)	Percent detected on physical examination	Percent with positive nodes
0 –0.5	20	2
0.51–1.0	42	15
1.1 –2.0	53	20
2.1 –3.0	85	65
3.1+	98	78

metastasized to the axillary nodes and only 40% could be detected on physical examination. Above that size, there was a steep increase in axillary nodal involvement. Detection rates for physical examination did not approach those of mammography until the cancers had reached a size of 2–3 cm, but by that time 65% had spread to the regional nodes (Feig et al. 1979). In addition, the accuracy of physical examination is also influenced by factors unrelated to the tumor itself. Physical examination is least accurate in deep lesions and those occurring in large breasts (Feig et al. 1977). These findings would indicate that combined screening by physical examination and mammography should be able to reduce breast cancer mortality far more than could be achieved by physical examination alone.

Based on results from the Cincinnati BCDDP, Moskowitz has estimated that annual physical examination could raise the relative survival of patients with breast cancer to 59% from the national average of 50% for women who were not screened. Combined screening by mammography and physical examination could increase the relative survival to 78% (Fox et al. 1978; Milbrath et al. 1981; Moskowitz and Gartside 1982).

Is Early Breast Cancer True Cancer?

Pathologic examination of mastectomy specimens from patients with breast carcinoma, retrospective analysis of previous biopsy material taken from patients in whom breast cancer later developed, and the prospective correlation of subsequent breast cancer risk with findings from previous breast biopsy all indicate that invasive ductal breast cancer, which represents 95% of all breast cancers, does not arise de novo from normal breast tissue but represents the culmination of a sequence of epithelial transformations (Fig. 4) (Kern and Brooks 1969; Gallager and Martin 1969a, b; Black et al. 1972; Humphrey and Swerdlow 1962; Ashikari et al. 1974; Moskowitz et al. 1977; Moskowitz 1980). Atypical hyperplasia is a necessary precursor to ductal carcinoma since all carcinomas must arise from atypical hyperplasia. However, most cases of atypical hyperplasia do not progress to cancer. Atypical hyperplasia may remain unchanged or regress to normal epithelial tissue. In this sense, atypical hyperplasia may be considered a nonobligatory precursor to carcinoma. Women with atypical hyperplasia proven by biopsy do not necessarily develop breast cancer, but they are at a fivefold increased risk.

Many sources of evidence suggest a causal relationship between in situ and invasive ductal carcinoma. Whole-organ sections of breasts with invasive ductal carcinoma have been found to contain multiple widely distributed foci of in situ and minimally invasive carcinoma (Gallager and Martin 1969a, b; Schwartz et al. 1980; Qualhein and Gall 1957; Morganstern et al. 1975). The conclusion that this relationship is not fortuitous is supported by the fact that in situ ductal carcinoma was not found in any of the breasts of 419 patients who underwent subcutaneous mastectomy for nonmalignant conditions (Pennisi et al.

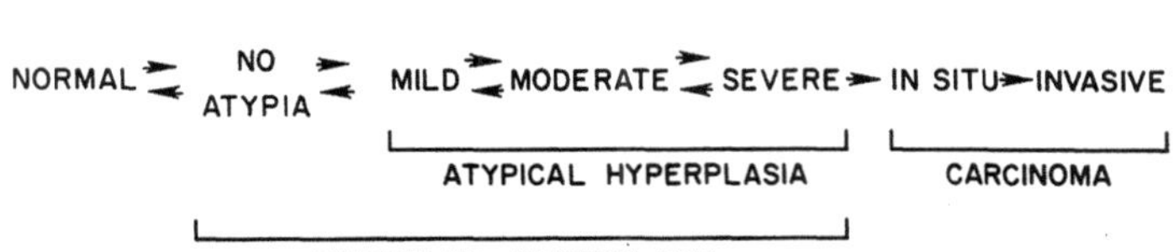

Fig. 4. Breast cancer development seen as a sequence of changes from normal epithelial tissue. The various stages of hyperplasia are reversible. Carcinoma represents committed malignant growth

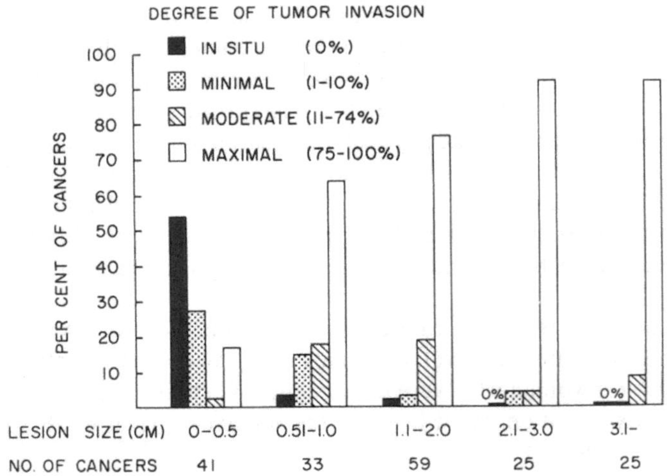

Fig. 5. Composition of each size-category of cancers detected on screening according to degree of tumor invasion. (After Feig 1979)

1977), and was discovered in only 1 of 776 autopsy subjects following death from conditions other than breast cancer (Sandison 1962).

Further evidence for the transition from in situ to invasive carcinoma may be obtained from serial sections of the cancers themselves. Their margins may be composed of various proportions of in situ and infiltrating growth (Silverberg and Chitale 1973; Feig et al. 1979) (Fig. 5). For most cancers, the change from in situ to invasive growth begins when the lesion is between 0–0.5 cm in size.

The bulk of evidence also suggests that most minimal carcinomas detected in screening are as aggressive as the larger cancers found in clinical practice. The major difference is in the stage of development, not in biologic potential. Most nonpalpable cancers display evidence of invasive growth at an early stage (Fig. 5). Among cancers measuring less than 0.5 cm, only half were in situ lesions; in the remaining half, invasive growth had already begun. Tumor invasion progresses rapidly so that it may be observed in 95% of cancers between 0.5 and 1 cm in size.

Furthermore, when ductal carcinomas detected in screening are graded histologically according to the method of Bloom (Bloom 1950a, b, 1957, 1964; Bloom and Field 1971), in which grade III lesions appear most anaplastic and exhibit the most aggressive behaviour, most small nonpalpable cancers are of grades II and III indicating moderate to high tumor aggressiveness. Although grade I lesions were mainly found in the smaller size categories detected in screening, even there they represent a minority of lesions (Feig et al. 1979). Although some well-differentiated grade I cancers detected in screening, such as tubular carcinomas, were once thought to be relatively indolent, they are now recognized as representing transition states to less differentiated cancers (Linell et al. 1980; Feig et al. 1978; Peters et al. 1980).

It is true that the term breast cancer encompasses tumors of different biologic capabilities, but both growth rate studies and survival studies suggest that there is no sizable group for which early detection is unnecessary. Breast cancers vary in their growth rates as observed in serial mammographic studies (Gershon-Cohen et al. 1963; Lundgren 1969; von Fournier et al. 1980). Survival rates for cancers of similar size vary according to their histologic grade

(Bloom 1950a, b, 1964; Bloom and Richardson 1957; Bloom and Field 1971). However, follow-up studies of breast cancer patients who refused treatment show that less than 5% were alive 10 years after the onset of symptoms (Bloom 1964). Although these data are based on large palpable lesions, if a significant fraction of untreated tumors were of low biologic potential this would have been reflected in a higher survival rate for untreated carcinomas.

It is impossible to observe directly the natural history of an in situ lesion since the excisional biopsy needed to determine its presence also removes it from further observation. However, due to the known multifocal nature of the disease, it can be assumed that many patients treated by excisional biopsy alone will have one or more remaining foci of intraductal carcinoma remaining. When such patients were studied by Betsill et al. (1978), seven of ten were found to develop a subsequent carcinoma in the same breast, with an average latent period of 10 years. Six of the seven carcinomas were invasive. Two of the patients died of metastatic carcinoma and two were known to be alive with metastases when last contacted. Similar findings have been obtained by other investigators (Haagensen 1971; Kraus and Neubecker 1962; Dean and Geschickter 1938; Farrow 1970).

By comparison, among patients treated by excisional biopsy for in situ lobular carcinoma, only 15% developed infiltrating carcinoma in the ipsilateral breast and an additional 15% eventually developed infiltrating carcinoma in the contralateral breast after a 20-year follow-up (McDivitt 1978; Rosen et al. 1978; Haagensen et al. 1978). Accordingly, there has been some debate as to whether this disease represents an extremely high-risk marker (more properly termed lobular neoplasia) rather than a true in situ carcinoma. However, in situ lobular carcinoma represents only 17% of in situ carcinomas detected in screening at the BCDDP (Beahrs et al. 1979).

This interpretation of in situ lobular carcinoma is in accordance with data from a subcutaneous mastectomy study (Pennisi et al. 1977). The relatively high prevalence rate 15% or 60/419) among patients who underwent subcutaneous mastectomy for benign disease indicates that in situ lobular neoplasia grows slowly and has a low potential for invasion. By inference, the observation that there were no cases of intraductal carcinoma among the same 419 patients, even though invasive ductal carcinoma occurs four times as often as invasive lobular carcinoma, indicates that intraductal carcinoma becomes invasive in a relatively short period of time so that the pool of in situ ductal carcinomas is continually depleted.

Additional evidence that minimal carcinomas evolve into advanced cancers unless intercepted at an early stage comes from comparing data from several screening programs in which different criteria for biopsy on initial (prevalence) screening were used. The Louisville BCDDP employed conservative mammographic criteria, which resulted in the detection of one cancer in every four to five biopsies. The Cincinnati and Milwaukee BCDDPs used a more aggressive approach. They were willing to accept a greater number of benign biopsies in order to detect a larger number of minimal cancers. More aggressive mammographic criteria were used so that lesions were biopsied even if their mammographic appearance suggested a low possibility of malignancy. A yield of one cancer in every ten biopsies was judged acceptable. This approach produced a higher prevalence rate in initial screening – 7.5 cancers/1,000 person-years at Cincinnati-Milwaukee vs 3.9 cancers/1,000 person-years at Louisville. As a result, the incidence of rate for advanced disease (stage II or higher) was 300% greater in Louisville than in Cincinnati – 1.12/1,000 person-years vs 0.36/1,000 person-years. All differences were statistically significant (Moskowitz 1979).

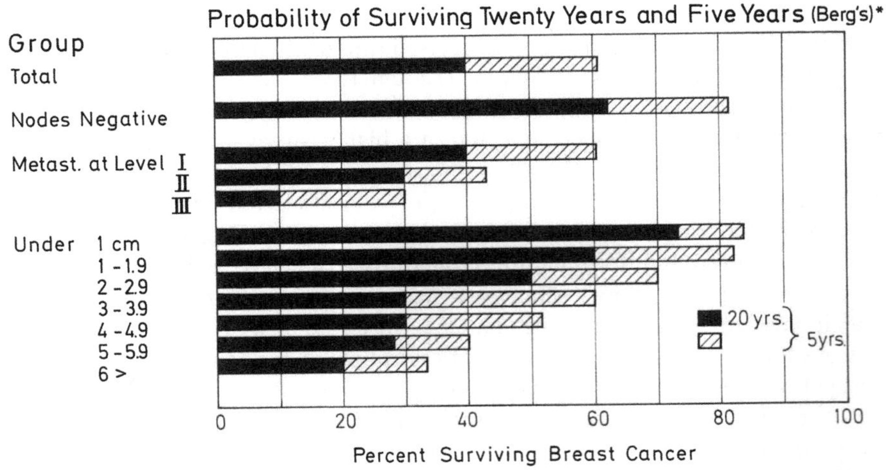

Fig. 6. Breast cancer survival 5 years and 20 years after treatment of 1,458 women by radical mastectomy. Patients are grouped according to lymph node status and lesion size. (After Seidman 1983; Berg and Robbins 1966)

Can Early Breast Cancer Be Cured?

Breast cancer survival is easily measured and clearly depends on lesion size and lymph node status at the time of treatment (Fig. 6). Breast cancer cure is less readily determined. Since breast cancer is a chronic disease, a patient may be alive 5 years after treatment but have occult metastases that will eventually lead to death. Nevertheless, the likelihood of cure can be more reliably documented over longer periods of time.

If survival is plotted as a function of time, the survival curve for breast cancer patients will initially decline at a steeper rate than that of the normal population. After approximately 20 years, according to Brinkley and Haybittle (1975), the slope of the survival curve for breast cancer patients will become less steep so that the curve is parallel to but lower than the survival curve for the normal population. These authors define cure in such terms since breast cancer patients surviving 20 years will have an overall life expectancy similar to that of the normal population. After 20 years, as for shorter periods of follow-up, survival rates will depend on the stage of disease at the time of initial treatment. However, as indicated by Brinkley and Haybittle's definition, 20-year survival rates are equivalent to cure rates. Their data show a 20-year actuarial survival rate of 48% for stage I cancers as opposed to 19% for stage II cancers. Similar data have been produced by others (Duncan and Kerr 1976; Bloom and Field 1971). Thus, diagnosis at an earlier stage of the disease would appear to result in a higher cure rate.

It is also possible that stage I cancers contain a significantly higher proportion of less lethal lesions. However, this explanation seems unlikely since Bloom and Field's data indicate that for cancers of the same histologic grade, 15-year survival rates for patients with stage I cancers are 22%–44% higher than rates for patients with stage II cancers (Bloom and Field 1971).

Long-term follow-up data indicate that the effect of lead time bias cannot be a significant explanation for improved survival. These analyses indicate that the lead time for early detection is no more than 2–3 years (Schwarz 1978; Hutchinson and Shapiro 1968), far too short to account for improved survival over periods of 10–20 years. The lead time can also be estimated from studies on breast cancer growth rates (Gershon-Cohen et al. 1963;

Lundgren 1969; von Fournier et al. 1980; Pearlman 1976; Philippe and LeGal 1968) and by a comparison of the prevalence to incidence rates using the method of Hutchinson and Shapiro.

The 5-year follow-up results on 6,030 women between 35 and 50 years of age screened by mammography and physical examination at the Cincinnati BCDDP constitute further evidence that early detection in younger women can favorably alter breast cancer mortality (Moskowitz and Gartside 1982). No breast cancer deaths were recorded in the 5-year follow-up; whereas seven deaths would have been expected in this period according to the national breast cancer mortality data. Although these results are statistically significant, they do not represent definitive proof of mortality reduction due to the absence of a randomized control group.

Some benefit from screening may also accrue for those cancers that metastasize prior to detection. Bond (1975) has shown by means of regression analysis that the removal of such cancers at a less advanced stage may both prolong the length of survival and improve the quality of survival even though the cancer has already spread beyond the breast. This improvement may be due to: (1) reduction in the rate of metastasis and/or (2) enhancement of host defense (Carter and Smith 1977). For such patients, breast cancer screening may not avert death, but it may alter the course of the disease. As with other chronic conditions, such as arteriosclerotic cardiovascular disease, the purpose of medical care is to prolong life rather than to effect a cure.

Benefit/Risk Analysis

Although incontrovertible proof of the benefit of screening women below the age of 50 years awaits results from the randomized clinical trials now underway in Sweden and Canada, such benefit is a reasonable expectation as indicated in the proceeding discussion. Specific values for the expected benefit and risk for mammographic screening can be calculated using the method of Seidman (1977) based on current BCDDP screening data and from our present knowledge of possible radiation risks. To estimate the benefit of screening for each age-group, he analyzed the number of cancers detected as well as the improvement in survival expected from early detection and determined the increased life expectancy per 1,000 women screened in each age-group.

To calculate risk, his results have been modified to reflect the most recent estimate of possible radiation risk and the current reduced mammographic dosage. Risk has been calculated separately using the doses of 0.1 rad for film screen mammography, 0.8 rad for xeromammography, and 0.4 rad, being the average between these two techniques. These reduced-dose techniques were used for a substantial portion of the BCDDP screenings (Bates and Demidecki 1979) and have been found to be as effective as the higher dose techniques used at the beginning of the BCDDP (Muntz et al. 1980; Dodd 1981).

The risk estimate of 3.5 excess cancers/million women/year/rad given by the National Cancer Institute for women aged 35 years and above at the time of exposure has been used to determine the annual risk that might occur after a latent period of 10 years (Upton et al. 1977). This risk is assumed to apply for each remaining year of the patient's life as determined by longevity tables. Survival rates for breast cancers caused by high doses of radiation have been found to be similar to those of naturally occurring breast cancers (Feig 1980), as expected, since they are pathologically indistinguishable (Dvoretsky et al. 1980).

Table 4. Estimation of life expectancy gains and losses from screening (modified from Seidman 1977 to assume risk factor of 3.5 excess cancers/million women/year/rad at the doses given)

Number of years of life expectancy per 1,000 women screened					
Age at entry (years)	Gain from		Loss per mammographic examination according to dose (rad)		
	Initial screening	Second annual screening	0.1	0.4	0.8
35–39	6.3	2.8	0.09	0.36	0.7
40–44	15.3	7.5	0.06	0.24	0.48
45–49	27.7	11.4	0.04	0.16	0.32
50–54	21.3	1.7	0.03	0.12	0.24
55–59	15.7	4.8	0.02	0.08	0.16

Survival rates for cancers that might possibly be caused by low-dose mammography have been assumed to be the same.

This risk estimate has been multiplied by the mean breast dose for a two-view mammographic examination to determine the number of years of life expectancy lost through radiation per 1,000 women screened. The results of these calculations are shown in Table 4. The benefit for both the initial and second annual mammographic screening of self-selected women at the BCDDP centers is seen to increase with age at the time of screening as expected since the incidence of naturally occurring breast cancers rises markedly with patient age (Seidman 1983). Benefit for the initial (prevalence) screening is greater than benefit for the second annual (incidence) screening. Benefit substantially exceeds risk in both the initial and second annual screening for all age-groups and, therefore, suggests that the annual screening of women aged 40 years and older would lead to a significant reduction in breast cancer mortality. These results support a screening schedule at annual intervals. This conclusion was also reached in a benefit/risk analysis of five annual screenings at the Cincinnati and Milwaukee BCDDP centers (Fox et al. 1978). Annual screening for women aged between 40 and 45 years is also supported by the mathematical model of Chiacchierini and Lundin (1979) if screening can be proven to reduce breast cancer mortality by at least 10%. As previously discussed, an analysis of BCDDP data indicates that the 40% mortality reduction proven for women above the age of 50 years in the HIP study can now be equaled or surpassed in younger women.

These estimates of benefit vs risk may represent minimum values, with the actual values being substantially greater. The risk at low doses may be nonexistent or only one-third that expected from linear extrapolation of high-dose data (Committee on the Biological Effects of Ionizing Radiation 1980). The risk to older women may be even less. Although the risk estimate of 3.5 excess cancers/million women/year/rad suggests that women exposed above the age of 30 years are only 45% as sensitive to radiation as younger women (Upton et al. 1977), recent data on American, Canadian, and Swedish women suggest that this value may be closer to 10%–20% (Boice and Monson 1977; Myrden and Hiltz 1969; Myrden and Quinlan 1974; United Nations Scientific Committee on the Effects of Atomic Radiation 1972; Baral et al. 1977; Miller and Howe 1981).

This chapter has attempted to summarize evidence regarding the screening of women below 50 years of age who are in the breast cancer age-group. Current data strongly suggest that screening with reduced-dose techniques can save lives in these women. Although this analysis does not provide incontrovertible proof for a reduction in mortality by screening these women, such data should be forthcoming from randomized screening trials now being conducted in Sweden. The case for screening these women is already so compelling that we must act now on the basis of the best available evidence so that lives will not be lost while awaiting results from these studies.

The foregoing analysis of benefits vs risks would support the following mammography policy:

1. Care of women with symptoms of breast cancer: Mammography is an essential part of the evaluation of the symptomatic patient and when optimally combined with physical examination offers a high degree of accuracy.
2. Screening of asymptomatic women:
   a) All women should be taught proper breast self-examination by the age of 20 years and should have an annual physical examination of the breast after the age of 35 years.
   b) The first, or baseline, mammograms should be obtained by the age of 40 years. An earlier age is preferable when there is a history of breast cancer or of premenopausal breast cancer in the patient's mother and/or sisters.
   c) Subsequent mammographic examinations should be performed at 1–2-year intervals, determined by the combined analysis of physical and mammographic findings and other risk factors, unless medically indicated sooner.
   d) Annual mammography and physical examination are recommended for all women over the age of 50 years.

References

1. Ashikari R, Hadju SI, Robbins GF (1971) Intraductal carcinoma of the breast (1960–1969). Cancer 28: 1182–1187
2. Ashikari R, Huvos AG, Snyder RE, Lucas JC, Hutter RUP, McDivitt RW, Schottenfeld D (1971) A clinicopathologic study of atypical lesions of the breast. Cancer 33: 310–317
3. Bailar JC (1976) Mammography: A contrary view. Ann Intern Med 84: 77–84
4. Bailar JC (1977) Screening for early breast cancer: Pros and cons. Cancer 39: 2783–2795
5. Bailar JC (1978) Mammographic screening: A reappraisal of benefits and risks. Clin Obstet Gynecol 21: 1–14
6. Baral E, Larrson LE, Mattson B (1977) Breast cancer following irradiation of the breast. Cancer 40: 2905–2910
7. Bates LM, Demidecki AJ (1979) Results of the Centers for Radiological Physics' measurements at the Breast Cancer Detection Demonstration Projects. In: Muntz EP, Logan WW (eds) Reduced dose mammography. Masson, New York, pp 123–130
8. Beahrs OH (1983) Comparative merits of mammography and physical examination. In: Feig SA, McLelland R (eds) Breast carcinoma: Current diagnosis and treatment. Masson, New York
9. Beahrs OH, Smart CR (1983) The Breast Cancer Detection Demonstration Projects as viewed by the clinician. In: Feig SA, McLelland R (eds) Breast carcinoma: Current diagnosis and treatment. Masson, New York
10. Beahrs OH, Shapiro S, Smart CR (1979) Report of the working group to review the National Cancer Institute – American Cancer Society Breast Cancer Detection Demonstration Projects. JNCI 62: 640–709
11. Berg JW, Robbins GF (1966) Factors influencing short and long term survivals following operations for breast cancer. Surg Gynecol Obstet 122: 1311–1316

12. Betsill WL, Rosen PP, Lieberman PH, Robbins GF (1978) Intraductal carcinoma. Long-term follow-up after treatment by biopsy alone. JAMA 239: 1863–1867
13. Black MM, Barclay TH, Cutler SJ, Hankey BG, Asire AJ (1972) Association of atypical characteristics of benign breast lesions with subsequent risk of breast cancer. Cancer 29: 338–343
14. Bloom HJG (1950a) Prognosis in carcinoma of the breast. Br J Cancer 4: 259–288
15. Bloom HJG (1950b) Further studies on prognosis of breast carcinoma. Br J Cancer 4: 347–367
16. Bloom HJG (1964) The natural history of untreated breast cancer. Ann NY Acad Sci 114: 747–754
17. Bloom HJG, Field JR (1971) Impact of tumor grade and host resistance on survival of women with breast cancer. Cancer 28: 1580–1589
18. Bloom HJG, Richardson WW (1957) Histological grading and prognosis in breast cancer. Br J Cancer 11: 359–377
19. Boice JD, Monson RB (1977) Breast cancer following repeated fluoroscopic examinations of the chest. JNCI 59: 823–832
20. Bond WH (1975) Natural history of breast cancer. In: Stoll BA (ed) Host defence in breast cancer. Year Book Medical Publishers, Chicago, p. 95 (New aspects of breast cancer, vol 1)
21. Brinkley D, Haybittle JL (1975) The curability of breast cancer. Lancet 2: 95–97
22. National Cancer Institute (1976) Cancer patient survival, a report from the Cancer Surveillance, Epidemiology and End Results (SEER) Program. DHEW Publication No. (NIH) 77-992, U.S. Department of Health, Education, and Welfare, Public Health Service, National Institutes of Health, Bethesda, Maryland
23. Carter D, Smith RRL (1977) Carcinoma in situ of the breast. Cancer 40: 1189–1193
24. Chiacchierini RP, Lundin FE (1979) Risk benefit analysis for reduced dose mammography. In: Logan WW, Muntz EP (eds) Reduced dose mammography. Masson, New York, pp 61–72
25. Committee on the Biological Effects of Ionizing Radiation (1980) The effects on populations of exposure to low levels of ionizing radiation. National Academy of Sciences, National Research Council, Washington, DC
26. Cramer DW (1978) The role of cervical cytology in the declining morbidity and mortality of cervical cancer. Cancer 34: 2018–2027
27. Dean L, Geschickter CF (1938) Comedo carcinoma of the breast. Arch Surg 36: 225–234
28. Dodd (1981) Radiation detection and diagnosis of breast cancer. Cancer 47: 1766–1769
29. Duncan W, Kerr GR (1976) The curability of breast cancer. Br Med J 2: 781–783
30. Dvoretsky PM, Woodard E, Bonfiglio TA, Hempelmann LH, Morse IP (1980) The pathology of breast cancer in women irradiated for acute postpartum mastitis. Cancer 46: 2257–2262
31. Farrow JH (1970) Current concepts in the detection and treatment of the earliest of the early breast cancers (The James Ewing Lecture). Cancer 25: 458–477
32. Feig SA (1980) Biological determinants of radiation-induced human breast cancer. CRC Crit Rev Diagn Imaging 13: 229–248
33. Feig SA, Shaber GS, Patchefsky AS, Schwartz GF, Edeiken J, Libshitz HI, Nerlinger R, Curley RF, Wallace JD (1977) Analysis of clinically occult and mammographically occult breast tumors. Am J Roentgenol 128: 403
34. Feig SA, Shaber GS, Patchefsky AS, Schwartz GF, Edeiken J, Nerlinger R (1978) Tubular carcinoma of the breast. Radiology 129: 311–314
35. Feig SA, Schwartz GF, Nerlinger R, Edeiken (1979) Prognostic factors of breast neoplasms detected on screening by mammography and physical examination. Radiology 133: 577–582
36. Feinleib M, Zelen M (1969) Some pitfalls in the evaluation of screening programs. Arch Environ Health 19: 412–415
37. Fox SH, Moskowitz M, Saenger EL, Kereiakes JG, Milbrath J, Goodman MW (1978) Benefit/risk analysis of aggressive mammographic screening. Radiology 128: 359–365
38. Frazier TG, Copeland EM, Gallager HS, Paulus DD, White EC (1977) Prognosis and treatment in minimal breast cancer. Am J Surg 133: 697–701

39. Gallager HS, Martin JE (1969a) The study of mammary carcinoma by mammography and whole organ sectioning. Cancer 23: 855–873
40. Gallager HS, Martin JE (1969b) Early phases in the development of breast cancer. Cancer 24: 1170–1178
41. Gershon-Cohen J, Berger SM, Klickstein HS (1963) Roentgenography of breast cancer moderating concept of "biologic predeterminism". Cancer 16: 961–964
42. Haagensen CD (1971) Diseases of the breast. Saunders, New York, pp 528–544, 586–590
43. Haagensen CD, Lane N, Lattes R, Bodian C (1978) Lobular neoplasia (so-called lobular carcinoma in situ) of the breast. Cancer 42: 737–769
43a. Howe GR, Miller AB, Sherman GJ (1982) Breast cancer mortality following fluoroscopic irradiation in a cohort of tuberculosis patients. Cancer Detect Prev 5: 175–178
44. Humphrey LJ, Swerdlow M (1962) Relationship of benign breast disease to carcinoma of the breast. Surgery 52: 841–846
45. Hutchinson GB, Shapiro S (1968) Lead time gained by diagnostic screening for breast cancer. J Natl Cancer Inst 41: 665–681
46. Kern WH, Brooks RN (1969) Atypical epithelial hyperplasia associated with breast cancer and fibrocystic disease. Cancer 24: 668–675
47. Kraus FT, Neubecker RD (1962) The differential diagnosis of papillary tumors of the breast. Cancer 15: 444–455
48. Letton AH, Mason EM (1981) Five-year-plus survival of breast screenees. Cancer 48: 404–406
49. Linell E, Ljungberg O, Andersson I (1980) Breast carcinoma, aspects of early stages, progression, and related problems. Acta Pathol Microbiol Scand [A] [Suppl] 272: 1–233
50. Lundgren B (1969) Observations on growth rate of breast carcinomas and its possible implications for lead time. Cancer 40: 1722–1725
51. Mausner JS, Shimkin MB, Moss NH, Rosemond GP (1969) Cancer of the breast in Philadelphia hospitals 1951–1964. Cancer 23: 260–274
52. McDivitt RW (1978) Breast carcinoma. Hum Pathol 9: 3–21
53. Milbrath JR, Moskowitz M, Bauermeister D (1981) Breast cancer screening. CRC Crit Rev Diagn Imaging 16: 181–218
54. Miller AB (1982) The national breast screening study: An opportunity for physicians. Can Fam Physician 28: 369–373
55. Miller AB, Howe GR (1981) A study of cancer following multiple fluoroscopies. Implications for the use of mammography in screening for breast cancer. Presentation at the Annual Meeting of the Royal College of Physicians and Surgeons of Canada, Toronto
56. Millis RR, Thynne GSJ (1975) In-situ intraduct carcinoma of the breast: a long term follow-up study. Br J Surg 62: 957–962
57. Morganstern L, Kaufman PA, Friedman NB (1975) The case against tylectomy for carcinoma of the breast. The factor of multicentricity. Am J Surg 130: 251–258
58. Moskowitz M (1979) Screening is not diagnosis. Radiology 133: 265–268
59. Moskowitz M (1980) Restructured data comparing screening approaches. Radiology 134: 262
60. Moskowitz M, Gartside PS (1982) Evidence of breast cancer mortality reduction: Aggressive screening in women under age 50. Am J Roentgenol 138: 911–916
61. Moskowitz M, Pemmaraju S, Russell P, Gardella L, Gartside P, deGroot I (1977) Observations on the natural history of carcinoma of the breast, its precursors, and mammographic counterparts: I. Natural history. Breast 3: 14–19
62. Muntz EP, Wilkinson E, George FW (1980) Mammography at reduced doses: Present performance and future possibilities. Am J Roentgenol 134: 741–748
63. Myrden JA, Hiltz JE (1969) Breast cancer following multiple fluoroscopies during artificial pneumothorax treatment of pulmonary tuberculosis. Can Med Assoc J 100: 1032–1034
64. Myrden JA, Quinlan JJ (1974) Breast carcinoma following multiple fluoroscopies with pneumothorax treatment of pulmonary tuberculosis. Ann R Coll Physicians Can 7: 45

65. Pearlman AW (1976) Breast cancer – influence of growth rate on prognosis and treatment evaluation. Cancer 38: 826–833
66. Pennisi VR, Capossi A, Perez FM (1977) Subcutaneous mastectomy data. A preliminary report. Plastic Reconstr Surg 59: 53–56
67. Peters GN, Wolff M, Haagensen CD (1980) Tubular carcinoma of the breast, clinical pathologic correlations based on 100 cases. Ann Surg 193: 138–149
68. Philippe E, LeGal Y (1968) Growth of 78 recurrent mammary cancers. Cancer 21: 461–467
69. Qualhein RE, Gall EA (1957) Breast carcinoma with multiple sites of origin. Cancer 10: 460–468
70. Rosen PP, Lieberman PH, Braun DW Jr, Kosloff C, Adair F (1978) Lobular carcinoma in-situ of the breast. Detailed analysis of 99 patients with average follow-up of 24 years. Am J Surg Pathol 2: 225–251
71. Sandison AT (1962) An autopsy study of the adult human breast. Natl Cancer Inst Monogr
72. Schwartz GF, Patchefsky AS, Feig SA, Shaber GS, Schwartz AB (1980) Multicentricity of nonpalpable breast cancer. Cancer 45: 2913–2916
73. Schwarz M (1978) An analysis of the benefits of serial screening for breast cancer based upon a mathematical model of the disease. Cancer 41: 1550–1564
74. Seidman H (1977) Screening for breast cancer in younger women, life expectancy gains and losses: An analysis according to risk indicator groups. CA 27: 66–87
75. Seidman H (1983) Breast cancer incidence, mortality, survival and prognosis. In: Feig SA, McLelland R (eds) Breast carcinoma: Current diagnosis and treatment. Masson, New York
76. Shapiro S (1977) Evidence of screening for breast cancer from a randomized trial. Cancer 39: 2772–2782
77. Silverberg SG, Chitale AR (1973) Assessment of significance of proportions of intraductal and infiltrating tumor growth in ductal carcinoma of the breast. Cancer 32: 830–837
78. Stoll BA (1976) Effect of age on growth pattern. In: Stoll BA (ed) Risk factors in breast cancer. New aspects of breast cancer, vol 2. Year Book Medical Publishers, Chicago, pp 129–148
79. Strax P, Venet L, Shapiro S (1973) Value of mammography in reduction of mortality from breast cancer in mass screening. Am J Roentgenol 117: 686–689
80. Tabar L, Gad A, Akerlund E et al. (to be published) Screening for breast cancer in Sweden. I. Results of the first round of screening. In: Feig SA, McLelland R (eds) Breast carcinoma: Current diagnosis and treatment. Masson, New York
81. United Nations Scientific Committee on the Effects of Atomic Radiation (1972) Ionizing radiation: Levels and effects, vol 2. United Nations, New York
82. Upton AC, Beebe GW, Brown JM, Quimby GH, Shellabarger C (1977) Report of the NCI ad hoc working group on the risks associated with mammography in mass screening for the detection of breast cancer. JNCI 59: 481–493
83. Venet L, Shapiro S, Strax P et al. (1975) Effect of screening on survivals. In: Gallager HS (ed) Early breast cancer, detection and treatment. Wiley, New York, pp 97–103
84. Von Fournier D, Kubli F, Bauer M, Schneider-Affeld F, Klapp J, Curland S (1980) Growth rate of 53 primary breast carcinomas with an observation time of 0.2–11 years. In: Nieburgs HE (ed) Prevention and detection of cancer, part II – Detection, vol 2 – Cancer detection in specific sites. Dekker, New York, pp 1711–1721
85. Wanebo HJ, Huvos AG, Urban JA (1974) Treatment of minimal breast cancer. Cancer 33: 349–357
86. Westbrook KC, Gallager HS (1975) Intraductal carcinoma of the breast. A comparative study. Am J Surg 130: 667–670
86a. Young JL Jr, Percy CL, Asire AJ (eds) (1981) Surveillance, epidemiology, and end results: Incidence and mortality data, 1973–1977. National Cancer Institute Monograph 57. National Cancer Institute, NIH Publication No. 81–2330

87. Zelen M (1972) Problems in the early detection of disease and the finding of faults. Bull Intern Stat Inst 44: 649–661
88. Zelen M (1976) Theory of early detection of breast cancer in the general population. In: Hueson JC, Mattheiem WH, Rozencweig M (eds) Breast cancer. Trends in research and treatment. Raven, New York, pp 287–300
89. Zelen M, Feinleib M (1969) On the theory of screening for chronic disease. Biometrika 56: 601–614

Multicentric Breast Carcinoma

R. L. Egan and M. B. McSweeney

Breast Imaging Center, Section of Radiology, Emory University School of Medicine,
1364 Clifton Road, Atlanta, GA 30322, USA

Separate deposits of carcinoma in the breast and the occurrence of distinctly different histologic types of carcinoma in the same breast have been recognized in 13%–75% of women with breast carcinoma (Cheatle and Cutler 1931; Egan et al. 1969; Egan 1970, 1982; Gallager and Martin 1969; Lagios 1977; Tellem et al. 1962; Morgenstern et al. 1975). Criteria for these categories have not been uniform, e.g., Lagios contends that a 3-cm distance between deposits is necessary for the sites separate to be considered as while Cheatle regards only a band of normal tissue, with no distance specified, between sites as being adequate. Most previous studies have relied on gross and microscopic examinations to establish multiple sites of carcinoma in the breast.

With mammographic radiographic detail, the breast can be examined in its entirety prior to removal for gross and histopathologic studies. The X-ray examination provides unlimited approaches in the evaluation of disease content and the variations related to diagnosis, treatment planning, and prognosis.

Our throughly correlated clinical, radiographic, and pathologic whole-breast studies with long follow-up periods of the subjects provide some insight into breast cancer. We sought explanations why 25% of stage I breast carcinomas act as stage II (Fisher et al. 1980), why many stage II lesions have as good a prognosis as stage I, and why 40% of women with breast cancer die at the rate of 25% per year and 60% die at the rate of 2.5% per year (Fox 1979).

Materials and Methods

At Emory University, a correlated clinical, radiographic, and pathologic approach for making whole-organ studies of breasts has been developed; it consists of freezing the breast, slicing it into serial sections, and radiographing the sections. Areas for microscopic study are selected by examination of the radiographs. Considering that ultradetail radiography permits a resolution of objects down to 50 μm, and even smaller, this approach is probably the nearest to a "whole-organ" study. All nonfatty tissues examined by X-ray were also studied by light microscopy since it was soon learned that fatty tissues on these radiographs contained no detectable glandular tissues. Avoiding the mounting of adipose tissue allowed technically easier, more detailed, and better quality preparations. Also, to us this proved to be a faster, less expensive, and more thorough approach than subserial sectioning, in which it is a matter of chance as to whether all the pathology is included (Egan 1970).

Intact specimens were obtained following needle biopsy and diagnosis, following positive axillary lymph node biopsy with positive clinical or X-ray findings in the breast (or strong

Recent Results in Cancer Research. Vol. 90

clinical and X-ray findings in the breast, especially in surgically poor-risk patients), and on some occasions following simple mastectomy – prophylactic and/or diagnostic, after a radical mastectomy for carcinoma or prior to prosthetic implant of the breast. Breasts containing a carcinoma detected by a cluster of calcifications not associated with a mass were routinely biopsied, the wound closed, paraffin-block studies carried out, and in 1–2 days a mastectomy performed.

The breast was neatly cut into about 20–40 sections, 5-mm thick, in the plane of the mediolateral mammogram. The sections were carefully laid out and numbered and X-rayed with 12 kV(p). No filter was added to a beryllium-window X-ray tube; we used a long target-film distance and extremely fine-grain industrial film with hand processing. The slicer radiographs were reviewed by the pathologist and radiologist. Each area of identifiable glandular tissue and suspected pathology was selected, fixed, and embedded in paraffin; 7-μm thick slides were prepared, stained by various appropriate stains, and studied both with the naked eye and by light microscopy. All cases were reviewed on at least three occasions by the radiologist, pathologist, and surgeon in conference; at least 2–3 was spent reviewing each case.

Complete studies on 161 whole breasts (156 patients) from 3 May 1965 to September 1969 were subject to a follow-up of over 10-years. The cases included: 15 with benign disease, one of which was bilateral; one male; two patients were lost to the follow-up; four simultaneous bilateral primary carcinomas; three initial primary carcinomas; 13 second primary carcinomas only; and 118 unilateral breast primary carcinomas. For this report, 118 cases of unilateral primary carcinoma were examined as a group as it was difficult to estimate the effect of the contralateral primary carcinoma on prognosis.

The criteria for multicentricity included: wide separation of foci – determined grossly, with noncancerous breast tissue intervening, radiographically, and microscopically; patterns of multiple areas scattered throughout much of the breast, or a sharp delineation of different histologic types. An intraductal carcinoma surrounded by or adjacent to duct carcinomas was regarded as one site and one type. An in situ lobular carcinoma in the same duct system as an intraductal carcinoma was regarded as a single focus. A large mass of carcinoma felt most likely to have resulted from coalescence and collapse into a single mass, made up of many distinguishable nodules, was considered unicentric unless distinct and well-separated foci were demonstrable.

Results

Distinct multiple sites of carcinoma were present in 72 cases (60%), multiple histologic types in 29 (25%), and multiple sites or multiple types in 82 (69%) (Table 1). With regard to the four classes relating to site and type of carcinoma, the cases were rather evenly distributed in stage I and stage II yet there was a decidedly better prognosis in carcinoma with a unicentric site and single histologic type (Table 2). The volume of tumor in the single-site, single-type carcinoma had no striking effect on the survival rate (Table 3). With multiple sites and types of tumor (as indicated in Table 4, Fig. 1), the trend was one of a poorer prognosis according to all clinical and X-ray findings, especially in tumors of greater volume. In 26 carcinomas with a volume of less than 0.5 cm^3, survival was 92% while with 21 cancers larger than 10 cm^3 (approximately equivalent to a diameter of 2.5 cm survival was 29%. Even in larger, unicentric, single-type tumors survival remained at 75%. Clinical signs of carcinoma signaled a poorer prognosis. Prognosis was not significantly associated with calcification or with positive intramammary lymph nodes. Intramammary lymph

Table 1. Number of sites and histologic types of 118 unilateral primary breast carcinomas

Site and type	Number	Total percentage of cases
Single site		
Single type	36	31
Multiple types[a]	10	8
Multiple sites		
Single type	53	45
Multiple types[a]	19	16
Total	118	100
Multiple sites/types	82	69

[a] All associated with duct carcinoma

Table 2. Stage of disease and 10-year survival of the 118 operable primary unilateral breast carcinomas

	No.	% 10-year survied	Stage 0		I		II	
			% in stage	% survived	% in stage	% survived	% in stage	% survived
Single site								
Single type	36	78	8	100	58	81	33	67
Multiple types	10	50	0	0	70	71	30	0
Multiple sites								
Single type	53	66	11	100	45	79	43	43
Multiple types	19	47	0	0	53	70	47	33
Total	118	65	8	100	52	74	40	40

Table 3. Total tumor volume and method of detection of the 118 carcinomas related to 10-year survival

	Volume in cm^3 < 2		> 2		Clin + X-ray +		Clin − X-ray +	
	No.	% survived	No.	% survived	No.	% survived	No.	% survived
Single site								
Single type	27	85	26	46	40	55	13	100
Multiple types	7	71	12	33	12	33	7	71
Multiple site								
Single type	22	82	14	71	30	73	6	100
Multiple types	5	60	5	40	9	44	1	100
Total	61	80	51	49	91	57	27	93

Clin +, *X-ray* +, clinical and X-ray evidence of cancer; *Clin* −, *X-ray* +, X-ray evidence but no clinical evidence of cancer

Table 4. Histologic types of carcinoma in the 118 unilateral carcinomas

	In situ	Duct	Duct and scir-rhous	Med-ullary	Lob-ular	Mu-coid	Adeno-carci-noma	Intra-cystic papillary
Single site								
Single type	2	20	7	5	2	0	0	0
Multiple types	0	4	3	2	1	3	0	2
Multiple sites								
Single type	4	32	14	1	2	0	0	0
Multiple types	1	20	4	1	0	2	3	3
Total	7	76	28	9	5	5	3	5

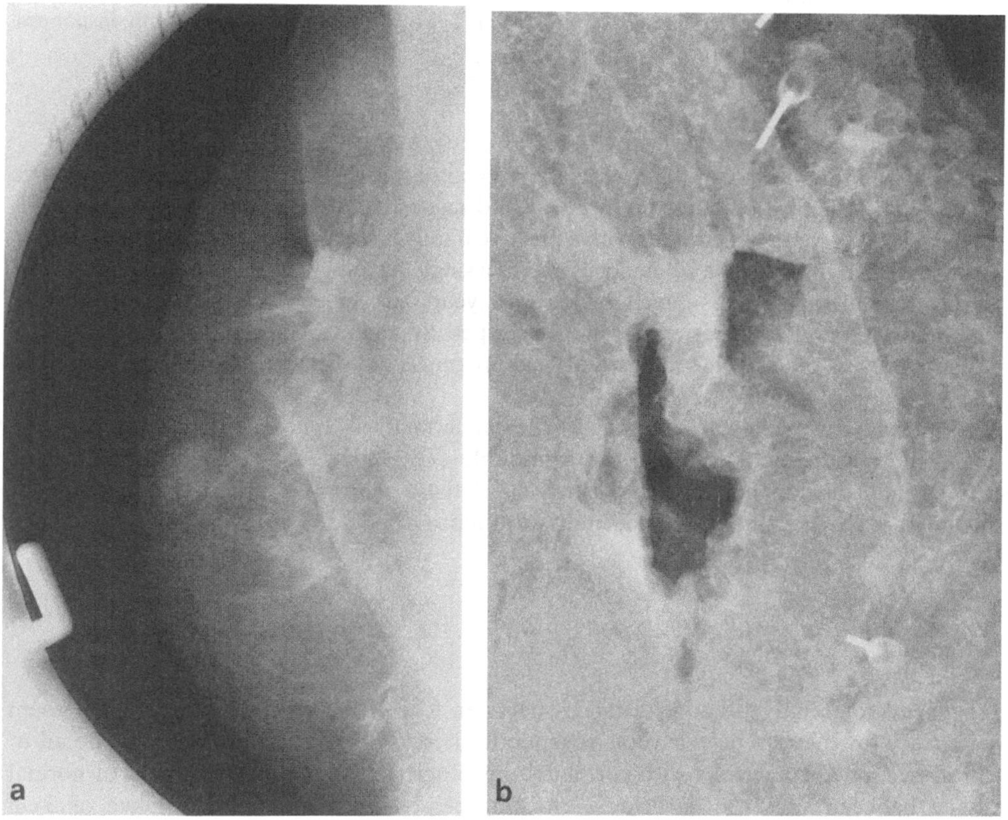

Fig. 1a, b. A 65-year-old woman who had discovered a lump in her left breast. **a** Mammogram shows at least four distinct sites of invasive carcinoma. **b** Radiograph of the breast specimen showing at least four sites of separate carcinoma foci. Histologically there were five invasive primary and multiple in situ duct carcinomas with multiple positive intramammary lymph nodes (one demonstrated here, *white lines*)

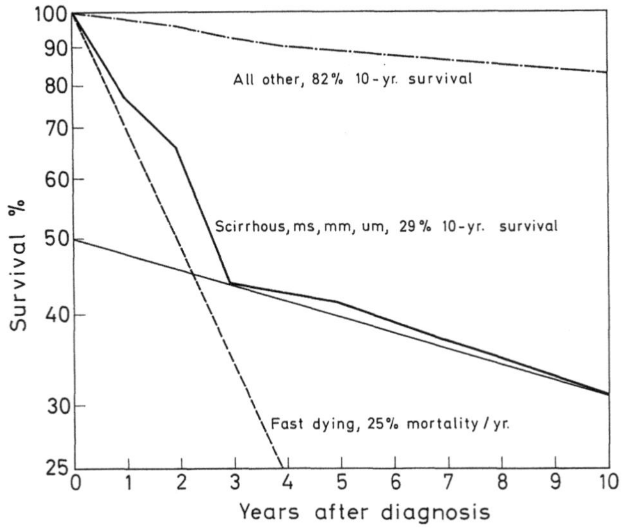

Fig. 2. Survival rates of multiple sites and/or types with a scirrhous element in breast carcinoma (*circles*) and all other breast carcinomas (*upper curve*). The subjects of the first group with the poorest survival have been plotted (*broken lines*)

nodes were present in 34 of the breasts (29%) and of these 11 (32%) contained metastatic carcinoma. Calcification detected by X-ray and suggestive of carcinoma was present in 79 breasts (67%). Nineteen patients with a positive family history of breast cancer had a better prognosis. Carcinomas as a single focus and of a single histologic type showed a high rate of survival in all age-groups (even beyond 70 years of age), which was in contrast to carcinomas in multiple sites and of multiple types. Stage II carcinomas and tumors with a volume greater than 10 cm^3 retained a good prognosis in unicentric, single-type lesions in the various age-groups.

The mortality of the single-site, single-type carcinoma was approximately 2.5% per year while the development of tumors with multiple sites and types is evident in a series of curves indicating higher mortality (Fig. 2). If these multiple-site and type carcinomas included a scirrhous element, the mortality approached 25% per year.

Discussion

The need for relatively large distances between foci of breast carcinoma did not seem necessary for them to be regarded as separate sites; using the fine radiographic detail of thinly sectioned specimens with correlated histologic study, the establishment of normal tissue between sites was sufficient. The requirement of a minimum distance of 3 cm between sites could preclude small breasts with multifocal carcinoma.

The breakdown of duct carcinoma into intraductal, comedo, invasive duct, and scirrhous carcinoma, even with the inconsistence of histologic and gross patterns, still provides a means of assessing prognosis. Definite and established desmoplasia was required for the designation of scirrhous carcinoma.

Contraction of breast tissues and shrinkage in the size of the breast is a frequent manifestation of breast carcinoma. It posed problems in this study as many large masses of carcinoma at one phase were probably a myriad of small masses. However, usually outside this main mass of highly invasive carcinoma there would be separate sites retaining the classification of multicentricity.

It is not necessary to assume that breast carcinoma changes morphologically with metastasis. When a metastatic growth is dissimilar to the known breast primary focus, it is more likely to have originated from a cell type in the same breast similar to that of the primary carcinoma, but one that has not been discovered. Axillary lymph node metastasis containing invasive duct carcinoma when the main mass in the breast was intracystic papillary or mucoid carcinoma was felt to be from an associated duct carcinoma in the same breast.

A definition of multicentricity of origin or location of breast carcinoma has not been established. This lack of uniformity in definition, variation in specimen preparation technique, and methods of study has produced a wide range of reported multicentric breast cancers. We relied on the Cheatle and Cutler (1931) definition that as long as normal ducts histologically separate tumor sites, each had developed de novo. We did not examine all breast tissue histologically but the incorporation of accurate, detailed radiography assured a near complete breast study, and structureless or fatty areas on the radiographs of sections that contained no tissue of histologic interest could be avoided. Without radiography, areas of in situ or microinvasive carcinoma would have gone undetected by palpation and inspection or incomplete subserial sectioning.

Many separate sites of invasive carcinoma could be seen coalescing to produce a single large tumor focus. Unless distinct foci were demonstrated, this was considered unicentric since peripheral growth could not be confidently excluded. Some larger, or mixed, unicentric carcinomas may have developed in this manner. Categorizing different cell types of contiguous carcinomas was difficult and required distinctly recognizable different cell types. Coalescence of tumor foci and/or collapse of breast tissues could explain a unicentric multiple-cell-type lesion.

Multiple separate carcinoma sites in 60% of the breasts suggest that breast cancer is a multicentric and, probably, a whole-organ, disease. The histologic characteristics of breast carcinoma may well reflect the biologic nature of the tumor and host resistance. There are no other similar series for direct comparison. Yet it is hoped that these observations may be sufficiently striking to arouse further investigation.

About 40% of newly diagnosed breast cancer patients die at the exponential rate of 25% per year (Fox 1979). This death rate is similar to that recorded in women with untreated breast cancer at the Middlesex Hospital in the late nineteenth and early twentieth centuries. The remaining 60% of the women with breast cancer die at the rate of 2.5% per year. The mortality curve of our women with unicentric single-type carcinoma superimposed on the 2.5% mortality curve and the death rate of the remaining women (multiple sites and types of carcinoma) with an element of scirrhous carcinoma approximated the 25% annual rate (Egan 1982).

Assignment of prognosis of breast cancer based on size, even though staged, is often tenuous. "Minimal" breast cancer encompasses lobular carcinoma in situ, noninvasive intraductal carcinoma, and invasive carcinoma, either lobular or ductal, forming a mass no greater than 0.5 cm in diameter. The term, "minimal" breast cancer, whether defined as less than 0.5 cm or less than 1 cm in diameter often is meaningless and misleading. Of the 118 subjects with unilateral carcinoma at stage I and 1 cm or more in diameter, 40 had a 74% 10-year survival rate while 16 with carcinomas at stage I and smaller than 0.5 cm had a

69% survival rate. In stage II, the "minimal" carcinomas had as poor a prognosis as the larger carcinomas, 45% compared with 40%, respectively. This alerts us to be wary of using "minimal" to connote assuredly curable cancer and realize that there are other prognostic factors besides size and stage.

Unicentric stage II carcinoma had a death rate of 33% while the multicentric mortality was 67%, a two fold difference (Table 2). With the use of these microscopic characteristics at the time of diagnosis, the biologic importance of the carcinoma could be established for understanding these diverse survival rates and for establishing logical treatment planning.

The clinical application of this time-consuming and expensive whole-breast study can be questioned. However, during thorough routine breast studies, multiple histologic types of carcinoma are demonstrated. The knowledge that multiple sites of breast cancer are common and are of great significance in prognosis may stimulate more thorough breast studies. Lagios (1977) has shown good results with a much less extensive procedure in his radiographic-pathologic routine study of breast cancer, which required only the added services of one technician. Schwartz et al. (1980) studying four sections from each breast quadrant and four sections from the retroareolar area demonstrated an incidence of 49.2% multicentricity of cancer in 43 breast specimens.

Conclusions

Multiple sites of breast carcinoma and multiple histologic types of carcinoma signal a poor prognosis. These findings reduce age of the patient, stage of disease, volume of tumor, and other clinical features to lesser indicators in the prognosis. Multiple sites of breast carcinoma in 60% of cancerous breasts suggest that this disease is at times multicentric in origin and could be a whole-organ process.

More extensive breast studies add valuable information about the multiple sites and histologic types of breast cancer and a routine could be established without prohibitive cost and effort.

References

1. Cheatle GL, Cutler M (1931) Tumors of the breast: their pathology, symptoms, diagnosis and treatment. Lippincott, Philadelphia
2. Egan RL (1970) Mammography and breast disease. Williams and Wilkins, Baltimore
3. Egan RL (1982) Multicentric breast carcinomas: Clinical-radiographic-pathologic whole organ studies and 10-year survival. Cancer 49: 1123–1130
4. Egan RL, Ellis JJ, Powell RW (1969) Team approach to study diseases of the breast. Cancer 23: 847–854
5. Fisher ER, Redmond C, Fisher B (1980) Pathologic findings from the National Surgical Adjuvant Breast Project (Protocol No. 4): VI. Discriminants for five-year treatment failure. Cancer 46: 908–918
6. Fox MS (1979) On the diagnosis and treatment of breast cancer. JAMA 241: 489–494
7. Gallager HS, Martin JE (1969) The study of mammary carcinoma by mammography and whole organ sectioning: early observations. Cancer 23: 855–873
8. Lagios MD (1977) Multicentricity of breast carcinoma demonstrated by routine correlated serial subgross and radiographic examination. Cancer 40: 1726–1934

9. Morgenstern L, Kaufman PA, Friedman NB (1975) The case against tylectomy for carcinoma of the breast. The factor of multicentricity. Am J Surg 130: 251–258
10. Qualheim RE, Gall EA (1957) Breast carcinoma with multiple sites or origin. Cancer 10: 460–468
11. Schwartz GF, Patchesfsky AS, Feig SA, Shaber GS, Schwartz AB (1980) Multicentricity of nonpalpable breast cancer. Cancer 45: 2913–2916
12. Tellem M, Prive L, Meranze DR (1962) Four-quadrant study of breast removed for carcinoma. Cancer 15: 10–17

Breast Cancer in the Younger Patient: A Preliminary Report

M. B. McSweeney and R. L. Egan

Breast Imaging Center, Section of Radiology, Emory University School of Medicine, 1364 Clifton Road, Atlanta, GA 30322, USA

Breast cancer occurring under the age of 35 years is not uncommon; it accounts for nearly 3% of all breast cancers (Langlands and Kerr 1979; Haagensen 1971). It is in this age-group that the diagnosis of curable breast cancer has the greatest potential for subject-years gained.

The diagnosis of early breast cancer in the younger patient presents a challenge to the surgeon and mammographer. Since carcinoma is less frequent at this age, cancer may not be considered in the clinical evaluation unless signs are classiv or advanced. There is a greater tendency to keep the patient under observation. The hesitancy in performing mammography on the symptomatic patient both from a fear of radiation and a misconception that all young patients have dense glandular tissue that would obscure lesions is unfortunate. Of malpractice suits in breast cancer about which we are consulted, 90% are in this age-group in connection with delays in diagnosis until an incurable stage has been reached.

The controversy in the literature regarding the effect of age on prognosis is unfounded. Breast cancer diagnosed in patients under the age of 35 years supposedly has a poorer prognosis than in other premenopausal breast cancer patients (Bloom 1964; Langlands and Kerr 1979; Sistrunk and MacCarty 1922). Berkson et al. (1957) contend that there is no diminished risk in the younger patient as long as the axillary nodes are not affected. Alderson et al. (1971) reported no effect of age on survival; some reports find a better prognosis in the younger patient (Mueller et al. 1978; Redding et al. 1979). These diverse opinions extend to the effects of coincident pregnancy and lactation as well as subsequent pregnancy on prognosis. Haagensen (1971) suggests that poorer prognosis in the younger patient is the result of more advanced disease upon first examination rather than different biologic aggressiveness.

Such reports spurred us to review our experience with breast cancer in young patients.

Materials and Methods

From 1963 to 1981, data was prospectively gathered on 43,000 clinical and mammographic studies performed on 8,000 patients referred to the Breast Imaging Center of the Robert Winship Clinic, the oncological clinic of Emory University Clinic. Patients with breast cancer diagnosed below the age of 35 years were selected from this patient population. Prospective clinical data and mammographic findings were reviewed and correlated with histopathology.

Recent Results in Cancer Research. Vol. 90

Results

Mammographic, clinical, and histopathologic data were available on the 27,000 breast examinations from 1963 to 1981. In these patients, 1,700 malignant and 5,300 benign lesions underwent histologic examination. Fenales under the age of 35 years accounted for 24.6% of patients undergoing mammography. Of the biopsy-proven carcinomas (7.5%), occurred in females under the age of 35 years. In the 74 patients with breast malignancy, there were 65 primary breast carcinomas, one metastasis from the opposite breast, one malignant cystosarcoma phylloides, one lymphosarcoma, three Hodgkin's lymphomas (one was a primary in the breast), one fibrosarcoma, and two melanomas. Four females with a carcinoma developed a second primary tumor in the opposite breast. The primary carcinomas were stage I lesions. The first primary carcinomas were of the infiltrating duct type while the second primary carcinomas included two infiltrating duct and two atypical medullary carcinomas.

Age at diagnosis ranged from 19 to 34 years with a mean of 30.01 years. Most patients showed no signs of known epidemiologic risk factors upon first examination (Table 1); 62 patients had a tumor mass, 59 of which were self-discovered (Table 2). The primary complaint of the younger patients with carcinoma was similar to that in all age-groups; the

Table 1. Epidemiologic risk factors in the 74 patients under the age of 35 years with breast malignancy

Risk factor	No. of patients
No known risk factors	42
Prior breast cancer	2
Prior ovarian cancer, melanoma, lymphoma	3
Family history breast cancer	13
Nulliparous	13
Cancer diagnosed during pregnancy	1
Cancer diagnosed during lactation	3
Prior mediastinal or chest therapeutic radiation	2
Total	79

Table 2. Chief symptoms of 74 patients under the age of 35 years with breast malignancy

Symptom	No. of patients
Mass discovered by patients	59
Mass discovered by physician	3
Discharge	3
Axillary adenopathy	3
Increase in breast size	1
Pain	2
Thickening	1
Unknown	2
Total	74

Table 3. Interval between noticing symptoms and diagnosis of malignancy

Interval	No. of patients
1–2 weeks	14
3–4 weeks	1
1–3 months	16
4–6 months[a]	14
7 months–1 year[b]	5
> 1 year	3[c]
Unknown	21
Total	74

[a] One patient was treated with antibiotics for 4 months
[b] Two patients underwent open biopsy, but in each case the surgeon biopsied only the productive fibrosis and judged the condition to be benign. A 4–8-month delay was caused because of the physician's error
[c] All three cases were patient delays

Table 4. Diagnosis of 74 breast malignancies

	X-ray positive	X-ray negative	X-ray equivocal	X-ray after biopsy[a]
Clinically positive	22	0	0	0
Clinically negative	16	11	2	6
Clinically equivocal	2	0	0	0
Examination post-biopsy[a]	41	11	2	20
Total				

[a] Elsewhere

primary complaint had been present for a period 2 weeks to 2 years (Table 3). Both physician and patient delay occurred treatment with regard to: five women on antibiotics were observed for 2 weeks to 4 months; two patients had inadequate incisional biopsies (the malignant tissue was not excised) and were not treated for 6 and 8 months; most patient delay was simply through failure to seek medical attention.

The primary breast carcinoma was of the infiltrating duct type in 42 patients, intraductal comedo in five patients, medullary carcinoma in ten, and invasive comedo in two. There was one case of each of the following – solid papillary, invasive lobular, inflammatory, tubular, and mucinous carcinoma and one case had more than one histologic type in one breast. All five lobular carcinomas in situ were associated with invasive duct or comedo carcinoma.

Mammography was postivie for malignancy in 41 of 54 females (76%) studied prior to biopsy; clinical examination was able to detect breast cancer in 22 cases (40%) – but was not necessarily the sole diagnostic method (Table 4). Clinical examination was not positive in any case in which the mammography result was negative or equivocal. Twenty women had undergone biopsies or mastectomies at other institutions prior to mammography. Treatment consisted of various regimens: 51 women underwent radical or modified radical

Table 5. Survival of 66 primary breast carcinoma patients related to axillary node status

Years after initial diagnosis	Negative	1–3 carcinomas	> 3 carcinomas	Unknown	Total
NED					
0–2	5	1	1	1	8
3–5	9	1	1	0	11
6–10	2	2	0	0	4
> 10	14	1	0	0	15
Metastases	3	4	1	0	8
Unknown	1	0	3	3	7
Died of disease after					
0–1	1	1	3	0	5
2–3	1	0	2	0	3
4–5	0	2	1	0	3
6–10	0	0	1	0	1
> 10	0	0	1	0	1

NED, no evidence of disease

mastectomy while 23 had combinations of surgery, radiation treatment, and chemotherapy. Survival was related to axillary node status (Table 5).

Discussion

In the Emory series, 8% of all breast carcinomas occurred in 25% of the women undergoing mammography. This number of breast cancer patients creates a large problem for both the surgeon and the mammographer. Compounding this problem is the difficulty in the clinical detection of these breast cancers as only 30% of the cancers were suspected clinically. Detection of breast cancer by mammography in young females requires more concentration but proves to of most value in females under the age of 35 years, being positive in 41 of 54 cancer cases (76%).

In the young females, only 15% of cases of breast cancer were actually inoperable, which is considerably lower than in other age-groups in this institution with its many referrals for inflammatory carcinomas as well as all types of inoperable breast cancers treated by radiation and/or chemotherapy.

All physicians examining the breasts of female patients must be constantly aware of the serious problem of breast cancer in young females. This series is small but so are other series in the literature. Some additional cases will eventually be added with increased follow-up. These data do serve to indicate the great value of mammography and early detection of breast cancer in young females.

Conclusions

The prognosis of breast cancer in younger patient depends upon the axillary node status. Mammography can be of great value in the diagnosis of breast cancer in the young patient. It must be widely used in symptomatic patients of this age-group. The accuracy of mammography in the detection of malignancy in patients under the age of 35 years is greater than that of physical examination. Radiographic overcalls (false-positive diagnoses) in the younger patient are only 1%. The greatest usefullness of mammography is in the salvage of the younger patient.

References

1. Alderson MR, Hamlin I, Staunton MD (1971) The relative significance of prognostic factors in breast carcinoma. Br J Cancer 25: 646
2. Berkson J et al. (1957) Mortality and survival in surgically treated cancer of the breast: a statistical summary of some experience of the Mayo Clinic. Proc Staff Meet Mayo Clinic 32: 645
3. Bloom HJG (1964) The natural history of untreated breast cancer. Ann NY Acad Sci 114: 747
4. Haagensen CD (1971) Diseases of the breast, 2nd edn. Saunders, Philadelphia
5. Langlands AO, Kerr GR (1979) Prognosis in breast cancer: the effect of age and menstrual status. Clin Oncol 5: 123
6. Mueller B, Ames F, Anderson GD (1978) Breast cancer in 3,558 women: age as a significant determinant in the rate of dying and causes of death. Surgery 83: 123
7. Redding WH, Thomas JM, Powles TJ, Ford HT, Gazet JC (1979) Age and prognosis in breast cancer. Br Med J 2: 1495
8. Sistrunk WE, MacCarty WC (1922) Life expectancy following radical amputation for carcinoma of the breast. A clinical and pathologic study of 218 cases. Ann Surg 75: 61

Bilateral Breast Carcinoma

M. B. McSweeney and R. L. Egan

Breast Imaging Center, Section of Radiology, Emory University School of Medicine, 1364 Clifton Road, Atlanta, GA 30322, USA

Introduction

Patients who have a history of carcinoma in one breast have an increased incidence of developing either primary or metastatic carcinoma in the opposite breast (Egan 1976; Haagensen 1971; Gutter 1976; Leis et al. 1965), and mammography contributes greatly to the detection of these lesions (Egan 1976; Gutter 1976). It is of significant prognostic value and imperative in clinical management to distinguish between bilateral primary carcinomas and metastasis from a primary carcinoma to the opposite breast. Nonsimultaneous bilateral breast carcinomas only occur after a patient survives a first primary carcinoma, but then subsequently develops a second, the first carcinoma having a relatively favorable prognosis. In contrast, metastasis from the opposite breast is a sign of advanced disease. Clinical differentiation of a second primary carcinoma versus metastatic carcinoma is frequently uncertain. Haagensen's (1971) criteria for diagnosis a primary carcinoma were that the primary be a solitary lesion and of a different histologic type from the other lesion, and that there be no distant metastases or evidence of local spread across the midline. However, since our whole-organ studies (Egan 1982) demonstrate that 70% of breasts with carcinomas are multicentric with or without multiple histologic types, insistence on a solitary site or different histologic type is an imprecise method of distinguishing primary from metastatic disease.

The pathologist, as well, may be unable to differentiate the two. The biopsy specimen represents a small area of the breast and may not include the optimum site for study. Different histologic types of carcinoma may be present in each breast; also, metastases from breast carcinoma may not be of the identical histologic type as the primary. The pathologist may not find an in situ component in the second breast, whether due to sampling error or absence of metastatic disease.

Mammography can accurately distinguish between primary and metastatic breast carcinoma (Egan 1972) (Table 1). Operable primary carcinomas, both contemporary and noncontemporary, show the primary signs of breast cancer, with or without the secondary signs. The spread of breast carcinoma to the second breast is usually across the sternum via the lymphatics, producing quite different mammographic findings. There is a diffusely edematous appearance of the breast, especially prominent in the subcutaneous tissues, with blurring of the trabeculae and venous margins, diffuse skin thickening, and visualization of the subcutaneous lymphatics. Metastases produce a diffuse increased density is the breast. No mass or malignant calcifications are present. These criteria correspond closely to the histopathologic criteria of Robbins and Berg (1964).

Our experience with bilateral breast carcinoma is presented and compared with the series of Haagensen (1971), Leis et al. (1965), and Robbins and Berg (1964).

Recent Results in Cancer Research. Vol. 90

Table 1. Mammographic features of primary breast carcinoma versus mestastasis from the opposite breast

Mammographic findings	Primary	Secondary
Nodule(s)	Usually present	0
Malignant calcification	± 50%	0
Skin thickening	None, local, or diffuse	Diffuse
Skin retraction	None, over mass, or nipple	0
Axillary nodes	±	±, often obscured
Parenchyma		
Density	Usually normal, may have diffuse density (advanced)	Diffuse denisty
Edema	Advanced	Present, may be first sign
Opposite breast	Normal or cancer	Absent or primary Ca
Nodule, single	Usually present	None
Nodule, multiple	May be present	Node distinct
Calcification	± 50%	None
Skin thickening	None local/diffuse	Usually diffuse, may be first sign

Materials and Methods

From 1963 to 1978 at the Emory University Clinic, 27,000 breast examinations by mammography and, when available, by histopathology took place. The females in this data group had been referred from the Robert Winship Clinic, the oncological unit of the Emory University Clinic. Histopathologic studies were performed by only a few pathologists. Clinical and mammographic data were obtained in a prospective manner.

Results

From 1963 to 1978, a total of 1,700 patients with primary operable carcinoma were studied by mammography and 97 of these had bilateral breast carcinoma. Carcinoma in the second breast was primary in 81 patients and metastatic in 16; in 22 patients there were simultaneous bilateral carcinomas (Table 2). Mammography proved highly effective in detecting the second carcinoma and was reliable in differentiating a second primary from a metastatic carcinoma. Of the second primary carcinomas, 35 were not associated with a palpable mass, all of these underwent mammography as a routine follow-up. The age upon diagnosis of the primary carcinomas is presented in Table 3. Of the patients with primary breast carcinoma, 81 were diagnosed as invasive duct, 16 intraductal, nine scirrhous, four mucoid, and two as medullary carcinomas; 21 were not otherwise specified (NOS) (Table 4). All lobular carcinomas in situ were associated with duct carcinomas.

The 81 primary carcinomas in the contralateral breasts occurred under the following circumstances: 31 were first detected by mammography in patients who had undergone a previous mastectomy; 23 occurred during the follow-up for a previous carcinoma and were diagnosed by the initial mammogram; 22 were simultaneous bilateral primary carcinomas; five developed bilateral noncontemporary carcinomas after normal initial bilateral mammograms. The bilateral simultaneous carcinomas were of comparable size. The

Table 2. Incidence of bilateral breast carcinoma

Author	Number of patients	Number of 2nd primary	Percent of 2nd primary	Number of simul-taneous	Percent simul-taneous	Percent total Ca simul-taneous
Emory Clinic	1,700	81	4.8	22	27.2	2.0
Haagensen	626	36	5.7	5	13.9	0.8
Leis et al.	611	49	8.0	2	4.0	0.3
Robbins and Berg	1,458	91	6.2	4	4.4	0.27

Table 3. Time interval in bilateral primary breast carcinoma

	Age at 1st primary (years)	Age at 2nd primary (years)
Simultaneous		
Median	53.5	53.5
Youngest	40	40
Eldest	80	80
Noncontemporary		
Median	49.3	53.9
Youngest	23	23
Oldest	81	86
Primary and metastatic		
Median	44.6	46.8
Youngest	23	25
Eldest	58	60

Table 4. Histologic types of primary breast cancer

	Duct	ID	Scir-rhous	Med-ullary	LCIS	Mucoid	NOS
Simultaneous, right	1	3	2		3		3
Simultaneous, left	11	1			2		5
Noncontemporary							
1st primary	40	4	2	1	4	2	3
2nd primary	29	8	5	1	5	2	10
Total	81	16	9	2	14	4	21

Some breasts had more than one type of carcinoma
ID, intraductal; *LCIS*, intraductal; *NOS*, not otherwise specified

second noncontemporary carcinomas were considerably smaller than the first and had fewer axillary lymph node metastases (Tables 5, 6). Of the second subsequent primary carcinomas, 40% were under 1 cm in diameter.

The development of second primary carcinomas and survival data are shown in Table 7. The second primary carcinoma occurred within 6 years of the first in 83% of the cases; in

Table 5. Size of primary breast carcinomas

	< 1 cm	1–1.9 cm	2–3.9 cm	4–10 cm	> 10 cm
Simultaneous, right	11	3	2	3	1
Simultaneous, left	9	3	3	5	0
Noncontemporary					
1st primary	7	6	11	2	1
2nd primary	22	15	13	2	3

Table 6. Axillary lymph node metastasis in 81 bilateral breast carcinomas

	None	Axillary lymph node metastasis
Simultaneous, right	15	7
Simultaneous, left	18	6
Noncontemporary		
1st primary	34	25
2nd primary	37	22

Table 7. Number of primary breast cancers

	Years after first cancer							
	0[a]	1[b]	2–4	5–6	7–12	12–18	> 18	Total
Emory Clinic	22	9	20	16	6	3	5	81
Haagensen	5	0	7	2	16	6	–	36
Robbins and Berg	4	10	24	11	27	13	7	96

[a] 0 = simultaneous
[b] 1 = 7–12 months after first cancer

Table 8. Condition of patients following diagnosis of second primary carcinoma

Years after 2nd primary	Dead	Alive	
		NED	Ca
0–1	13	10	1
1–2	7	6	0
2–3	5	7	3
3–4	3	6	1
4–6	1	6	1
6–10	2	14	1
11–15	1	2	0
Total	32	51	7

NED, no evidence of disease

the remaining 17% of cases it was spread over 23 years (Table 7). Four years after diagnosis of the second primary carcinoma, 28 of the 32 deaths had occurred and only six patients were alive with metastatic disease (Table 8).
There were 16 metastatic carcinomas from the opposite breast; seven patients had undergone mastectomy prior to being entered into the study; eight of the 16 patients had a primary carcinoma on the initial mammogram; and one patient had simultaneous carcinomas bilaterally.

Discussion

The incidence of bilateral breast carcinomas in the four series was remarkably similar (Table 2). Yet, the incidence of simultaneous bilateral carcinomas at the Emory University Clinic detected by mammography was two to seven times greater than in the series relying on clinical examination alone. There were no cases of second primary cancer within 6 months of the diagnosis of the first carcinoma in these patients examined by mammography at the clinic. It is, thus, assumed that mammography detected the second primary carcinoma in many cases 6 months to 3 years prior to it becoming clinically evident. All of the second simultaneous primary breast carcinomas were detected by mammography.
Mammography, by providing recognition of more simultaneous bilateral breast carcinomas, leads to early treatment of the second carcinoma (Fig. 1). Mammography was more efficient in detecting the second carcinoma than clinical examination and even prophylactic mastectomy, as practiced by Leis et al. (1965), and was as efficient as Urban's (1967) bilateral breast biopsies, if lobular carcinomas in situ are excluded. Since 83% of the second primary carcinomas at the Emory University Clinic were detected within the 6th postmastectomy year and the remaining 17% within 23 years, mammography is helpful in

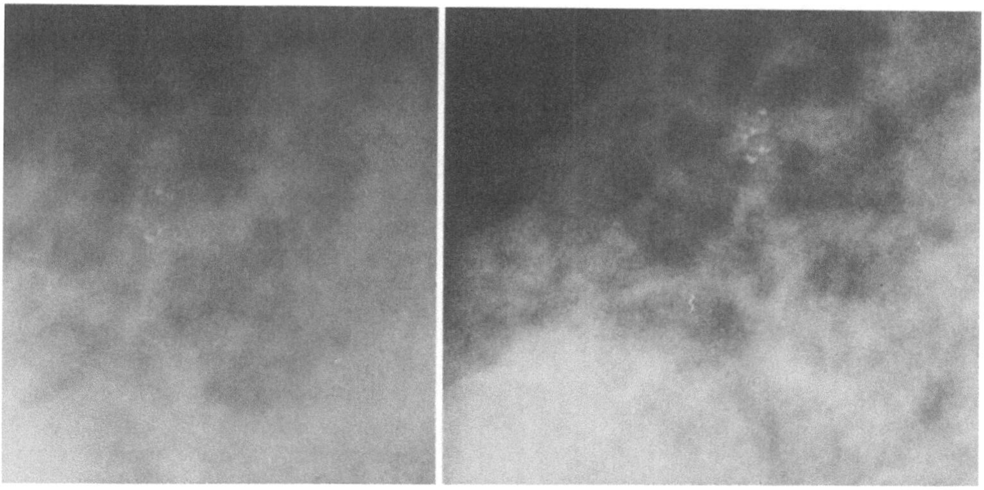

Fig. 1. Routine mammogram of a 49-year-old woman 1974. There were punctate calcifications in the upper inner quadrant of the left breast highly suspicious of carcinoma. Pathology: multifocal intraductal papillary and comedo with invasive comedo carcinoma. Two axillary lymph nodes contained metastasis. On routine follow-up in 1981, another cluster of punctate calcifications appeared in the left breast. This was a noninvasive multifocal comedo carcinoma

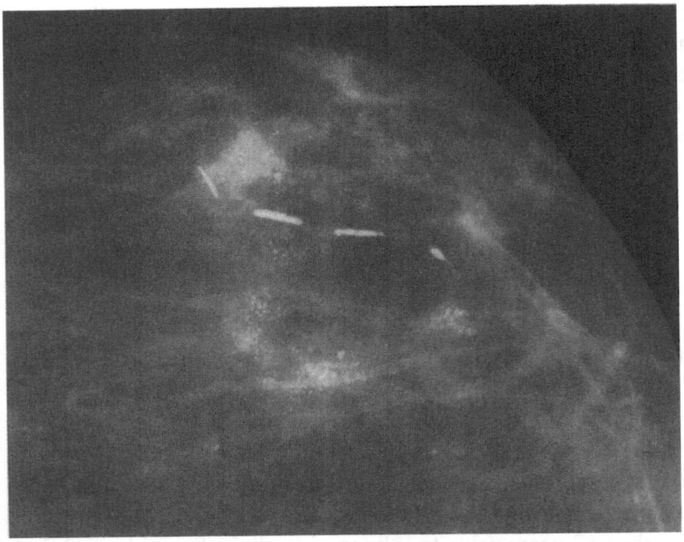

Fig. 2. Mammogram of a 79-year-old woman upon routine follow-up 30 years postmastectomy for infiltrating carcinoma of the opposite breast. This second primary carcinoma, manifested stippled calcification, was nonpalpable and proved to be a comedo carcinoma with minimal invasion. Prognosis was excellent

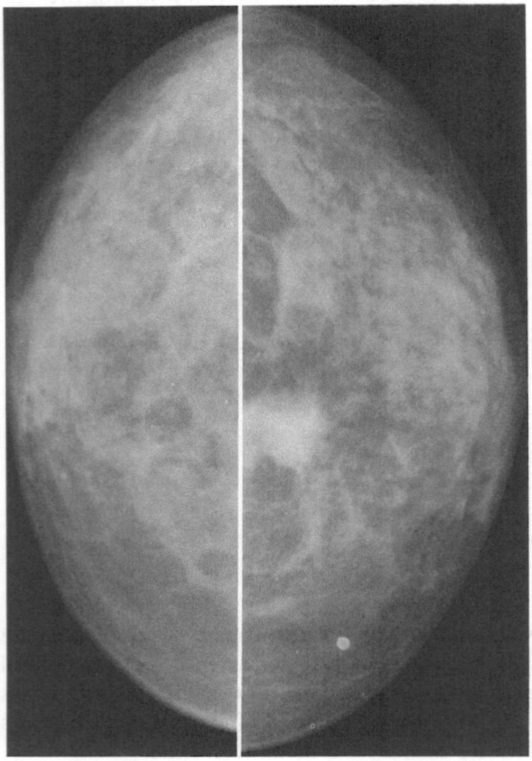

Fig. 3. Mammogram of a 65-year-old woman who had upon examination an upper central mass in the left breast. The right breast was normal under physical examination. Mammography revealed two highly spiculated contiguous carcinomas containing fine central calcifications; 2 cm lateral to these was a 7-mm moderately invasive carcinoma. In the upper outer quadrant of the right breast, there were two clusters (radiographically carcinoma) of stippled calcifications not associated with a mass. Pathology of left breast: multifocal invasive duct carcinoma with productive fibrosis; pathology of right breast: multifocal comedo and papillary carcinoma with one site of microinvasion; all axillary lymph nodes were without tumors

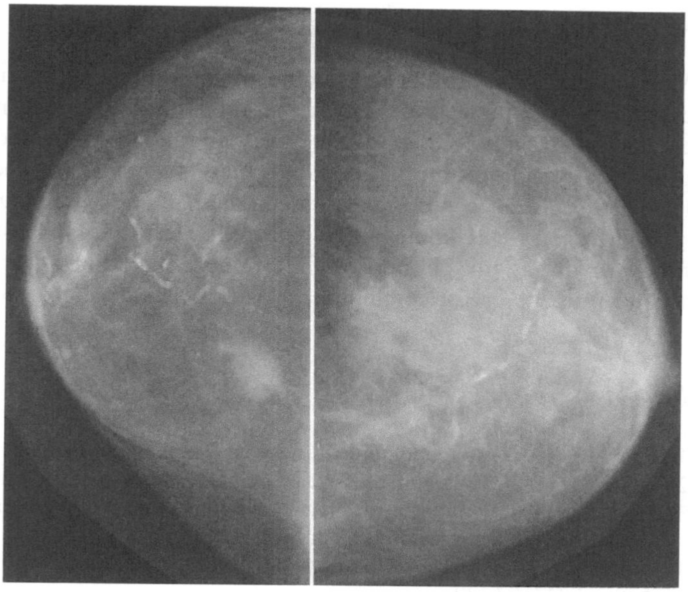

Fig. 4. Mammogram of a 77-year-old woman with 1-week history of upper central mass in the left breast, clinically malignant. In the clinically normal right breast, routine mammography revealed a 1.2-cm moderately invasive carcinoma with stippled calcification in the lower inner quadrant. Both were invasive duct carcinomas, stage 1

predicting the decreased risk for the second primary carcinoma after the 6-year follow-up.

Only 11% of the first primary carcinomas were less than 1 cm in diameter, whereas one-third of the second primary carcinomas were less than 1 cm. With the first primary carcinoma, all but two patients had signs or symptoms of breast cancer, but one-half of the second primary carcinomas were detected during routine follow-up examinations (Figs. 2, 3). A mass was palpable in 89% of the primary carcinomas and in only 30% of the second primary carcinomas. The 62% clinically occult second primary carcinomas diagnosed by mammography demonstrate the value of close follow-up, including mammography, during at least the first 6 years after mastectomy (Table 7, Fig. 4).

Four years after diagnosis of the second primary breast carcinoma is the important point in prognosis. Of the 32 deaths, 28 had occurred by then, and only two of six patients with cancer were still living after 4 years. Four years after the second primary carcinoma, 41% of the patients were still alive (Table 8).

Carcinoma in the second breast is today a second primary in at least 75% of cases, this being a conservative estimate. In the 1950s, the 10-year salvage rate of cases with breast cancer in world centers was 25%. Today's data indicate that over 50% of breast carcinoma cases can be cured. Early diagnosis of a second primary carcinoma by mammography and prompt treatment can increase the salvage by at least 150% (50% × 75% = 37.5%; 37.5% ÷ 25% = 150%).

Conclusions

Mammography is extremely valuable in finding and differentiating a second primary carcinoma from metastasis. Carcinoma in the opposite breast is usually a second primary carcinoma, it is not necessarily metastasis, and should be treated accordingly. If the second primary carcinoma is properly treated, there should be marked increase in survival of at least 150%. The second primary carcinoma has a specific natural history: Almost all the second primary carcinomas were detected within the 6th postmastectomy year, a close follow-up during this period is, therefore, essential; and 4 years after the diagnosis of the second primary breast carcinoma, prognosis is extremely good.

References

1. Egan RL (1972) Mammography, 2nd edn. Thomas, Springfield
2. Egan RL (1976) Bilateral breast carcinomas: role of mammography. Cancer 38: 931–938
3. Egan RL (1982) Multicentric breast carcinomas: clinical-radiographic-pathologic whole organ studies and 10-year survival. Cancer 49: 1123–1130
4. Gutter Z (1976) Cancer of the remaining breast: radiologic contribution to diagnosis. Can Med Assoc J 114: 27–30
5. Haagensen CD (1971) Diseases of the breast. Saunders, Philadelphia
6. Leis HP, Mercheimer WL, Black MM, DeChabone A (1965) The second breast. NY State J Med 2460–2468
7. Robbins GF, Berg JW (1964) Bilateral primary breast cancers. Cancer 17: 1501–1527
8. Urban JA (1967) Bilaterality of cancer of the breast. Biopsy of the opposite breast. Cancer 20: 1867–1879

The Radiographic Appearance of Normal and Metastatic Axillary Lymph Nodes

N. Bjurstam

Department of Diagnostic Radiology, University of Göteborg, Sahlgren's Hospital, 413 45 Göteborg, Sweden

The radiographic appearance of lymph nodes is of interest for two main reasons: 1. Lymph nodes are frequently visible on mammograms. They are probably the most common discrete mass found in the breast (Wolfe 1977). They may be located anywhere in the breast but occur most often in its axillary tail. 2. The preoperative assessment of lymphatic dissemination in breast cancer is of prime importance for the classification and proper planning of treatment. The presence of lymph node metastases is a very strong prognostic marker in breast cancer. In the clinical staging of breast carcinoma, interpretation of the findings of axillary palpation plays an important role. However, the palpation of the axilla is the most difficult part of the clinical examination and the clinical examination of the axilla is rather inaccurate (Johnsén et al. 1975).
Mammography offers a complement to clinical examination in the evaluation of axillary lymph nodes. Lymph nodes in the axillary tail of the breast are visualized on films in three-view mammography in a large number of cases. If special views of the axilla are obtained, lymph nodes are visualized in almost all cases (Bjurstam 1978).

Anatomy

Haagensen (1971) divided the axillary lymph nodes into six groups. According to him, the central nodes are the largest and most numerous. The central nodes lie embedded in fat in the center of the axilla and are the nodes most easily palpated and most easily projected freely on films when special views of the axilla are obtained. These nodes are also those in which metastases are most often found (Haagensen 1971). In Haagensen's series, this group was involved in 90% of cases of axillary lymph node metastases.

Materials and Methods

Our subjects comprised a consecutive series of 1,303 females with breast symptoms and included 177 females with primary breast carcinoma. In 130 of these, radical mastectomy was performed. In 50 of the 130 radical mastectomy specimens (38%), metastatic lymph nodes were found in the histopathologic examination.
Besides the three standard views of the breast, the patients were examined with one film of each axilla. During the exposure of the film, as hard a compression as possible was exerted on the axilla in order to displace the lymph nodes laterally so that they were projected free of the thoracic wall.

Recent Results in Cancer Research. Vol. 90

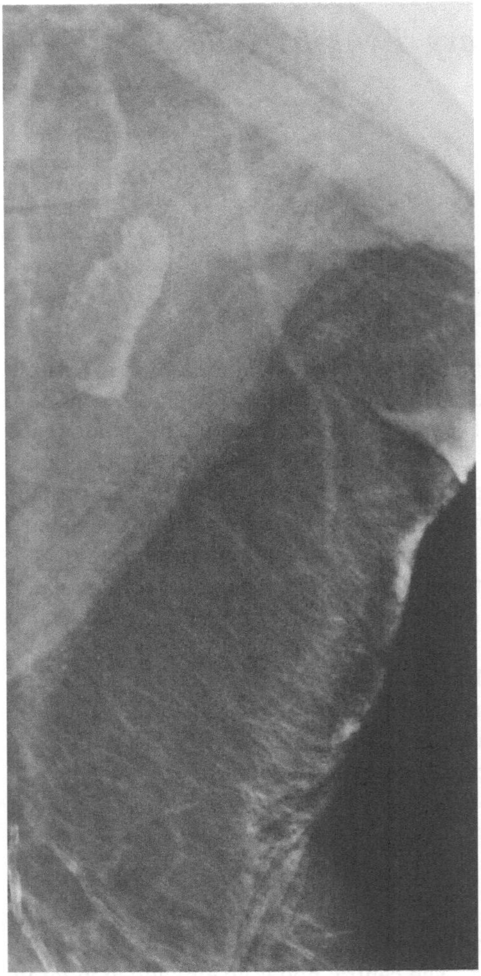

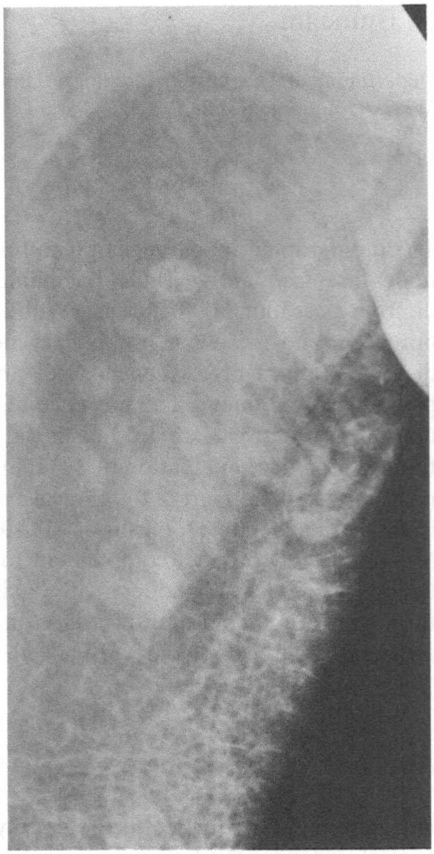

Fig. 1 (Left). Fatty replacement of an axillary lymph node measuring 30 mm

Fig. 2 (Right). Normal axillary lymph nodes

The lymph nodes were measured on the films and the largest diameter of the largest visible lymph node in each axilla was recorded. The attenuation of the nodes, their shape and margins, and the occurrence of fatty replacement (Fig. 1) was also noted. No correction was made for geometric enlargement.

Results

In most cases, four to eight lymph nodes were projected on the film (Fig. 2). This should be compared with the results of the pathologic examination of the dissected axilla in which, in the present series, an average of 21 lymph nodes were found.

Table 1. Distribution in percent of lymph nodes of different size in 2,119 axillae in different age-groups in patients without carcinoma

Radiographic size (mm)	Age-groups		
	≦ 35 years	35–54 years	≧ 55 years
≦ 5	28	17	8
6–10	58	60	56
11–15	14	19	26
> 15	1	4	11

Table 2. Radiographic size of the largest node compared with histopathologic examination in 130 radical mastectomy specimens

Size (mm)	Diagnosis by microscopy		
	No metastases (%)	Metastases in 1–3 lymph nodes (%)	Metastases in > 3 lymph nodes (%)
≦ 10	56	50	32
11–20	41	42	58
> 20	3	8	11

Table 3. Percentages of axillae with fatty replacement of lymph nodes in different age-groups in patients with carcinoma

Age-groups (years)	%
≦ 35	7
35–54	27
≧ 55	54

Size

The size of the largest lymph node in patients without carcinoma in different age-groups is presented in Table 1. The results demonstrate that the size increases with age. In only 15% of patients under 35 years of age did the largest lymph node exceed 10 mm, compared with 37% of patients aged 55 years or more. Lymph nodes measuring more than 20 mm were only occasionally found and then only in patients aged 45 years or more.
The radiographic sizes of the largest lymph nodes in the 130 radical mastectomy specimens are given in Table 2. Metastatic lymph nodes were only slightly larger than nodes without metastases. In only 11% of axillae with more than three lymph node metastases did the diameter of the largest lymph node exceed 20 mm.

Fatty Replacement

Fatty replacement of lymph nodes was quite common and increased with age (Table 3). Only a few per cent of the axillae in patients aged 20–29 years contained nodes with fatty replacement compared with 50% in the age-group 60–69 years. Fatty replacement was very common in the largest nodes suggesting that fatty replacement may cause the enlargement. Nodes with fatty replacement may sometimes reach a considerable size, in the present series occasionally up to 30 mm (Fig. 1).

Other Abnormalities

The most frequent sign of metastatic lesion is homogeneous nodes with increased attenuation, which was found in 71% of the axillae with more than three lymph node

Table 4. Radiographic appearance of axillary nodes compared with histopathologic examination in 130 radical mastectomy specimens

Appearance	Diagnosis by microscopy (in %)		
	No metastases (n = 80)	Metastases in 1–3 lymph nodes (n = 12)	Metastases in > 3 lymph nodes (n = 38)
Irregular shape	1	25	42
High attenuation	5	33	71
Fatty replacement	43	25	13

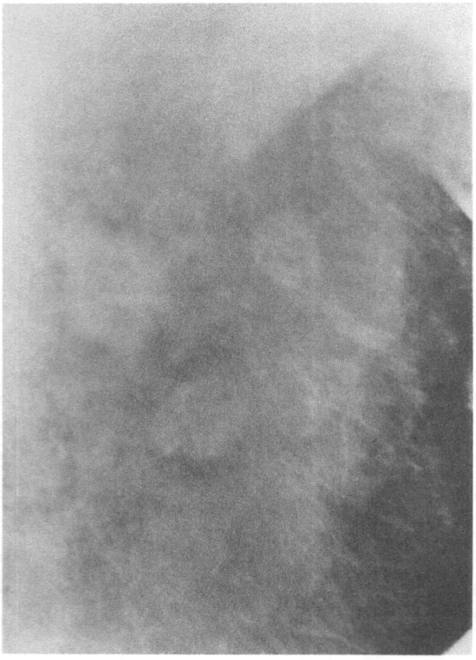

Fig. 3. Metastatic lymph nodes with irregular borders

metastases (Table 4). Irregular nodes occurred in 42% of cases in the same group (Fig. 3).
A combination of high attenuation and irregular shape almost invariable signified metastatic disease. Of axillae with perinodal metastatic growth, 75% had one or more nodes with high attenuation and 50% had irregular nodes. Nodes without metastatic involvement showed increased attenuation in only 1% of the axillae and irregular nodes only occurred in rare cases.
Calcifications, which are important indications of primary breast carcinoma, were found in 3% of the axillae with metastases and then only in advanced disease with, in most cases, diffuse malignant growth in the axilla. The calcifications were of the same type as those in the primary tumor.

Discussion

It is evident that no distinct radiographic indication of metastatic involvement of the lymph nodes exists. Most metastatic lymph nodes are rounded and sharply circumscribed and

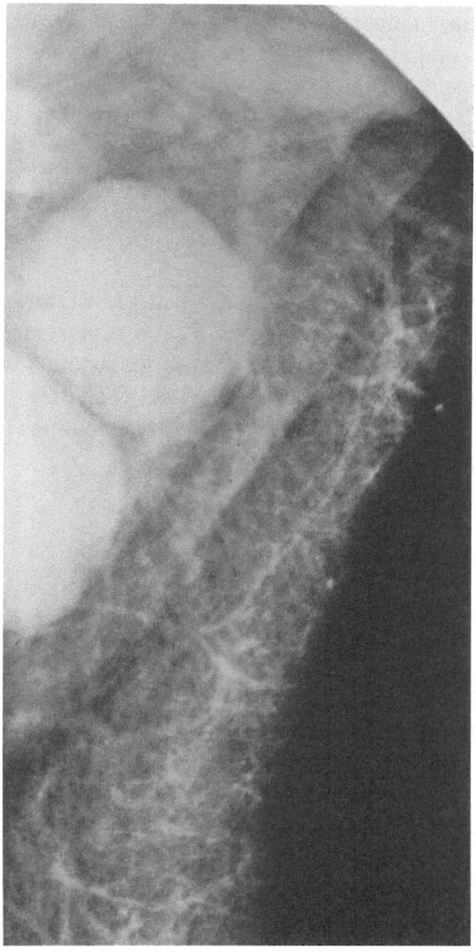

Fig. 4. Enlarged metastatic lymph nodes

their size does not markedly differ from that of normal nodes. It is only in advanced metastatic disease that the lymph nodes become irregular in shape with less distinct borders. The most important early abnormalities indicating metastatic disease are homogeneous nodes with increased attenuation. However, the same abnormalities can be found in patients with inflammatory nodes, primary lymphoid hyperplasia, and lymphoma. In patients with rheumatoid arthritis, homogeneous, enlarged nodes with increased attenuation are also a common finding (Bjurstam 1978; Andersson et al. 1980).

Despite the fact that no distinct radiographic indication of metastatic involvement of the lymph nodes exists, radiography of the axilla is a more accurate method than clinical examination in diagnosing metastatic involvement (Bjurstam 1978). In the present series, metastatic disease was diagnosed correctly in 70% of cases by radiography compared with only 42% by clinical examination. However, the false rate was higher with radiography – 32% compared with 15% by palpation. When the axilla was considered as clearly involved by radiography, there was no false positive diagnosis.

There are only a few reports on the radiographic appearance of metastatic lymph nodes. Leborgne et al. (1963) described metastatic nodes as "rounded shadows varying in size, having uniform density and circumscribed borders." They also pointed out that metastatic nodes do not generally possess any characteristics that permit then to be distinguished from other pathologic processes in the lymph nodes. Kalisher (1975), on the other hand, stated that metastatic nodes are generally larger (> 25 mm) with high attenuation and lobulated or angular margins; they tend to be matted together. This is not in agreement with the results in the present series. Metastatic lymph nodes were only occasionally larger than 25 mm (Fig. 4). Most metastatic lymph nodes were rounded or ovoid and they were matted together only in very advanced disease.

Conclusions

Normal lymph nodes are usually less than 10 mm in diameter, ovoid, or lobulated with low or moderate attenuation. Fatty replacement is common, especially in older women. No distinct radiographic signs of metastatic involvement exist. Most metastatic lymph nodes are sharply circumscribed and their size does not markedly differ from that of normal nodes. The most important abnormalities indicating metastatic disease are homogeneous nodes with increased attenuation.

References

Andersson I, Marsal L, Nilsson B, Sjöblom KG, Wollheim FM (1980) Abnormal axillary lymph nodes in rheumatoid arthritis. Acta Radiol [Diagn] (Stockh) 21: 645

Bjurstam N (1978) Radiography of the female breast and axilla. Acta Radiol [Suppl] (Stockh) 357: 107–117

Haagensen CD (1971) Disease of the breast, 2nd edn. Saunders, Philadelphia

Johnsén C, Bjurstam N, Hedberg K, Hultborn A, Johansson NT, Peterson LE (1975) Breast disease. A clinical study with special reference to diagnostic procedures. Acta Chir Scand [Suppl] 454: 55

Kalisher L (1975) Xeroradiography of axillary lymph node disease. Radiology 114: 67

Leborgne R, Leborgne F, Leborgne JH (1963) Soft tissue radiography of the axilla in cancer of the breast. Br J Radiol 36: 494

Wolfe JN (1977) Xeroradiography. Uncalcified breast masses. Thomas, Springfield

*Evaluation of New Imaging Procedures for Breast Cancer**

M. Moskowitz, S. A. Feig, C. Cole-Beuglet, S. H. Fox, J. D. Haberman, H. I. Libshitz, and A. Zermeno

Breast Cancer Detection Center, University of Cincinnati, Cincinnati, OH 45267, USA

Since breast cancer will affect one of 11 American women during their lifetime, it is a major target of medical research. Mammography has been in the forefront of this effort because of accumulating evidence that early detection improves prognosis and because of the demonstrated ability of mammography to detect cancer at nonpalpable stage (Baker et al. 1982). Its widespread use has been tempered by the issue of possible risk from low doses of ionizing radiation as well as by the fact that although more accurate than any other detection method, including physical examination, it may still find only 80%–90% of breast cancers (Baker et al. 1982).

These factors have served to stimulate some medical investigators and manufacturers of medical equipment to conduct and support studies of alternative breast imaging procedures such as telethermography, graphic stress thermography, cholesterol plate thermography, ultrasound, and diaphanography. For several reasons, these studies have not always had the rigorous evaluation they deserve. In some cases, commercial incentives have led to the hasty marketing of equipment before its accuracy (or lack of accuracy) was fully known. In other instances, personal and professional motives have caused some investigators to announce a research "breakthrough" based on poorly designed and/or poorly analyzed studies. Companies may provide these investigators with professional forums and research funds at a time when government grants are in short supply. Thus, the investigators may become unwitting partners in unscientific misadventures.

These "medical advances" can then be offered to patients and even some referring physicians who lack the specialized knowledge to evaluate their claims. Many patients seek reassurance that they do not have a breast cancer yet hesitate to undergo a mammogram because they have heard from the news media about the possible radiation risk. They are quick to seize on claims for a "reliable", but "safe" alternative test, and they are perfect victims for deception.

That many women are highly aware of breast cancer yet unnecessarily apprehensive of the medical X-ray exposure is ironic. The potential tragedy is that large numbers of tiny cancers could be lost to early detection through such misguided apprehension. The risk may be much greater than the theoretical risk from properly executed mammography (Fox et al. 1978; Moskowitz 1981; Moskowitz et al. 1976).

Evaluation of new imaging modalities has been relatively inefficient in the past. Through trial and error, new modalities have found some level of acceptance by the medical community. The process has been expensive, time consuming, and nonscientific. In terms of breast disease, however, this may not be its main failure. If a new method, such as

---

* This paper was originally published in the American Journal of roentgenology (vol. 140 pp. 591–594, 1983) and is republished here with kind permission

thermography, ultrasound, computed tomography (CT), or diaphanography, is not proven to detect very small, highly curable breast cancer, its wide use may delay diagnosis significantly and lead to otherwise avoidable loss of life. Diagnostic imaging procedures that do not detect lesions at an earlier stage than current clinical practice do nothing but add unproductive expense to the cost of medical care and set attitudes that may be difficult to change. For example, the widespread implementation of thermography before its role in breast cancer detection was firmly determined led to unrealistic expectations, followed by rejection of this technique. Yet, it is entirely possible that thermography may have a useful role in risk-factor analysis, prognosis, and possibly in detection, but because of the haphazard process used for its evaluation its proper role as an imaging procedure has not been defined. Many such problems could be avoided if minimum guidelines for the clinical evaluation of any new breast imaging modality were adopted. This paper describes the basic process, the kinds of data that should be gathered, and the reporting sequence prior to the general distribution and sale of expensive equipment. The goal is to organize the process and, more importantly, to emphasize certain necessary steps that have been frequently bypassed because of exigencies of time or money. Indeed, this outline might form a framework for evaluating new imaging modalities for other areas of the body as well.

Definitions

A *diagnostic* test is defined as one that provides sufficient information to permit therapeutic intervention. For the patient with a palpable breast mass, the definitive diagnosis is established by histology and/or aspiration. Imaging procedures such as mammography or ultrasound are not in themselves diagnostic when they function to provide the initial indication for biopsy. But they may be diagnostic if they affect a clinical decision against biopsy. For example, ultrasound can differentiate cysts from solids, and biopsy may not be performed. But even here, when feasible, aspiration should be done.

Screening may be defined as detection of breast cancer in an asymptomatic person or persons with the *goal* of *lowering* diagnostic threshold at the time of detection. This patient examined may be at any level of risk based upon epidemiologic factors, which may be known but which do not localize or establish the presence of disease. Important in the concept of screening is the requirement of lowering threshold of detection significantly below the current clinical threshold. The clinical threshold for breast cancer detection at this time in the United States may be defined as 50%–60% stage I disease.

When mammography is used to evaluate a palpable breast mass, it also serves as a screening procedure for the remainder of the breast and the opposite breast. Ultrasound, as a diagnostic procedure for determining whether a palpable mass is cystic or solid, may be warranted from data which indicate its effectiveness for that purpose. However, the use of ultrasound only, to the exclusion of mammography, would not be warranted unless both were equally sensitive as screening modalities. Even if ultrasound were not intended as a screening modality, its substitution for mammography in the evaluation of a palpable mass would be tantamount to that purpose.

Evaluation Process: Introduction

The *specific roles* for a screening procedure may be stated as: (1) Detection of breast masses; (2) differentiation of cystic or solid lesions; (3) differentiation of benign from malignant lesions; (4) detection of malignant microcalcifications; (5) detection of 5 mm invasive cancers and/or cancers that are wholly in situ ductal or in situ lobular.

Results should be specified according to these roles, to lesion size, and also according to palpable and nonpalpable lesions. The performance of the new modality must be clearly understood by the clinician who requests these procedures as well as by the radiologist who interprets them.

Evaluation of the new modality requires that it be examined independently and in combination with existing methods in an objective nonbiased fashion. A truly blind study of a new modality must be both interpretively and *technically* blind. Not only must the interpretation be made without knowledge of findings from any other modality, but the *technician* should perform the examination in a similar manner. Additionally, patients examined by the new modality should not be preselected by clinical examination or any other imaging modality since this will lead to biased results. For example, if ultrasound is advocated as a replacement for mammography, patients should not be selected for ultrasound on the basis of a palpable mass.

Evaluation Process: Methodology

Phase 1: Preliminary Evaluation and Training

The purposes of this phase are to determine if a new instrument has any potential; to develop data to refine operating procedures, environmental requirements, and clinical configuration; to develop criteria for interpreting the study. This is primarily a developmental phase.

Once a new imaging method has passed the development phase its safety for humans must be determined. If the range of risks seems acceptable, the first phase of clinical testing can be entered. Clinical testing is essentially retrospective. Information from the new modality is compared with pathology. Criteria for distinguishing normal, benign, and malignant pathology are developed. Any potential for localizing abnormalities can also be evaluated. While efforts should be made to include as many cases of early disease as possible, this phase will generally be conducted on clinically detected breast cancer. For the most part, these cancers will be relatively far advanced. This testing will be performed on patients referred with symptoms, usually a palpable breast lump. All patients coming to biopsy, however selected, as well as a population of normal females will be examined with the instrument. This will result in three groups of subjects: (1) biopsy-proven malignant cases classified by stage; (2) biopsy-proven benign cases; and (3) cases negative on physical examination and mammography, and assumed to be normal.

The criteria for positivity and negativity are clearly established. If the instrument seems to separate clearly benign from malignant disease, it has the potential for a diagnostic test and could be a screening test as well. If it cannot distinguish benign and malignant disease, but can distinguish biopsy-suitable patients from normals while maintaining a high true positive rate for malignant disease, it has the potential to be a screening test. Assuming that the instrument is to be a screening tool, it is important to test its ability to detect stage I and, perhaps, minimal breast cancer. If it cannot detect any stage I cancers available in this phase, it will not have any potential as a screening tool.

This phase is primarily for internal use. Publication of the results should *not* be made in conjunction with commercial proposals. Any data analysis, published or not, should assign confidence limits to all results. These confidence limits should reflect the distribution of any determinate about the means, the number of cases in each class, and the number of features used. *This phase of the study will determine if a device has no potential.* It *cannot measure the degree* to which a device may be clinically useful. If this phase is successful, individual physicians will then be selected from other institutions for a period of training in the interpretation of the information generated from the new modality. These individuals will then be tested; a minimum standard defined and acceptable to the initial investigators must be achieved. Once this pool of independent interpreters from different institutions is obtained, the next phase of the study can begin.

Phase 2: Clinical Suitability

The purposes of this phase are initially to determine how the new device functions as a screening device compared with the current modalities in evaluating the transferability of the modality and in fixing environmental requirements. Transferability and environmental requirements are often overlooked. Experience gained in phase 1 should be used to fix the design of the instrument, procedures for its use, and any environmental requirements. By placing the instrument in other institutions in this second phase, the maturity of the device can be tested.

The nature of this phase of the study may best be described by the following critical points:

1. The device must be used on a population of patients who will not be selected for biopsy as well as on those who will be. The test cannot be used only on those patients who are *known* to have a suspicious lump.
2. The results can play *no* role in the management of the patient. The results should not be interpreted on site nor, in fact, should the results be available to the attending physician until the entire study project is completed.
3. No information should be given to those interpreting the information other than the name and age of the patient, *until* the study is completed and the results are in.
4. Each patient will receive a clinical examination, mammographic examination, and evaluation with the new modality. After appropriate management is selected for the patient, the mammograms of all patients examined will be independently read in a blind fashion by the other observers in the program *away from the original locality*. Modality X will similarly be independently read elsewhere. The images will be distributed in a round robin fashion and evaluated for technical quality and inter- and intraobserver agreement will be scored. The stage at detection for each modality will be determined. The sensitivity and specificity for each modality will be compared.
5. The patient should not be charged for examination by the new modality.
6. If there is any alteration of the interpretive criteria for the instrument during this phase, the entire study must begin all over again. If, after the data are made available, new algorithms are noted, which, perhaps, will increase the positive rate for early cancers, the entire phase 2 must be repeated using the new algorithms.

The results of this phase will determine if stage I and some minimal cancers are detectable and at what cost in terms of false positives. A negative study here, i.e., failure to detect the stage I and minimal breast cancers that are currently being detected otherwise would indicate that the instrument has very little potential as a screening procedure. It is not likely that a test which can not detect a significant portion of the minimal breast cancers and stage I breast cancers currently found in a routine workup would detect a significant number of other "occult" minimal cancers.

The data should be analyzed in a manner that yields the least possibility of being misconstrued and keeps in mind the purpose of the new modality. For instance, if the new modality is advocated as a replacement for mammography, then the significant statistic is the percent of mammography-positive, clinically negative cancers found by the new modality according to lesion size. If the new modality is advocated for its ability to differentiate cystic from solid lesions, then its ability in this function should be given according to lesion size.

If this blind study shows that the instrument can detect a reasonable number of minimal and stage I breast cancers at an acceptable cost, then a phase 3 study to determine its use as a screening tool would be justified. In other words, if the results are positive, the instrument is still viable, but not proven as a screening tool.

We believe that phase 2 can be performed at a reasonable cost in any relatively high-volume diagnostic setting, but it must be *blind.* The enthusiastic use of new instruments by zealous advocates is perhaps the single greatest reason for their ultimate failure and delay in determining their appropriate clinical role.

Phase 3: Clinical Verification of Screening Function

The objective here is to verify the usefulness of the instrument in detecting breast cancer by clinical stage compared with currently available screening modalities. This stage provides the type of data necessary to estimate its value in the clinical screening role. To maximize the number of minimal breast cancers and allow an adequate evaluation of this most important function, a large number of asymptomatic persons would have to be enrolled. It is not necessary that these persons be of low risk or unselected in terms of risk factors. One could accept into the study self-selected symptomatic patients, and to maximize the yield of minimal breast cancers, high-risk females would be encouraged to attend. The study should be done in areas where there is a relatively high mortality rate and/or incidence of breast cancer rather than in a low-incidence/mortality area.

Based on the experience of the Breast Cancer Detection Demonstration Project (BCDDP), we estimate that for every 10,000 patients screened initially (prevalence screen), approximately 30 minimal breast cancers should be found.

In our opinion, it would be unreasonable to expect those supporting the development of a new modality to wholly underwrite the costs of the phase 3 screening procedure. It would also be improper to charge patients for, or base patient management decisions on, an unproven modality. Since the instrument would be tested against the best presently available modalities, i.e., physical examination and mammography, the problem could be solved as follows:

1. The new modality could be engrafted into a currently ongoing screening program funded by some other source. The costs of the new modality added to the screening program would be absorbed by the company producing it.
2. It could be performed in a center where females are screened, for whatever reason, by physical examination and mammography and treated accordingly. Under these circumstances, the patient would be paying for the mammogram and physical examination, but not for the new instrument screening. We would recommend that if this course be taken that the screening already be in place and not be established just for the purpose of using the new instrument.
3. An alternative course is to establish an entirely new screening program using the currently accepted modalities plus whatever new modalities may be available. This entire screening program could then be funded by a national body such as the National Cancer Institute.

Table 1. Standard error chart

Assumed true-positive rate	Assumed number of cases						
	10	15	20	25	30	35	40
90%	9.5%	7.7%	6.7%	6.0%	5.5%	5.1%	4.7%
85%	11.3%	9.2%	8.0%	7.1%	6.5%	6.0%	5.6%
80%	12.6%	10.3%	8.9%	8.0%	7.3%	6.8%	6.3%
75%	13.7%	11.2%	9.7%	8.7%	7.9%	7.3%	6.8%
70%	14.5%	11.8%	10.2%	9.2%	8.4%	7.7%	7.2%
65%	15.1%	12.3%	10.7%	9.5%	8.7%	8.1%	7.5%
60%	15.5%	12.6%	11.0%	9.8%	8.9%	8.3%	7.7%
55%	15.7%	12.8%	11.1%	9.9%	9.1%	8.4%	7.9%
50%	15.8%	12.9%	11.2%	10.0%	9.1%	8.5%	7.9%

To use this table, one enters at the row corresponding to the assumed true-positive rate for any stage cancer, say 75%, and crosses over the columns until one arrives at the number of cases at that stage, for example, 30. The standard error is then 7.9%. This means that there is a less than 2.3% chance that the true-positive rate would be less than 59.2% (75%−2 × 7.9%) if the trial were repeated. This assumes that the results are normally distributed. It would be also mean that there would be only 5% chance that the true-positive rate would be less than 62% (75%−1.65 × 7.9) if the test were repeated.

Another example would be as follows: If one wants to show that there is only a 5% chance that the true-positive rate for minimal cancer is less than 80%, how many minimal cancers are needed? If one assumes that the new test will yield almost a 90% true-positive rate, this is 10% over the target; 10% divided by 1.65 (for the 5% tail) yields a standard error of about 6% or about 25 minimal cancers. Actually, one would need more like 30 so there could be three positive misses and still have 90% true-positive. If the instrument yielded 85% true-possitive, it would take more than 40 cases to prove 80% at the 5% level.

The table can also be used for the false-positive rate. To obtain the standard errors for a false-positive rate of 10% one enters the table on the 90% true-positive rate row. For 15%, one uses the 85% row, for 20%, the 80% row and so or. This is a minor consideration since there are usually many negative cases

Whatever route is selected to obtain patients, they all should undergo mammography, clinical examination, and the new study. Clinical management decisions should be based on the results of the mammogram and physical examination. The results of the new modality interpretation should not be available to the investigators, and the clinical details should not be made available until all decisions have been made and recorded independently. The duration of this phase would be approximately 1 year in order to collect sufficient cases. (To determine the number of cases and/or patients needed, see Table 1.) Another 2 years would be necessary to collect and collate all the pathology and follow-up data. And probably another 6 months to 1 year would be required to arrive at an interpretation of the data. This *must* be a blind study of both mammography and the new modality and in each case interpretation should be performed away from the site of clinical study for comparison purposes.

Of major interest would be the true-positive rates on minimal, stage I, and stage II cancers, as well as the false-positive rates on normal cases. The true-positive rates on so-called clinically "occult"cancers, negative on physical examination, would also be of interest. If a negative result for detection of early disease is soon obvious, the degree of failure need not be quantified, and the study can be aborted at that point. If the results of mammography and the new modality appear to be similar, and if, in combination with physical examination, it seems to lower the stage of detection significantly over nonscreened thresholds, it is not unreasonable to assume that the test can indeed identify smaller more highly curable lesions.

Phase 3 follow-up for each individual enrolled in the prevalence should be carried out for 1, possibly 2 years. This is particularly important in evaluating the significance of "false positives." If the number of cancers occurring within 1–2 years of a screening that are negative to the standard tests (physical examination and mammography) but positive to the new modality and if the false-positive rate as a whole for the new modality is reasonably low, the new modality may function as a significant risk indicator. If the instrument is thought to be a risk marker, its specificity/sensitivity for biopsy-proven proliferative disorders could also be monitored.

Once again, as in phase 2, if criteria should change during phase 3, all cases used to establish new criteria would be considered invalid for this phase.

Conclusion

The authors believe that the method outlined is a rational way to evaluate new modalities such as ultrasound, thermography, diaphanography, CT, and nuclear magnetic resonance (NMR) for possible roles in breast cancer diagnosis and/or screening with specific regard to: (1) transferability of technology; (2) transferability of diagnostic criteria among different institutions and radiologists; (3) ability of the new modality to complement or replace mammography and clinical examination; and (4) the threshold size for detection of early cancer. This information must be known before any new modality can be considered for possible use in diagnosis or screening.

The introduction of new modalities in a less rigorous manner could have devastating results. Mammography is a well-established method of detecting small, clinically occult breast cancers. If it were to be replaced by a less sensitive method that had not been adequately tested to determine its true sensitivity, substantial numbers of breast cancers could be lost to early detection and cure. Thus, a supposed "step forward" could really be a step backward.

References

1. Baker L et al. (1982) Breast cancer detection demonstration project: Five year summary report. CA 32: 19–225
2. Fox S, Moskowitz M, Saenger EL et al. (1978) Benefit/risk analysis of aggressive breast cancer screening. Radiology 128: 359–366
3. Moskowitz M (1981) Mammographic screening: significance of minimal breast cancer. AJR 136: 735–738
4. Moskowitz M, Milbrath J, Gartside P et al. (1976) Lack of efficacy of thermography as a screening tool for minimal and stage I breast cancer. NEJM 295: 249–252

Microfocal Spot Magnification Mammography

L. Tabár

Department of Mammography, Falun Central Hospital, 79182 Falun, Sweden

Direct radiographic magnification increases the diagnostic information content of the radiogram. It has, therefore, been used in different fields of radiology (Ablow et al. 1969; Doi et al. 1976; Genant et al. 1975; Gordon et al. 1973; Greenspan et al. 1967; Hayt et al. 1973; Tabár and Dean 1982) and its value has also been realized in mammography (Doi 1977; Sickles et al. 1977; Sickles 1977). This technique requires that the following technical parameters should be properly selected and matched: (1) Size of the focal spot; (2) contrast and resolution of the screen-film system; (3) size of air-gap between the object and the film; (4) quality of X-ray beam; (5) size of the target. All the factors that play a basic role in image quality (resolution, noise, contrast) are affected when the direct radiographic magnification technique is used. In addition, the lesion is enlarged.

Doi (1977) has summarized the most important technical advantages of magnification mammography as compared with contact images:

1. *Sharpness effect.* The resolution is increased with magnification. The explanation of this is that the effective unsharpness of the screen-film system is reduced when the X-ray pattern is enlarged. The resolution increases by a factor equal to the degree of magnification.
2. *Noise effect.* Noise is greatly reduced (by a factor equal to the degree of magnification squared). The X-ray pattern is enlarged, but the noise of the screen-film system remains unchanged. This means that the "effective noise" is reduced relative to the original object size. This leads to improved visibility of the X-ray pattern.
3. *Air-gap effect.* By using an air-gap, the scattered radiation is reduced, which directly leads to increased contrast of the X-ray pattern. The size of air-gap should exceed 15 cm.
4. *Visual effect.* Perception (visual recognition) and analysis of small details on the radiograms (microcalcifications, etc.) improve considerably when the image is enlarged, the contrast is increased, and the effective noise is reduced.

Direct-magnification mammography (× 1.5, × 2.0) provides images superior to conventional contact mammograms. The increased resolution and the reduced noise lead to increased diagnostic information content. This is of great importance for the radiologist. The more accurate diagnosis directly leads to better patient management. First of all, many patients can avoid biopsy because magnification images provide a more precise distinction between malignant and benign breast diseases than conventional mammograms. This has special importance in screening programs.

The value of microfocal spot mammography has been repeatedly emphasized in the literature with regard to breast microcalcifications (Haus et al. 1979; Sickles 1977, 1979, 1980). Magnification mammograms greatly facilitate the analysis of the *form, density,*

Recent Results in Cancer Research. Vol. 90

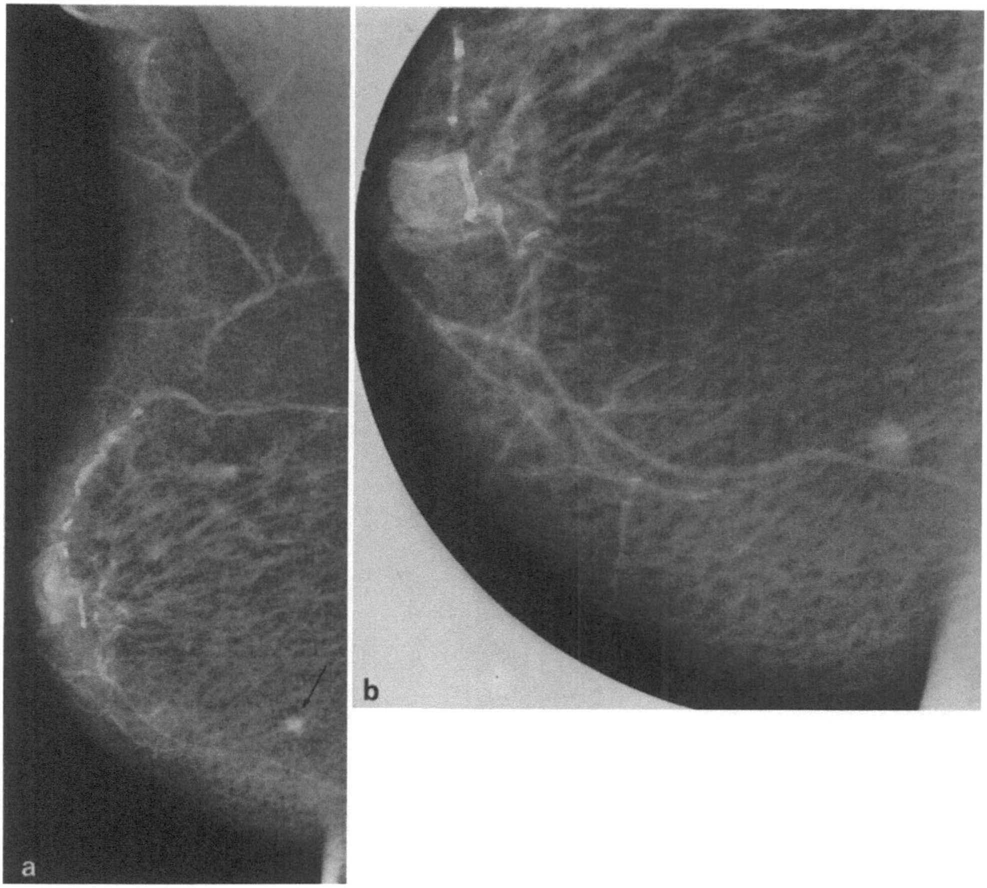

Fig. 1. a Right breast, mediolateral oblique projection. A small tumor shadow is seen in the lower half of the breast *(arrow)*. **b** Magnification view, mediolateral oblique projection. Small tumor mass surrounded by spicules. Mammographically malignant. Histology – infiltrating duct carcinoma; size – 4 × 4 mm. No axillary lymph node metastases. (In all figures, the microfocus magnification images were taken using the mammography system Mam 2, Elscint Inc.)

number, and *distribution* of microcalcifications. However, it should be emphasized that this technique has great value in the correct preoperative diagnosis of breast lesions without calcifications as well. Contour analysis of tiny circumscribed tumors or the demonstration of translucent, circular, or tubular structures within a stellate lesion (Fig. 3) can be crucial in the preoperative diagnosis. Our ultimate goal is to detect breast cancer in its earliest possible stages. Properly performed mammography lowers the diagnostic threshold considerably. However, breast cancer in its earliest stages often does not exhibit the well-known mammographic characteristics on contact mammograms. This may result in uncertainty in interpretation and leads to an increased number of unnecessary biopsies. Direct magnification mammography provides improvement in this new situation by increasing the diagnostic information content of the mammograms.

There is an additional benefit to be gained using magnification mammography. More and more women demand breast-conserving surgery instead of mastectomy. Under these

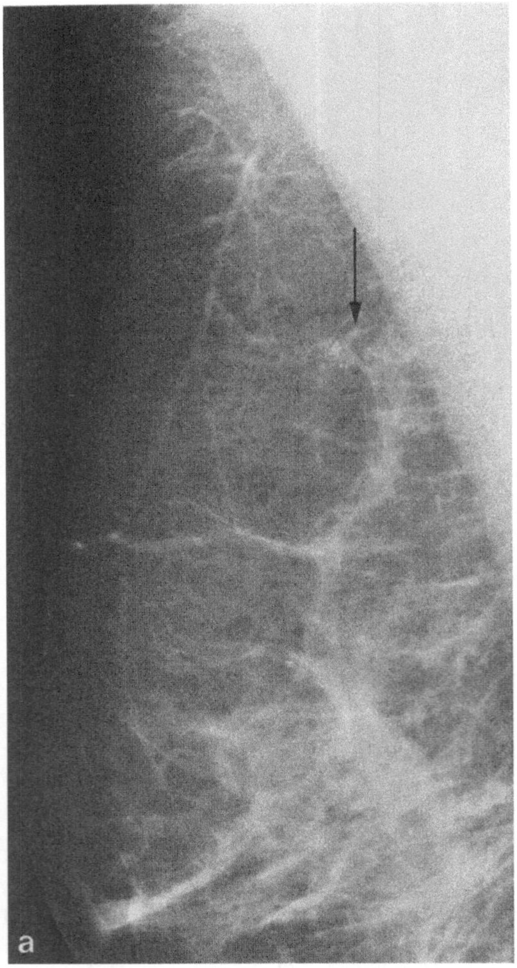

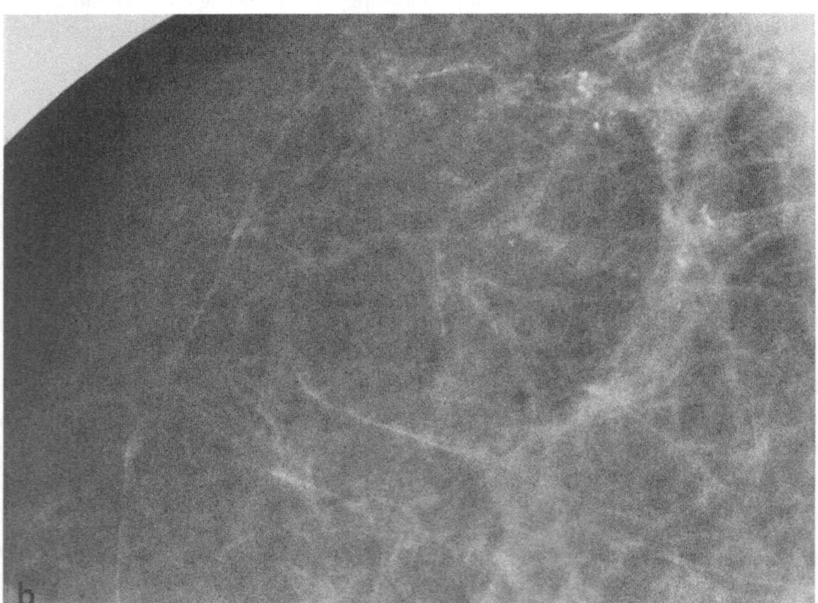

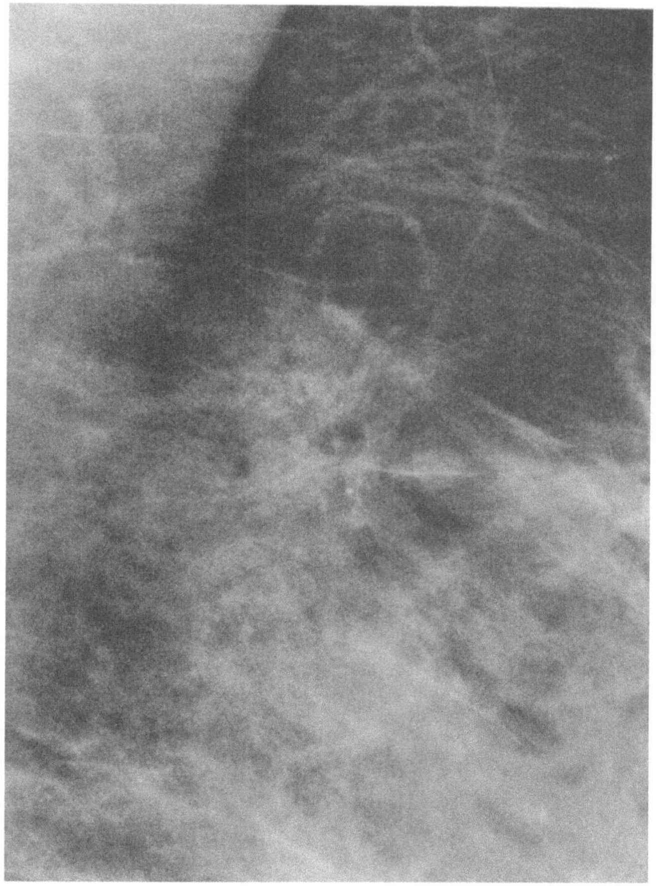

Fig. 3. 46-year-old asymptomatic woman, first screening examination. No palpable tumor in the breasts upon physical examination. Mammography, magnification view, detail picture of the mediolateral oblique projection – a stellate tumor is seen with faint calcifications. There is an oval translucency near the center of the lesion and the stellate structure is formed by radiating, radiolucent linear structures. Typical mammographic appearance of sclerosing duct hyperplasia. Histology – sclerosing duct hyperplasia. No evidence of malignancy

circumstances, the clinician is increasingly concerned to know whether the detected tumor is multifocal (multicentric). Magnification mammography is of great value in detecting the presence of additional cancer foci. It provides valuable information for the clinician and pathologist.

Although magnification mammography provides a picture quality superior to standard mammography and results in increased information content of the image, it remains an adjunct to conventional mammography. This is because magnification mammograms require three to four times the radiation dose of conventional mammograms. But in at least 70% of those selected cases in which the definitive radiographic diagnosis cannot be made with standard mammography, direct-magnification mammography gives invaluable help in revealing the nature of the lesion (Sickles 1979). The analysis is better, the diagnosis is better, consequently patient management is better.

Fig. 2. a Asymptomatic 61-year-old woman. First screening examination. Right breast, mediolateral oblique projection. A cluster of calcifications is seen in the upper half of the breast *(arrow)*. No associated tumor. **b** Magnification view, mediolateral oblique projection. The granular and casting type calcifications are mammographically diagnostic of ductal cancer. Histology – intraductal cancer in situ

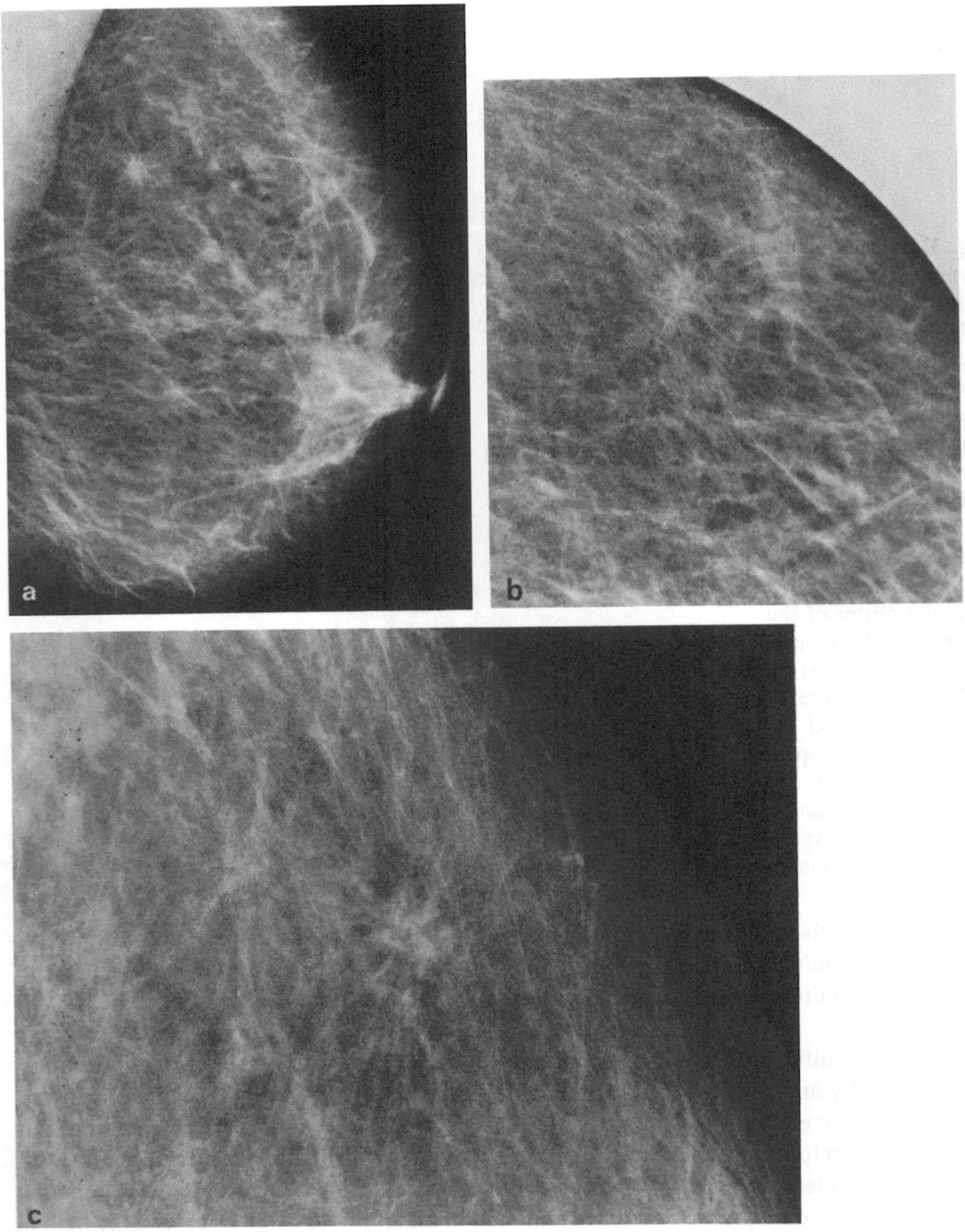

Fig. 4. a A patient aged 65 years. First screening study, asymptomatic. Mammogram of the left breast, mediolateral oblique projection. A small tumor is seen in the upper half of the breast. **b, c** Magnification views, oblique and crainocaudal projections – stellate lesion, mammographically malignant. Histology – infiltrating ductal carcinoma; size – 9 mm. No axillary lymph node metastases

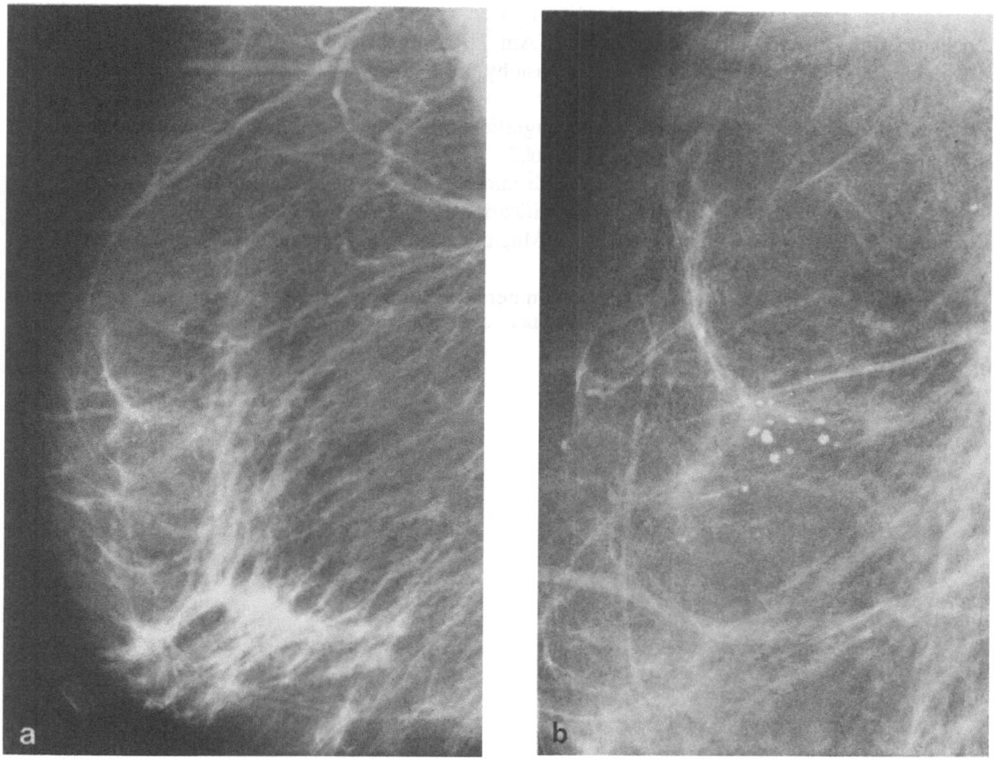

Fig. 5. a A 57-year-old asymptomatic woman upon screening examination. No palpable tumor. Mammogram of the right breast, mediolateral oblique projection; a cluster of calcifications is seen without associated density. **b** Magnification view, mediolateral oblique projection – round and oval, sharply outlined, smooth bordered, clustered calcifications with fairly high, uniform density. Mammographically benign type calcifications. Histology – ductectasia with large, intraluminal calcifications. No evidence of malignancy

References

1. Ablow RC, Greenspan RH, Gluck L (1969) The advantages of direct magnification technic in the newborn chest. Radiology 92: 745–750
2. Doi K (1977) Advantages of magnification radiography. In: Logan WW (ed) Breast carcinomas. Wiley, New York, pp 83–92
3. Doi K, Genant HK, Rossmann K (1976) Comparison of image quality obtained with optical and radiographic magnification techniques in fine-detail skeletal radiography: effect of object thickness. Radiology 118: 189–195
4. Genant HK, Doi K, Mall JC (1975) Optical versus radiographic magnification for fine-detail skeletal radiography. Invest Radiol 10: 160–172
5. Gordon SL, Greer RB, Weidner WA (1973) Magnification roentgenographic technic in orthopedics. Clin Orthop 91: 169–173
6. Greenspan RH, Simon AL, Ricketts HJ et al. (1967) In vivo magnification angiography. Invest Radiol 2: 419–431
7. Haus AG, Paulus D, Dodd GD, Cowart MS et al. (1979) Magnification mammography: evaluation of screen-film and xeroradiographic techniques. Radiology 133: 223–226

8. Hayt DB, Perez LA, Blatt CJ et al. (1973) Direct magnification intravenous pyelography in the evaluation of medullary sponge kidney. Am J Roentgenol 119: 701–704
9. Sickles EA (1977) Magnification mammography. In: Logan WW (ed) Breast carcinomas. Whiley, New York, pp 177–184
10. Sickles EA (1979) Microfocal spot magnification using xeroradiographic and screen-film recording systems. Radiology 131: 599–607
11. Sickles EA (1980) Further experience with microfocal spot magnification mammography in the assessment of clustered breast microcalcifications. Radiology 137: 9–14
12. Sickles EA, Doi K, Genant HK (1977) Magnification film mammography: image quality and clinical studies. Radiology 125: 69–76
13. Tabár L, Dean PB (1982) Magnification immersion radiography: Better soft tissues visualization in the hands. Fortschr Röntgenstr 136: 444–448

Special Techniques in Mammography

M. B. McSweeney, P. Sprawls, and R. L. Egan

Breast Imaging Center, Section of Radiology, Emory University School of Medicine, 1364 Clifton Road, Atlanta, GA 30322, USA

Introduction

Conventional film-screen mammography has proven to be a highly effective procedure for the diagnosis of a variety of breast diseases. However, there are several specific factors that limit image quality and the ultimate sensitivity of the examination. In many instances, the objects (calcifications, soft-tissue masses, etc.) associated with pathologic processes produce low-contrast images which might be near the threshold of visibility. Therefore, any modification of the procedure that can increase object contrast has the potential of increasing examination sensitivity.
Three specific factors that can reduce contrast and visibility in conventional mammography are: (1) Scattered radiation from the breast; (2) diffusion of light (blurring) within the intensifying screen; and (3) reduced film contrast within image areas receiving either low or high exposures corresponding to the toe and shoulder region of the film's characteristic curve. We have investigated methods designed to reduce the image-quality limitations listed above. These specific imaging methodologies and clinical applications are described in this and the following two papers.

Application of Grids in Mammography

Introduction

The visualization of small calcifications in soft-tissue structures requires adequate resolution of the receptor system and optimum contrast. Contrast is degraded both by partial penetration of the beam through breast structures and by the presence of scattered radiation. Conventional film-screen mammography utilizes the low-energy characteristic radiation from a molybdenum target to minimize penetration but until recently little was done to reduce scattered radiation.
Grids are now available that can be used for mammography. We have investigated the effects of such a grid on image contrast, visibility of small structures, and patient exposure.

Materials and Methods

All studies were performed on a Picker Mammorex, 0,6-mm nominal focal spot, molybdenum target with molybdenum filtration. The Kodak Min-R film-screen system or

Recent Results in Cancer Research. Vol. 90

the Kodak OM-1 film with the Min-R screen were used as receptors. The mammographic grid had a 5 : 1 grid ratio, fiber interspaces, and a carbon covering. Studies were conducted using a variable-thickness phantom, which simulated the range of compressed breast sizes normally encountered in mammographic practice. The Egan phantom (Egan and Fenn 1968) was also used in the evaluation of calcification visibility. The technique was then applied to patients undergoing mammography.

Results

The effect of object thickness on contrast was evaluated utilizing the variable-thickness phantom. Contrast was quickly reduced as object thickness increased (Fig. 1). However, using the grid, contrast was improved at all breast thicknesses normally examined in mammography.

The effect of contrast on calcification visibility is shown in Fig. 2. As breast size and density increase, the threshold of visibility is raised so that only the larger calcifications are visible. Using a grid, it is possible to extend a given level of visibility to larger breast sizes.

The effect of contrast as kilovolt peak increases from 25 to 35 kV(p) is shown in Fig. 3. Contrast diminishes with increasing kilovolt peak with and without grid use. However, for a given kilovolt peak, contrast is significantly improved with grid use.

With grid use, surface exposure values are increased. Relative values for patient exposure using the Min-R system are summarized in Fig. 4.

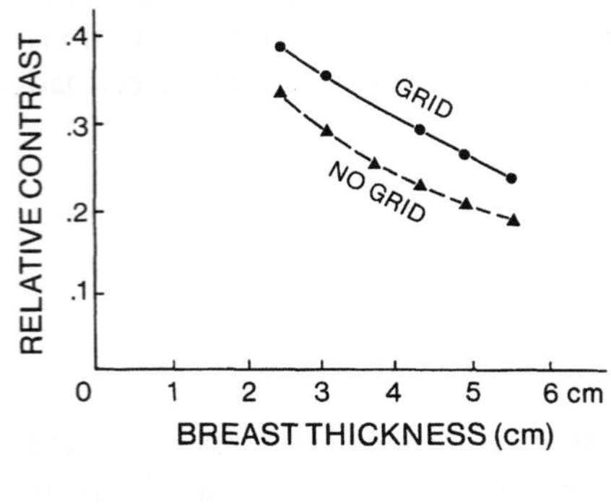

Fig. 1. Effect of object thickness on contrast. Grid use improves contrast at all thicknesses

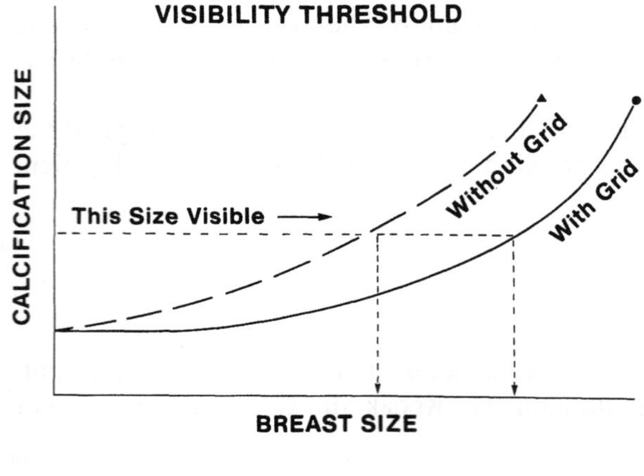

Fig. 2. Grid use extends the range of breast thickness in which small calcifications are visible

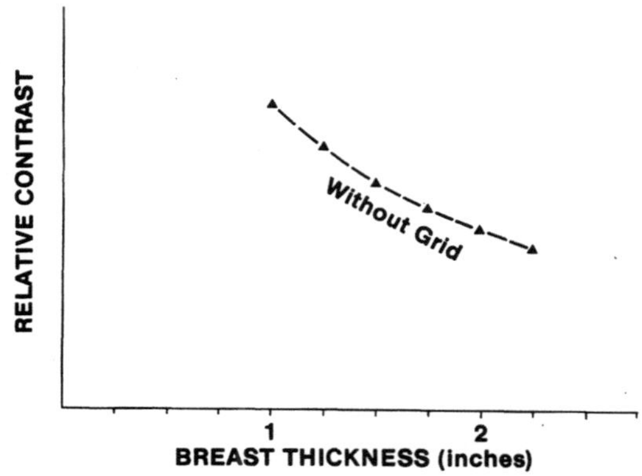

Fig. 3. Effect of kilovolt peak on contrast

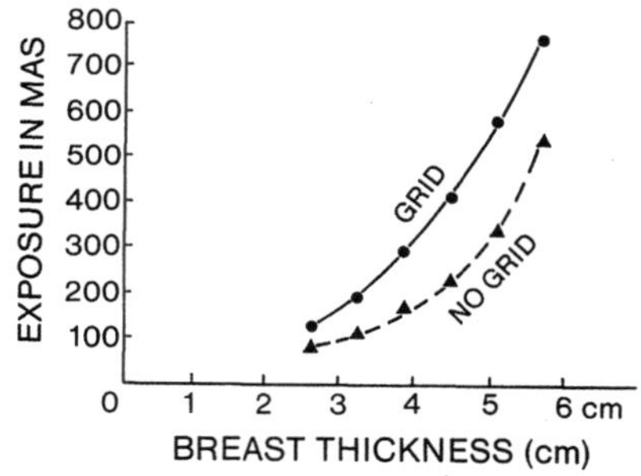

Fig. 4. Exposure related to breast thickness

Discussion

The application of grid techniques to mammography has only been introduced recently (Barnes 1979; Dick and Mutz 1978; Friedrick and Weskamp 1978; Jost 1979; Lammers and Kuhn 1979; Egan et al. 1983). Because of the breast composition and the low kilovolt peak levels used in mammography, scatter was once thought to be of negligible importance with respect to mammographic image quality. It has been demonstrated (Barnes and Brezovick 1977, 1978; Barnes 1979; Jost 1979) that radiation passing through the breast to the receptor contains a significant amount of scattered radiation, as much as 40%–85% of the primary radiation. Thus, scattered radiation is a major factor in the reduction of image contrast. Grids suitable for mammography have only recently become generally available. Conventional radiographic grids produce too much hardening of the beam to be useful in mammography. With the development of the fiber interspace, carbon-covered grids became possible that allow 70% primary beam transmission application in mammography (Friedrick and Weskamp 1978).

The amount of scattered radiation in a mammographic image is dependent upon breast size and the relative amount of fat to fibroglandular tissue within the primary beam. Breast thickness determines the intensity of scattered radiation at a specific point within the image. In conventional film-screen mammography, optimum contrast is obtained by using low kilovolt peak values, the characteristic radiation from molybdenum anodes. However, there is partial penetration of this low-energy radiation throughout the breast, yielding less than mximum contrast. Scattered radiation further degrades contrast. A 40%–80% range

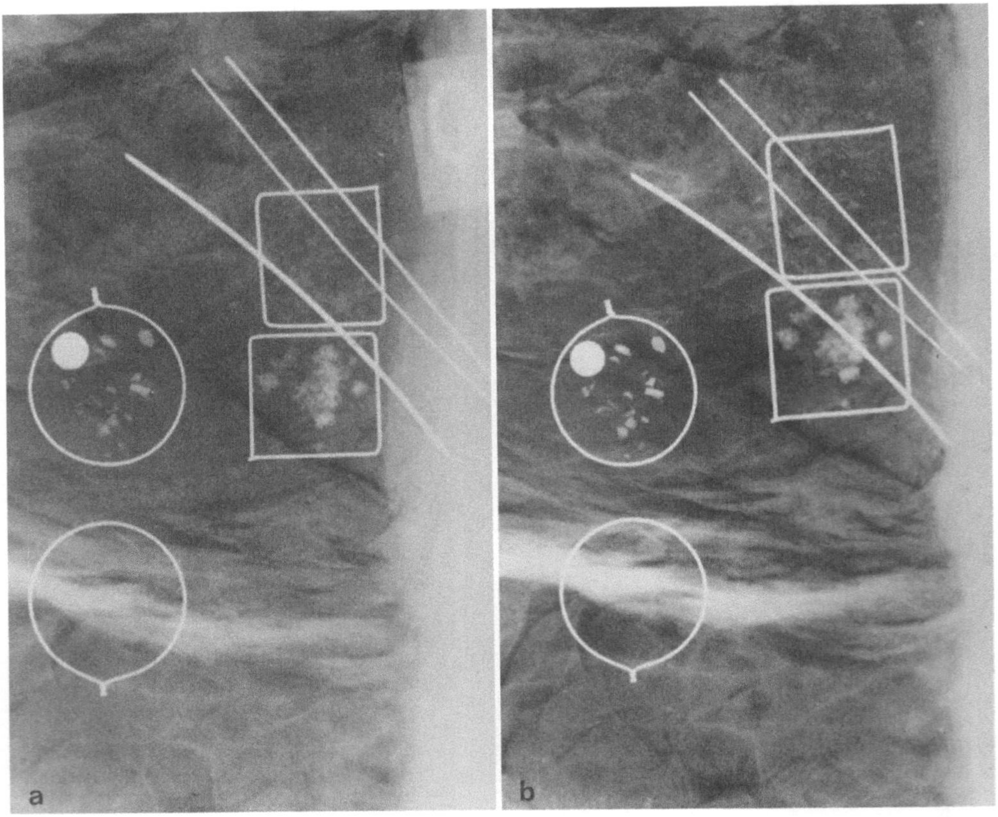

Fig. 5. a Phantom with small simulated calcific flecks within wire-enclosed square area. Standard film-screen technique. **b** Introduction of grid improves contrast and visibility of simulated calcium. *MAS,* milliampere seconds

of scattered radiation will reduce image contrast by 30%–45% (Barnes 1979; Jost 1979).

For inherently low-contrast objects within the breast, the presence of scattered radiation can significantly alter the visibility threshold. Using a grid can reduce the amount of scattered radiation reaching the image receptor and produce a higher level of image contrast (Fig. 5). The effectiveness of a grid to restore contrast increases in proportion to the amount of scattered radiation present. Our measurements indicate that for a 1-in.-thick breast, the grid produces a 20% increase in contrast and for a 2-in. breast the grid increases the contrast by 30%. It has been reported that the use of a grid can increase contrast by as much as 100% under maximum conditions (Dick and Mutz 1978).

A mammographic grid improves contrast at all breast thicknesses normally encountered in a clinical setting. Using a grid, thicker sections can be imaged with the same contrast as thinner sections without the grid (Fig. 6). Through the ability to maintain contrast in thicker objects, one can extend the range of breast thicknesses within which calcifications and soft tissue fibrils may be visualized. Without the grid, it is necessary for calcifications to be larger in a thick breast in order to be visible. By removing scattered radiation, it is possible to increase calcification visibility. Soft-tissue fibril visibility is also increased but

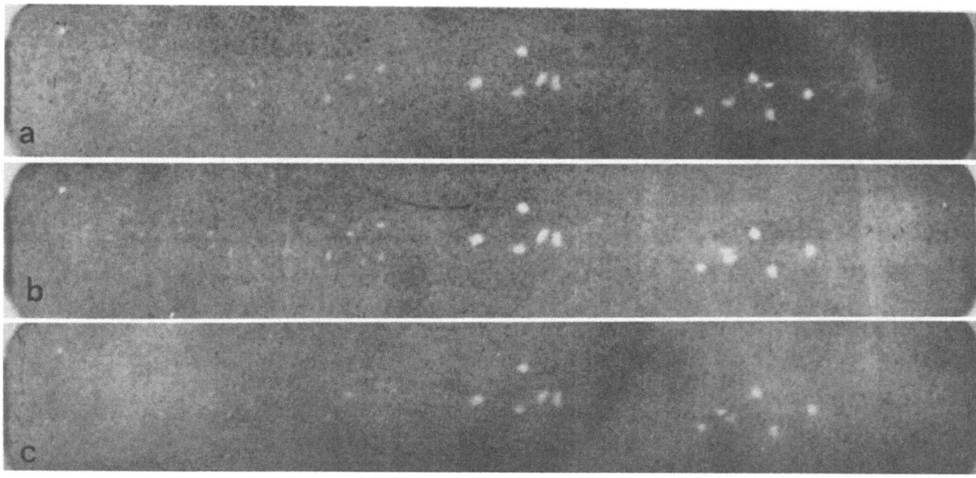

Fig. 6. a There are five clusters of calcifications. Phantom thickness is 1 in. **b** Phantom thickness of 2 in. results in decreased visibility of calcifications. **c** Use of grid with 2-in. phantom results in improved visibility of calcifications

not to the degree seen with calcification, as has been reported by Stanton and Logan (1979).

Although grid-augmented mammography improves image quality, patient exposure is increased. The increased radiation is necessary because of the 30% primary radiation absorbed by the grid. A second factor is the removal of scatter exposure of the receptor. The amount of scatter is a variable, increasing with breast thickness and density. Therefore, with larger breast thicknesses, scatter will be greater, grid absorption greater, and patient exposure increased (Fgi. 4). Reduction of patient exposure is desirable and may be accomplished in one of two ways. Increasing the kilovolt peak from the usual mammographic value of 25–27 kV(p) to 30 kV(p) will decrease the skin dose although the glandular dose will be reduced to a lesser extent because of beam hardening. Substituting OM-1 film for the Min-R film-screen system will reduce exposure by half. The reduced latitude and increased noise with OM-1 film can be tolerated because of improved contrast with grid use.

Conclusions

Grid-augmented mammography results in improved image quality through scatter reduction. The enhanced contrast permits greater visibility of small calcifications, particularly important in larger, thicker breasts.

The increased patient exposure in using a grid may be compensated by employing more sensitive film-screen systems and by a modest increase in kilovolt peak. Visibility of small calcifications and soft tissue structures remains improved with the modifications. It remains to be demonstrated whether the improvement in image quality with grid use makes a significant difference in diagnostic accuracy.

References

1. Barnes GT (1979) Characteristics of scatter. In: Logan WW, Mutz EP (eds) Reduced dose mammography. Masson, New York, pp 223–242
2. Barnes GT, Brezovick IA (1977) Contrast: Effect of scattered radiation. In: Logan WW (ed) Breast carcinoma – The radiologist's expanded role. Wiley, New York
3. Barnes GI, Brezovick IA (1978) The intensity of scattered radiation in mammography. Radiology 126: 243–247
4. Dick CE, Mutz JW (1978) New method for the experimental value of X-ray grids. Med Phys 5: 133–140
5. Egan RL, Fenn JO (1968) Phantoms for evaluating mammography techniques and mammographic detail. AJR 102: 936–940
6. Egan RL, McSweeney MB, Sprawls P (1983) Grids in mammography. Radiology 146: 359–362
7. Friedrick W, Weskamp P (1978) New modalities in mammographic imaging: Comparison of grid and magnification techniques. Medicamundi 23: 29–46
8. Jost G (1979) Evaluation of grid technique in mammography. In: Logan WW, Mutz EP (eds) Reduced dose mammography. Masson, New York, pp 253–258
9. Lammers W, Kuhn H (1979) Improved image quality in mammography by means of scattered radiation grids. Electromedia 47: 2–10
10. Stanton L, Logan WW (1979) Mammography with magnification and grids: Detail visibility and dose measurements. In: Logan WW, Mutz P (eds) Reduced dose mammography. Masson, New York

Magnification Mammography

M. B. McSweeney, P. Sprawls, and R. L. Egan

Breast Imaging Center, Section of Radiology, Emory University School of Medicine, 1364 Clifton Road, Atlanta, GA 30322, USA

Introduction

The sole mammographic indication of a noninvasive carcinoma is frequently the presence of a cluster of small (0.1–1 mm) stippled calcifications (Egan 1972). The contrast and visibility of these small calcifications can be severely reduced by blurring within the imaging system. The three potential sources of unsharpness within the conventional mammographic system are: (1) Patient motion; (2) finite size of focal spot; (3) light diffusion within the receptor (intensifying screen).

In practice, motion blurring is maintained at a relatively low level by patient compression and short exposure times. In the absence of motion, the blur within a mammographic image is typically a combination or composite of focal-spot and receptor blur. The contribution from each of these two sources depends on the size of the focal spot, the thickness and transparency of the intensifying screen, and the actual location of the breast with respect to the receptor and focal spot. When the breast is positioned near the receptor, as in conventional mammography, the receptor makes its maximum contribution to the total image blur. However, if the breast is separated from the receptor, as in magnification mammography, the effective receptor blur is reduced. This reduction in effective blur occurs because the image is magnified or enlarged relative to the inherent blur within the receptor. There is, however, a serious limitation to this approach: As breast-receptor separation (magnification) is introduced, focal-spot blur increases (Fig. 1). An improvement in image quality is realized only if a small focal spot is used and the separation distance (magnification) is adjusted to within the optimum range.

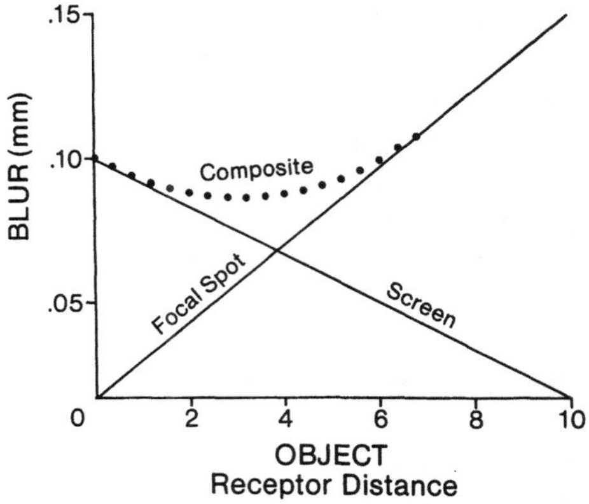

Fig. 1. Relative contribution of focal spot and screen blur as a function of object-receptor distance

Recent Results in Cancer Research. Vol. 90

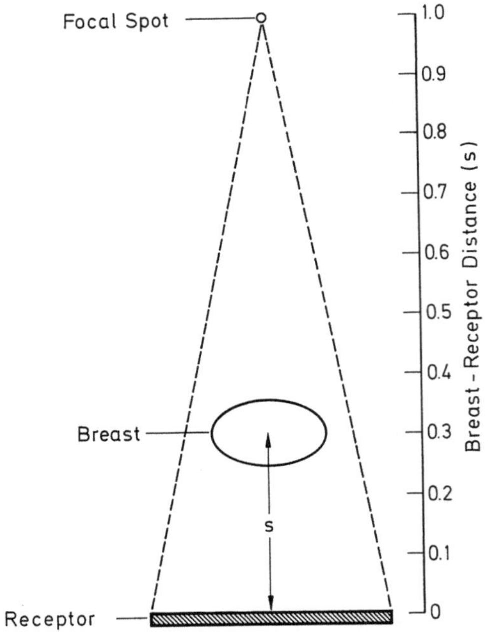

Fig. 2. A scale for expressing the location of the breast in magnification mammography

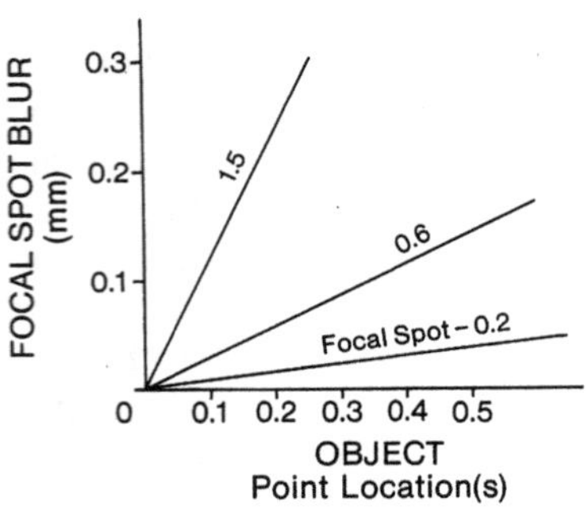

Fig. 3. Relationship of focal spot, screen, and composite blur to object (breast) location

For the purpose of blur analysis, it is desirable to describe object (breast) location by means of a scale extending from the receptor to the focal spot, as shown in Fig. 2. The effective blur from both the focal spot and the receptor are linear functions of object location (Sprawls 1977). This is illustrated in Fig. 3. Also shown in this figure is the composite blur value at different breast-receptor separation distances. A characteristic of the composite blur is that it initially decreases with separation, reaches a minimum value, and then begins to increase as the focal-spot blur begins to predominate. The separation distance (magnification) that produces minimum blur depends on the inherent blur value of the receptor and the size of the focal spot.

Materials and Methods

A Radiological Sciences, Inc. (RSI) microfocus X-ray tube with a 0.1-mm nominal (0.18-mm measured) focal spot was used. The receptor was a Kodak Min-R film-screen system with an inherent blur value of 0.16 mm. With this system, optimum image quality was obtained with a magnification of × 1.5–2.

Results

The improvement in image quality produced with magnification is demonstrated using an Egan breast phantom (Egan and Fenn 1968). The image in Fig. 4a was made with a magnification of × 1.5. The image in Fig. 4b was made with the phantom located at the receptor surface so that there was very little magnification. It has been photographically enlarged to permit critical comparison with the magnified image (Fig. 3a).

In addition to reducing receptor blur, magnification can improve image quality by increasing overall contrast under conditions of high magnification. The effective noise level is also reduced.

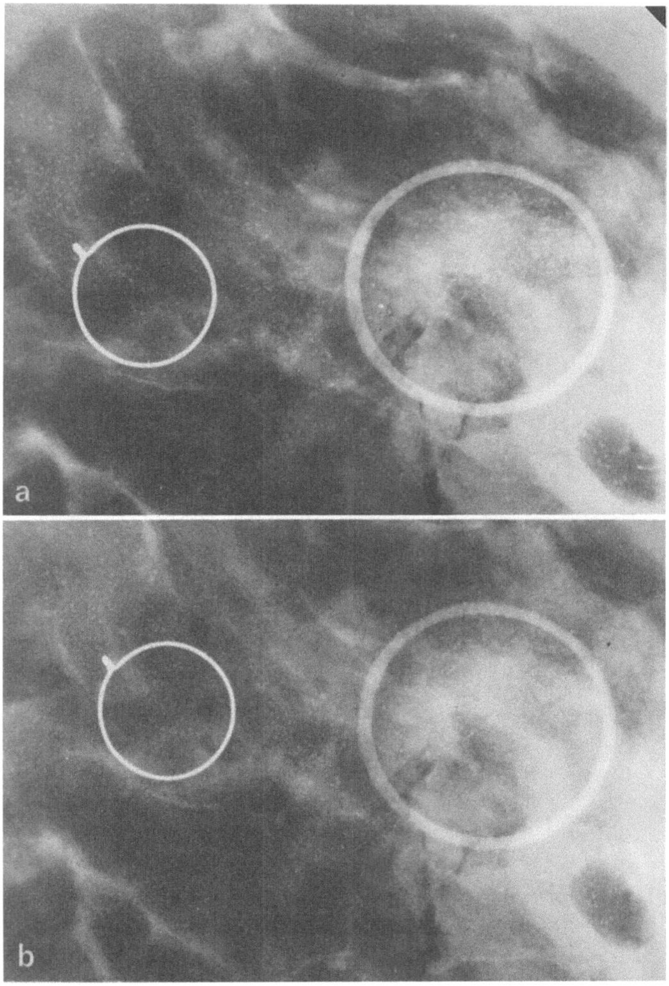

Fig. 4. a A breast phantom image made with the magnification technique. **b** An image produced without magnification

Conclusions

Magnification mammography utilizing a microfocus tube provides increased visibility of small calcifications when used with screen-film receptors. However, there are several factors that limit its general application. These include a diminished field of view and increased patient exposure.

References

1. Egan RL (1972) Mammography, 2nd edn. Thomas, Springfield
2. Egan RL, Fenn JO (1968) Phantoms for evaluating mammography techniques and mammographic detail. AJR 102: 936–940
3. Sprawls P (1977) The physical principles of diagnostic radiology. University Park Press, Baltimore, Maryland, pp 201–210

Enhanced-Image Mammography

M. B. McSweeney, P. Sprawls, and R. L. Egan

Breast Imaging Center, Section of Radiology, Emory University School of Medicine, 1364 Clifton Road, Atlanta, GA 30322, USA

Abstract

A blurred-mass subtraction technique has been developed for mammography, which enhances small-object contrast and visibility throughout the breast area. The procedure is easy to implement and requires no additional exposure. Perception of low-contrast objects is improved by eliminating extreme light- and dark-image areas. Contrast of structures within certain portions of the breast is increased by compression into the high-contrast portion of the film characteristic curve. Detail visibility is also increased by the edge enhancement produced by this process. This paper describes the enhancement process and gives an analysis of its capabilities and limitations.

Introduction

In mammography, accurate diagnosis often depends on the visibility of small, low-contrast objects within the breast image. There are many factors that contribute to the reduced contrast and visibility of these small objects. The factors include X-ray penetration of the objects, scattered radiation, and image blurring produced by the finite size of the focal spot and thickness of the intensifying screen. One factor that is especially significant in certain radiographic examinations, including mammography, is the limited capability of the film to develop maximum contrast over an extended range of exposure values.

The image-processing procedure of blurred-mask subtraction can be used to increase the contrast and visibility of small objects in certain portions of the breast. It is useful for producing a complementary image, which gives improved visualization in very dense areas of the original mammogram. It is especially suited to applications that require reproduction for instructional purposes and publication.

Materials and Methods

The procedure for producing an enhanced mammogram is illustrated in Fig. 1. The procedure is a two-step process. The first step is production of a blurred mask by copying the original mammogram through a piece of glass or clear plastic. The glass diffuses the light, producing a blurred image. Glass thickness determines the amount of blur. A thickness of 3 mm was used for the majority of films.

The Kodak Min-R system or OM-1 film with a Min-R screen was used for the original mammograms, DuPont subtraction film for the blurred mask, and DuPont subtraction

Recent Results in Cancer Research. Vol. 90

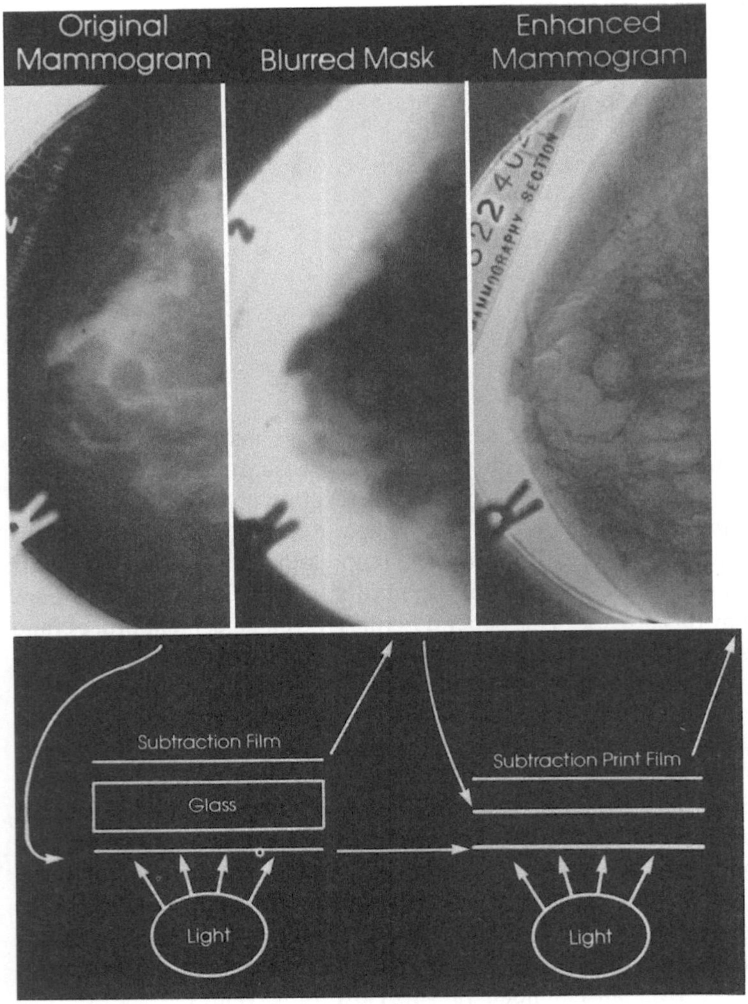

Fig. 1. Procedure for blurred-mass subtraction technique

print film for the final transparency. A standard DuPont Cronex printer was used. All films were processed in a 90-s processor.

Exposure times for making the blurred mask ranged from 1 to 3 s, varying with the mammographic density and with the thickness of the plastic. The exposure is adjusted to give a mask density that complements the density of the original mammogram. When the mask is placed over the mammogram in the second step, the combined densities are essentially the same throughout the image area and have a value of approximately 1.5 density units.

The second step in the procedure is the subtraction of the blurred-mask image from the original mammogram using subtraction print film for the final image. The mask and mammogram were optically aligned; exposure times ranged from 2 to 4 s, depending upon mask and original film density.

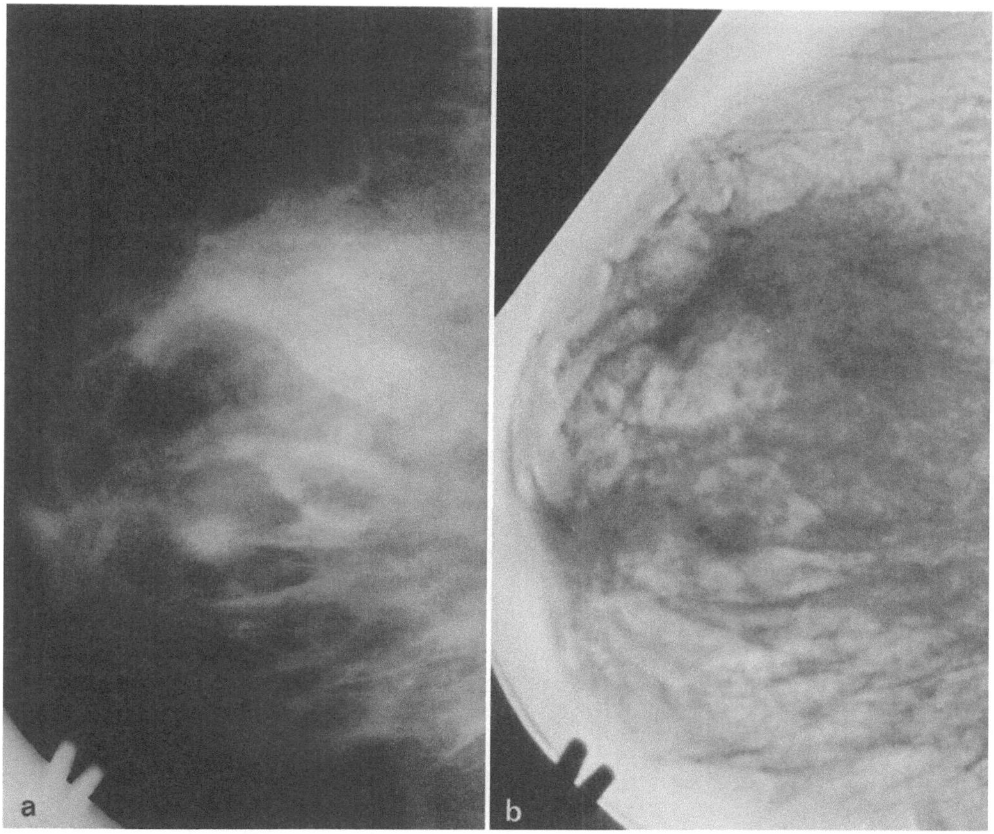

Fig. 2. **a** Conventional mammography. Dense breast tissue with cyst. **b** Enhanced mammography reveals improved visualization and additional cysts

Results

Subtraction of the background density is achieved if the combined densities of the original mammogram and mask are approximately equal throughout the breast. The subtraction results in a background of uniform density over which small objects are superimposed. Figure 2 demonstrates a breast containing dense nodular fibroglandular tissue in the upper half and two cysts at nipple level. Subtraction of the background density results in improved visualization of the known cysts as well as the demonstration of many others that were not seen on the original mammogram (Fig. 2b). Small-object detail is preserved, allowing visualization of fine trabeculae and calcification. Note that the enhanced mammograms are reversal images.

Enhancement of boundaries is achieved through this form of image processing and this type of edge effect may aid in the visualization of structures such as calcifications, fibrils, or masses. The breast in Fig. 3a contains dense fibroglandular tissue with visualization of an occasional cyst. Superimposed over the low-density region of the mammogram is a lobular carcinoma that could easily be overlooked. The edge-enhancement effect produces a low-density halo around the carcinoma spicules, which are now easily identified (Fig. 3b).

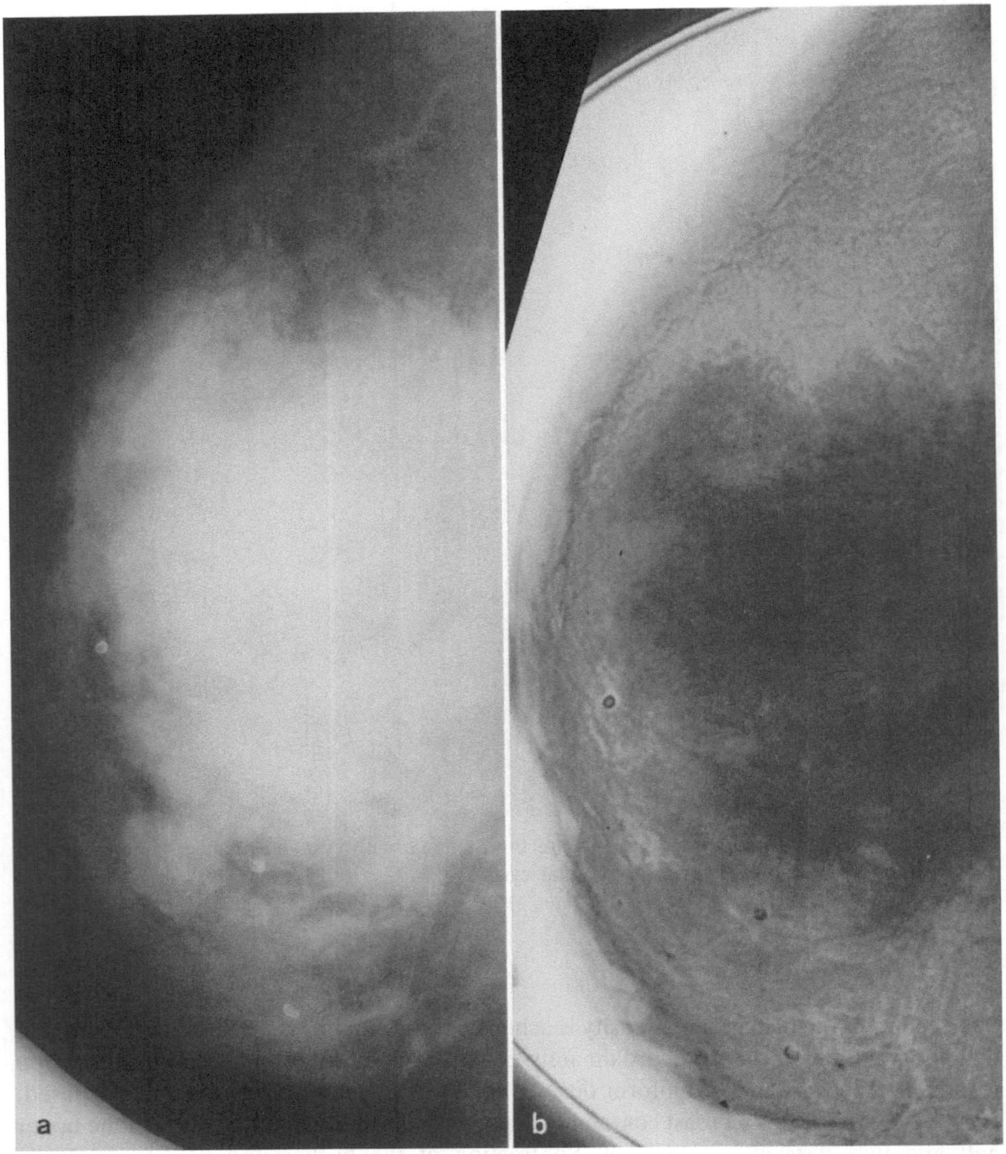

Fig. 3. a Conventional mammography. Carcinoma superimposed over low-density areas difficult to see. **b** Enhanced mammogram. Improved perception of carcinoma

By using proper light exposure when making enhanced mammograms, the wide range of densities present on the original film is compressed into a desired range for easy viewing and reproduction. Figure 4a demonstrates extreme density differences produced by the prostheses, resulting in low radiographic density, and by overlying fat and subcutaneous tissue, which produced areas of high density. Visibility of structures in the high-density areas is suboptimal, even when viewed with a high-intensity light source. In Fig. 4b, the

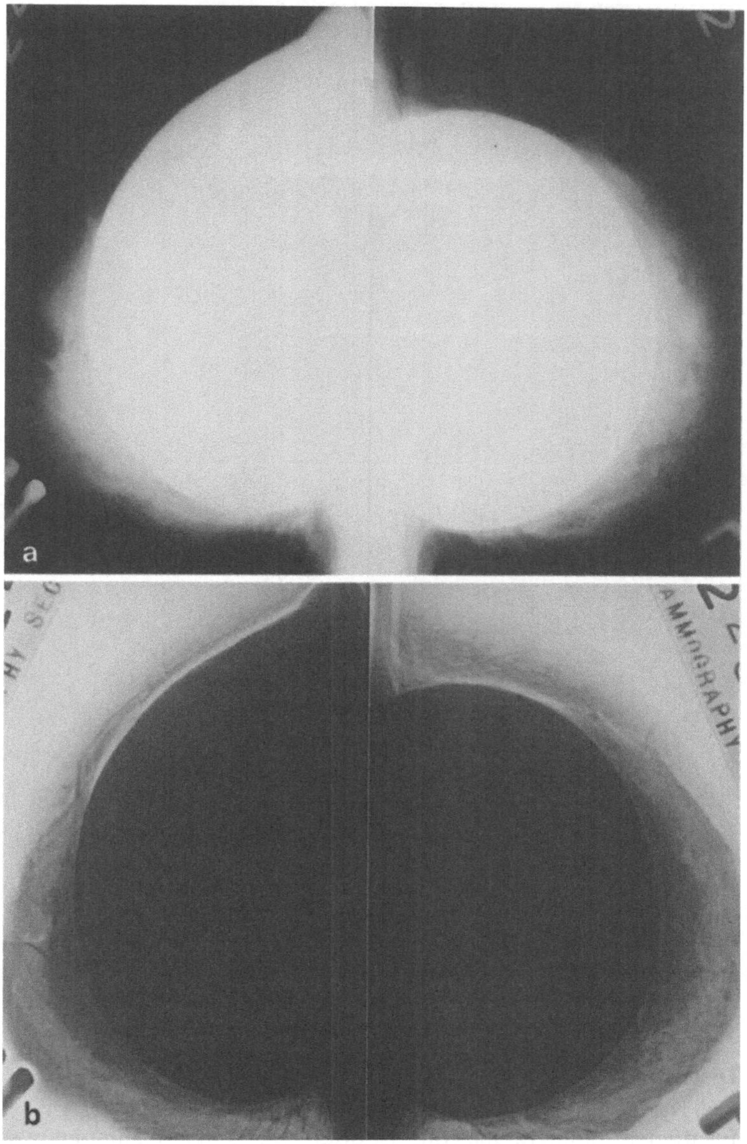

Fig. 4. a Conventional mammogram. Bilateral augmentation mammoplasty and reconstruction. **b** Enhanced mammogram. Improved visibility of subcutaneous structures

subcutaneous structures are readily visible and may be viewed on a conventional viewbox.

The blurred-mass subtraction technique is most useful in the high-density, or overexposed, regions of mammograms. Mammography film will record densities greater than 2.5 density units, which is considered the upper limit for viewing radiographs. Therefore, the information present in the high-contrast areas but not readily visible may be salvaged. The technique is not so successful in the lower-density areas in which no significant density differences are recorded.

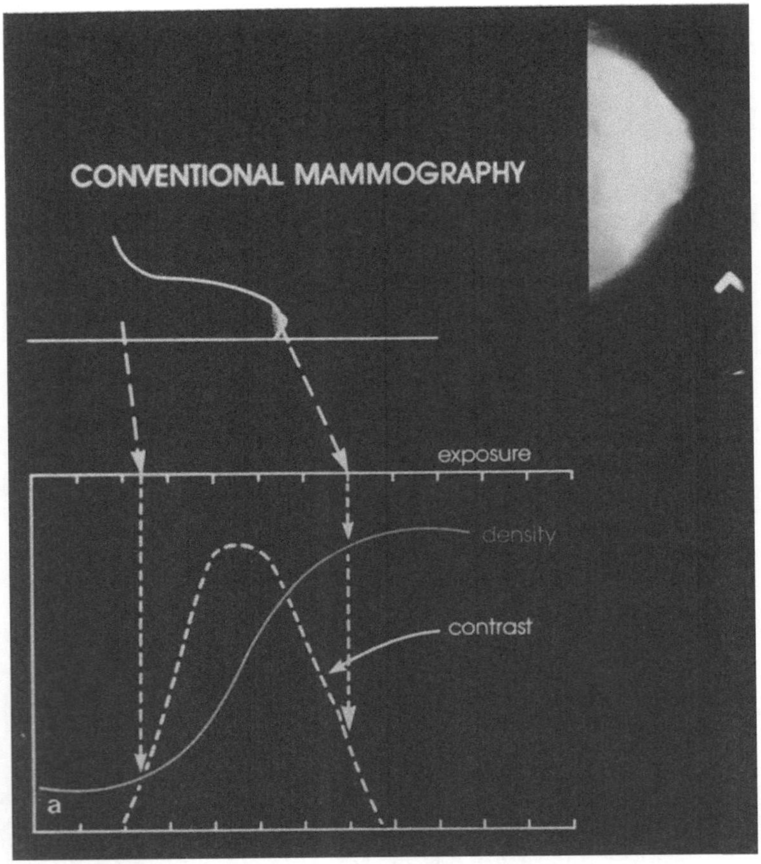

Fig. 5. a The natural variation in breast thickness and density produces an exposure range that exceeds the film's limits for optimum density and contrast. The apex of the contrast curve represents maximum contrast. The mammographic exposure range exceeds the narrow apex. **b** Conventional film-screen mammogram. Optimum contrast is not achieved in very light or very dark areas of the image

Discussion

Insufficient radiographic contrast often results in a mammogram's inability to display the small structures that are necessary for detection of small lesions and adequate interpretation. The variation in thickness and density found in many breasts often produces an exposure range that exceeds the limits of the film for recording maximum contrast.

There have been numerous attempts to improve radiographic contrast with photographic techniques. The subtraction technique was described by Ziedses des Plantes in 1935 (quoted by Davidhoff 1966) but not applied to mammography. Reversal contrast printing has been found useful in overexposed mammograms (Chait and Hale 1971; Dronkers and Van Der Zwagg 1974; Galkin et al. 1979; Orloff 1978), but this process does not create an edge enhancement or uniform density background. Mauer et al. (1951) reported a triple-masking technique using four film emulsions. This complex procedure required critical alignment and an exact matching of densities at each step. Kattan et al. (1973)

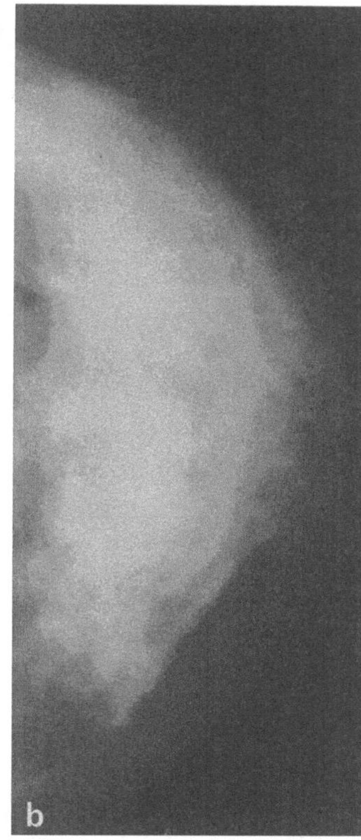

Fig. 5b. Legend see p. 84

described an undersubtraction technique for the production of negatives and subsequently a blurred undersubtraction technique for enhancing radiographs (1981). These techniques are not widely used in mammography, possibly because of the time involved and complexity of the procedures.

Figure 5 illustrates conditions often present in conventional mammography that can limit image contrast. The general relationship between film density and exposure is shown in the form of a conventional film characteristic curve. The amount of contrast that the film will produce is determined by the slope of the characteristic (density) curve at each specific exposure value. The second (contrast) curve shows the relative contrast value as it relates to the basic characteristic curve. The point to be made here is that the maximum film contrast is limited to a relatively small range of exposure values. When a thick or dense portion of the breast produces a relatively low film exposure, that portion of the image is recorded with relatively low contrast as indicated in Fig. 5. The thin portions of the breast near the surface produce relatively high exposures, which result in a very dark or dense image with reduced contrast. The contrast and visibility of small objects is at a maximum when they are recorded near the midportion of the film characteristic curve, which corresponds to a background film density of approximately one density unit. At this point, the objects are recorded with maximum contrast and the film can be viewed with conventional viewbox illumination. However, this condition of optimum contrast and visibility is limited to a relatively short range of film exposures.

In an enhanced mammogram, small objects are recorded on a more uniform background density. A specific characteristic of the enhancement process is that it extends the exposure

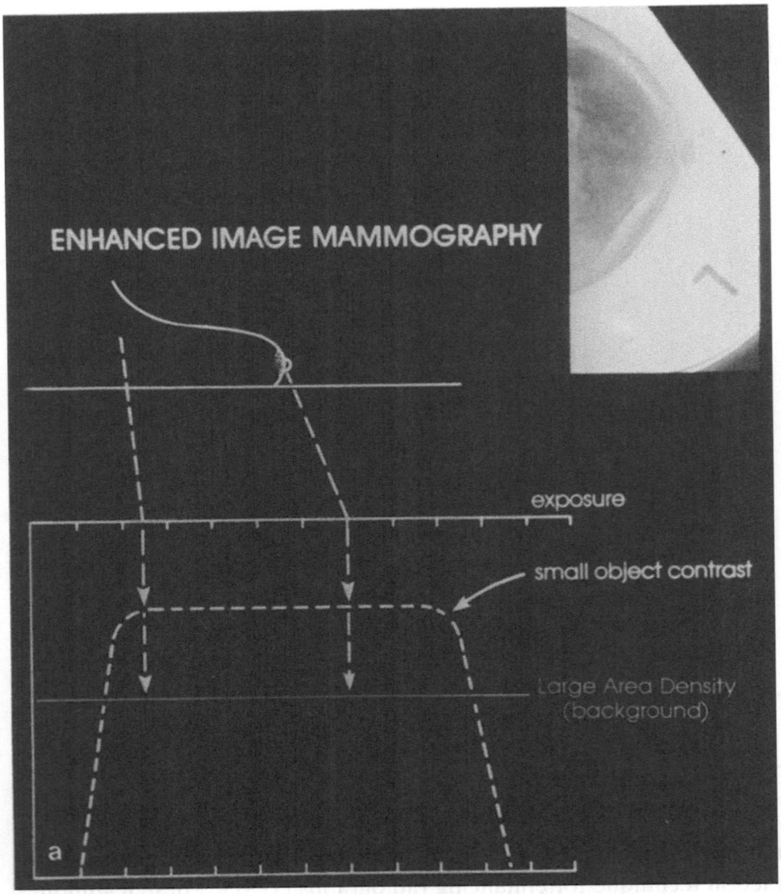

Fig. 6. a In an enhanced mammogram, small objects are imaged with increased contrast and visibility on a uniform-density background. The range of exposures that result in optimum contrast is expanded as reflected in widening of the contrast curve apex. **b** Enhanced image of mammogram in Fig. 5a. Note improved visibility of subcutaneous area and ability to see through dense fibroglandular tissue

range over which maximum film contrast can be produced, as illustrated in Fig. 6. A second characteristic of this process is that the visibility of some objects is increased by edge enhancement. The way in which it enhances edges is illustrated in Fig. 7. Attention is first directed to the film density profile for the small object shown at the top of the figure. In the original image, the profile is well defined and corresponds to the size and shape of the original object. The height of the profile in the blurred image shows that the contrast is reduced and the size of the image becomes larger than the original object.

When the blurred image is subtracted from the original image, the enhancement of boundaries and edges is achieved. In the actual area of the object, the contrast of the original image exceeds that of the blurred image and will be recorded above the average background density level. However, outside the immediate area of the object, when the blurred image is subtracted it creates an area with a density below that of the average background level. This tends to emphasize the edge or the boundary of the object and has the property of increasing visibility.

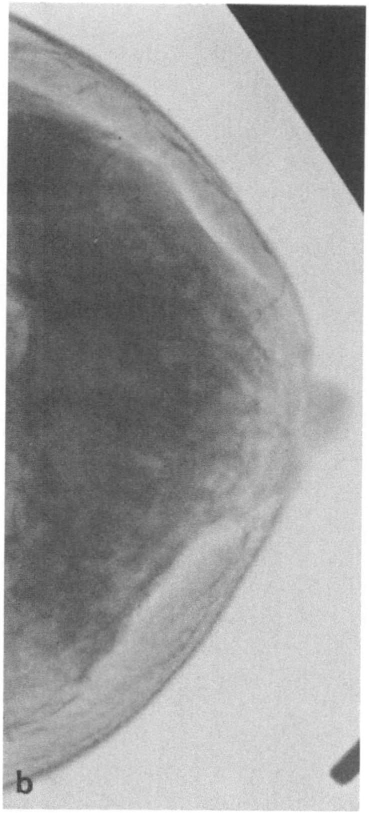

Fig. 6b. Legend see p. 86

A significant loss of resolution cannot be tolerated in mammography. Dronkers and Van der Zwagg (1974), using reversal contact printing, reported no observable difference in small-detail visibility even with magnification factors of × 50. In comparing enhanced mammograms with the original films, we have not encountered any loss of small-object definition.

A practical application of the enhancement technique is in the preparation of prints for publication, slides, copies, and other teaching material. Reproduction of mammograms is difficult because of the relatively low contrast frequently present in portions of the film. It is impossible to reproduce adequately the fine mammographic detail that can be viewed only with a magnifying lens and hot light. The uniform background density, improved small-object visibility, and edge enhancement achieved through this photographic process can improve the quality of reproductions.

Summary

The objective of enhanced-image mammography is to produce a complementary image that will produce improved visualization, particularly in very dense areas of the breast. The original mammogram is preserved and should be interpreted with the enhanced image. Edge enhancement aids in improved perception. Enhanced mammography is particularly

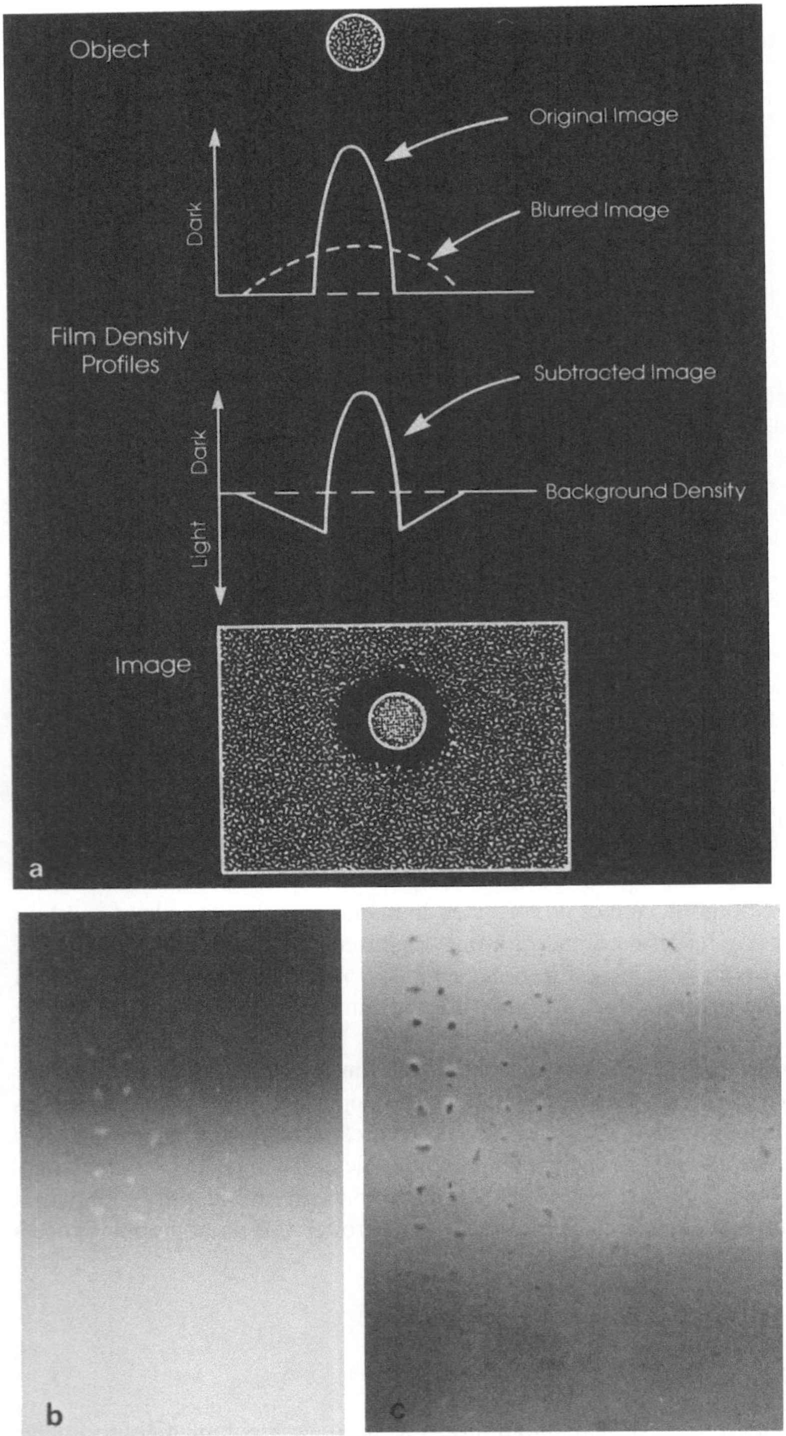

Fig. 7. a Production of edge enhancement. **b** Latitude phantom with simulated calcific flecks, Min-R film-screen. **c** Enhanced image of latitude phantom. Note extended range of calcium visibility into the high- and low-density regions and the edge enhancement of the calcifications

useful in preparing reproductions for publications and slides. The enhancement technique is easy and inexpensive to produce. No specialized equipment is necessary. Enhanced-image mammography requires no additional patient exposure.

References

1. Chait A, Hale J (1971) Positive prints of dense roentgenograms. Radiology 101: 331–334
2. Davidhoff LM (1966) Neuroradiology: reflections of a neurosurgeon. Radiol Clin North Am 4: 3–9
3. Dronkers DJ, Van Der Zwagg H (1974) Photographic contrast enhancement in mammography. Radiol Clin Biol 43: 521–528
4. Galkin BM et al. (1979) Contrast enhancement of low dose mammograms. In: Logan WW, Mutz PE (eds) Reduced dose mammography. Masson, New York, pp 281–295
5. Mauer RE, Yule Jac, Cornwell WS (1951) A masking technique for making radiographic paper duplicates. Med Radiogr Photogr 27: 121–125
6. Kattan KR, Caplan MC, Felson B (1973) A method for improving roentgenographic illustrations for publication – blurred undersubtraction (BUS). Med Radiogr Photogr 49: 21–22
7. Orloff TL (1978) Contrast enhancement of mammograms. Med Radiogr Photogr 54: 38
8. Ziedses des Plantes BG (1935) Subtraktion. Eine röntgenographische Methode zur separaten Abbildung bestimmter Teile des Objekts. Fortschr Röntgenstr 52: 69–79

Breast Sonography and the Detection of Cancer

R. L. Egan, M. B. McSweeney, and F. B. Murphy

Breast Imaging Center, Section of Radiology, Emory University School of Medicine, 1364 Clifton Road, Atlanta, GA 30322, USA

Introduction

By 1956, X-ray examination of the breast had so improved that it had become a routine complement to physical examination of the breast. While these two procedures have remained the standards for breast cancer detection, each has its limitations. During the past two decades, additional methods for detecting breast cancer have been sought. These have included attempts to improve the radiographic technique, thermography, infrared scanning, light transmission, radioisotope scanning, galactography, pneumocystography, utilization of the Doppler effect, computed tomographic (CT) scanning, heavy-particle imaging, and nuclear magnetic resonance (NMR).

With the development of ultrasound imaging, the breast was one of the first organs to be studied. Wild and Reid (1952) evaluated breast masses by the A-mode technique. This was followed by Howry et al. (1954) in the United States, Jellins et al. (1971) in Australia, and Kobayashi (1975) in Japan. These investigators demonstrated the potential of differentiating breast cysts from solid lesions. However, the clinical application of breast sonography did not follow due to limitations of the available ultrasound equipment and expertise. Kobayashi reviewed these earlier developments in breast sonography up to 1975.

Improvements in ultrasound equipment and imaging techniques led to the clinical application of ultrasound studies in the pelvis and abdomen. Ultrasound scanning of the breast with standard contact equipment was investigated as a method for evaluation of palpable breast diseases. Cysts, in particular, could be identified and differentiated from solid tumors. The introduction of a specially designed water path by Egan and the Magnaflux Corporation in 1963 provided a method of examining the entire breast using tomographic scans.

An Australian company, Ausonics, developed the Octoscan, an eight-transducer body scanner. This was used to study the breast with considerable success. A smaller version with four transducers, two on each side of the breast with variable angles and a changeable Z-axis, overcame many of the technical problems of imaging the cone-shaped breast.

Life Instruments approached breast sonography by using a scanner with three transducers in a single head, each of the three transducers being focused at a different level. Other water-path breast units have been designed for Johnson and Johnson, Fry, Baum, and Toshiba, in addition to the design of hand-held small-parts scanners.

Viewing the great number of images recorded on tape, disc, or photographic emulsions has posed problems. One approach has been to reduce a large number of images to a small size and record these on a film disc to be viewed in sequence at varying speeds. Images recorded on video tapes can be replayed in diverse ways. Another approach has been to record the

Recent Results in Cancer Research. Vol. 90

images on video tape, transfer the images onto a disc, and view them from the disc. Images of both breasts are then viewed simultaneously. The image can be digitalized and fed into a computer to be viewed in many ways, in various combinations, and utilizing reconstruction and other postprocessing advantages. Image quality is degraded when transferred to photographic disc or dual-review disc, although there is improved ease of viewing.

These technical problems with breast sonography have in recent years commanded so much attention that establishing criteria for the presence of breast abnormalities with their specific changes or the efficacy of the clinical application of breast sonography became secondary. In fact, there was a highly competitive course to produce the epitome in nonionizing breast screening. Johnson and Johnson planned a clinical trial of breast sonography but quickly aborted that effort. Claims, without substantiation, abounded that ultrasound was the superior imaging technique in dense breasts, in follow-up examinations, in pregnant women, and in women fearful of radiation. The meager data on breast sonography can confirm none of these claims. Instead, it should be emphasized that breast sonography in its present state can only be complementary to physical examination and mammography.

During this period of development of breast sonographic units, there were other efforts to establish the characteristics of breast structures and disease. Schneck and Lehman (1982) studied the sonographic anatomy of the breast by correlation of sonographic images with gross and microscopic breast materials. Kroll et al. (1982) carried out correlated X-ray, clinical, ultrasound, and, when available, pathologic studies of the breasts of 7,500 females. Cole-Beuglet (1982), Fry and Harper (1979), and others performed combined studies on breast imaging. However, no controlled clinical protocol comparing sonographic and X-ray studies of the breast has been done.

Thus, we designed a protocol to evaluate breast sonography. The primary aims were: (1) to establish the relative accuracy of breast sonography in the detection of breast diseases; (2) determine its complementary value to physical examination and mammography; and (3) select the types of breasts in which it would be potentially most useful.

Materials and Methods

In the Emory University Breast Imaging Center, 15–22 females daily, usually with a breast problem, were referred for routine mammography over a period of 6 months. Many of these women were referred from the Robert Winship (Oncologic) Clinic of the Emory University Clinic; some were referred by physicians elsewhere in the Emory Clinic. Approximately 50% of the referrals were from physicians outside Emory University.

The Ausonics and Life Instrument sonography units, designed especially for examination of the breast, were used. With both units, the examination was carried out in the prone position with the breasts suspended in a water bath. The Life Instrument unit provided a fixed programed examination and was operated at 3.5 MHz. Each breast was scanned in a transverse fashion from the infraclavicular to the inframammary areas. Supplemental single-pass scans from the lateral and then the medial aspects of the breast followed. The four transducers of the Ausonics system at 4.2 MHz could be used singly or in various combinations. There were provisions for a split-screen, full-screen compounding, single- or multiple-transducer single pass, and rotational scanning. With the Ausonics unit, compression could easily be added, but this was difficult with the Life Instrument unit. If possible, compression was added only after a routine scan was made. Dual viewing was provided for both systems.

Since only 10–12 subjects could easily be scanned per day, they were examined when a room and a technician were available. All the females in this study were scanned after the mammographic examination. Women with obvious abnormalities on mammography were encouraged to wait for breast sonography so that histologically proven cases could be accumulated. Although the Life Instrument unit was installed 2 months after the Ausonics system, an attempt was made to obtain near-equal numbers of patients on each unit. The protocol had to be limited to 6 months. The first 2 months were utilized in installing the equipment, developing the breast sonography technique and routine, and becoming familiar with the equipment and interpretation of the images. Only 4 months, then, remained to evaluate the procedure. Each month, one radiologist interpreted the mammograms, with no more clinical information than the age of the patient, and recorded the findings on an appropriate form. The other radiologist interpreted the breast sonograms and recorded the results. After this the two radiologists reviewed the studies together and compiled a clinical report. At the end of each month, the roles of the radiologists were reversed.

The Emory Clinic and the Grady Memorial Hospital patient charts were reviewed. Letters were sent to each external referring physician and in many instances follow-up was carried out by telephone. Each sonographic study was rated for its relative clinical benefits as: (1) no benefit; (2) slight benefit; (3) great benefit; or (4) adverse effect.

Results

A total of 786 patients were included in the last 4 months of the study protocol. During this period and during a 1-month follow-up, there were 77 biopsies with 31 proven carcinomas. The age of the patients, breast complaints, history of breast cancer, and previous surgery (Table 1) were considered average for the Breast Imaging Center except for a tendency for younger women to undergo breast sonography. On clinical examination, there was a failure to detect 11 (36%) carcinomas, with 20 benign lesions categorized as malignant. On sonography, seven carcinomas were not detected and ten benign lesions were labeled as carcinomas. With mammography, six carcinomas were not detected while eight benign lesions were classified as carcinomas (Tables 2–4).

Table 1. Age, symptoms, family history, and prior surgery in 786 study patients

Age (years)	No. patients	Symptom				Family history	Prior surgery		
		Thickening[a]	Mass	Discharge	Other		Aspiration	Biopsy	Mastectomy
< 30	42		16	5	13	9		6	3
31–40	151	4	41	4	32	50	10	18	7
41–50	194	9	25	3	51	37	7	35	20
51–60	208	4	27	1	39	53	9	69	26
61–70	126	2	14	2	32	15		17	25
> 70	55		8		13	4		6	15
Total	786	19	131	15	180	168	26	151	96

[a] Subjects complaining of a "fullness" or "thickening" in the breast

Table 2. Age of patients, biopsy results, and diagnosis of 786 patients

Age (years)	No. patients	No. biopsies	No. malignancies	Clinical examination			Mammography			Ultrasound		
				Pos.	FP	FN	Pos.	FP	FN	Pos.	FP	FN
< 30	42	8	0	0	8	0	0	1	0	0	0	0
31–40	151	14	2	1	8	1	1	3	1	0	0	2
41–50	194	11	5	3	6	2	2	3	3	2	1	3
51–60	208	14	4	3	6	1	3	5	1	1	1	3
61–70	126	20	13	7	7	6	12	1	1	9	0	4
> 70	55	10	7	6	2	1	6	2	1	3	1	4
Total	786	77	31	20	37	11	24	15	7	15	3	16

Pos., positive; *FP*, false-positive; *FN*, false-negative

Table 3. Relative clinical usefulness of breast sonography in 786 patients and number of breasts with cysts not otherwise detected

Age (years)	No. patients	Usefulness			No. cysts found
		Slight	Great	Detrimental	
< 30	42	34	6	0	2
31–40	151	74	20	0	22
41–50	194	88	15	0	11
51–60	208	84	12	1	5
61–70	126	40	14	0	1
> 70	55	18	10	1	0
Total	786	338	77	2	41

Table 4. Relative accuracy of detection of carcinoma by physical examination, mammography, and breast sonography using by Ausonics and Life Instruments units

	31 Ca			US	
	Clinical examination	Mammography	US	Aus-22 ca	Life-9 ca
Pos.	63%	75%	47%	68%	0%
FP	4.7	1.9	0.4	0.6	0
FN	37	25	53	32	100

Ca, carcinoma; *US*, ultrasound; *Pos.*, positive; *FP*, false-positive; *FN*, false-negative

The usefulness, or complementary value, of breast sonography was judged to be of some value in 338 patients, of decided value in 77 patients, and of no value in 368 patients. In two cases, it may have resulted in a delay in treatment; in one case, it was the sole positive finding leading to biopsy and the diagnosis of carcinoma (Fig. 1).

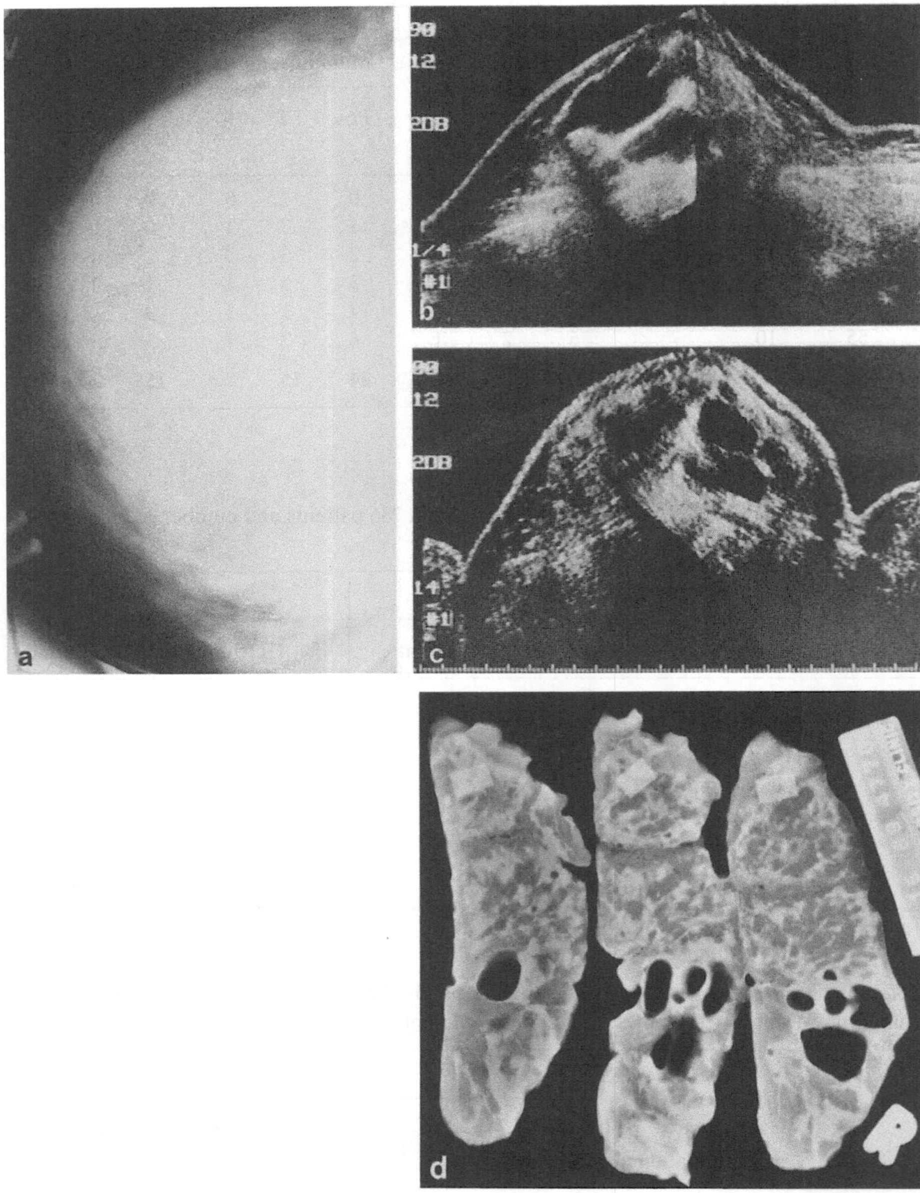

Fig. 1a–d. A 45-year-old female. Attempted needle aspiration of right breast mass resulted in ecchymosis. **a** Mammogram of right breast showing dense glandular tissue, no discrete mass. **b, c** Ultrasound visualization showing demarcated anechoic masses with increased through transmission. Multiple cysts throughout the breast; no other abnormalities. **d** 5-mm slicer section radiograph for demonstration of numerous cysts

Fig. 2a, b. A 34-year-old female right breast mass. **a** Mammogram demonstrates well-demarcated mass with notch. Impression – solid mass, probably fibroadenoma. **b** Ultrasound visualization through mass showing simple cyst. Cyst was aspirated

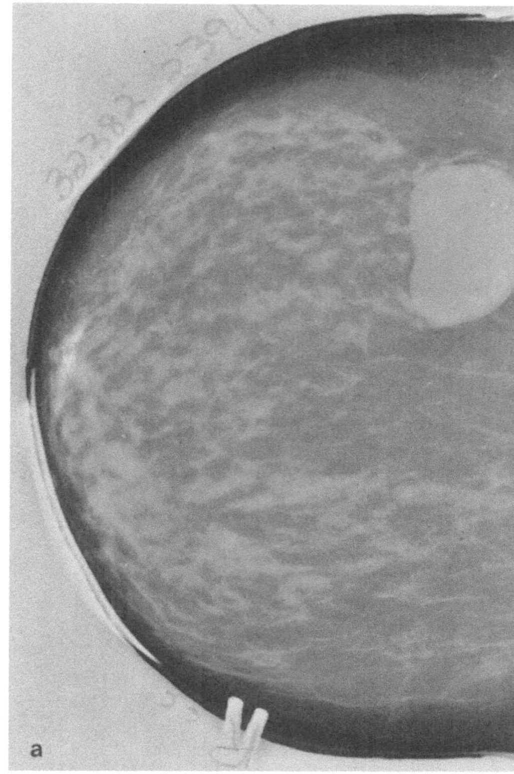
a

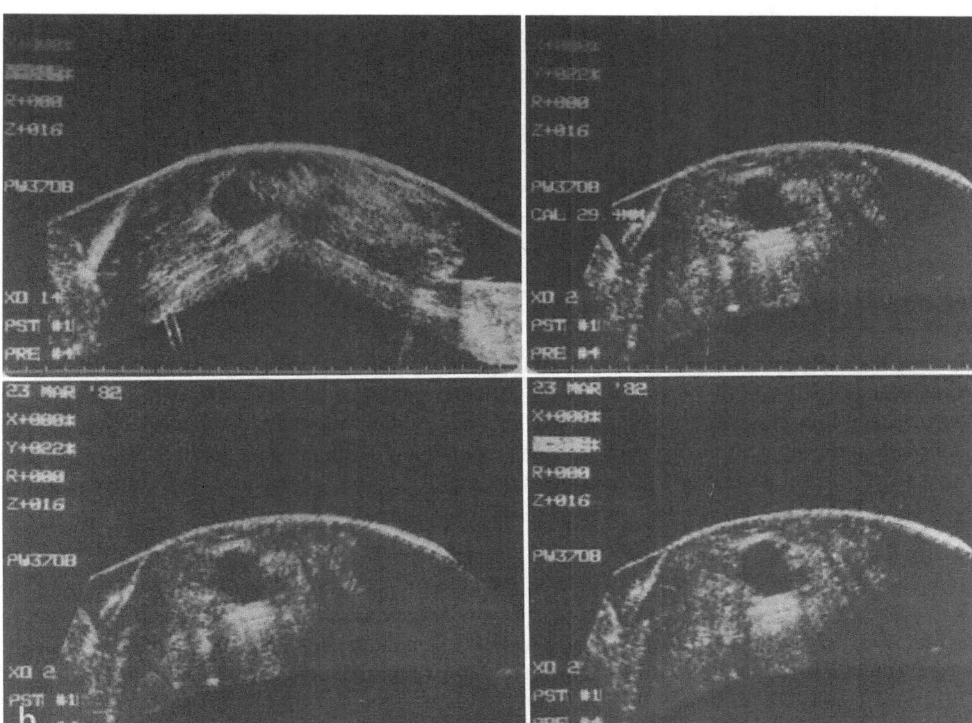
R+000
Z+016
PW3708
XD 1
PST #1
PRE #4
Y+022*
R+000
Z+016
PW3708
CAL 29 MM
XD 2
PST #1
PRE #4
23 MAR '82
X+000*
Y+022*
R+000
Z+016
PW3708
XD 2
PST #1
b
23 MAR '82
X+000*
R+000
Z+016
PW3708
XD 2
PST #1
PRE #4

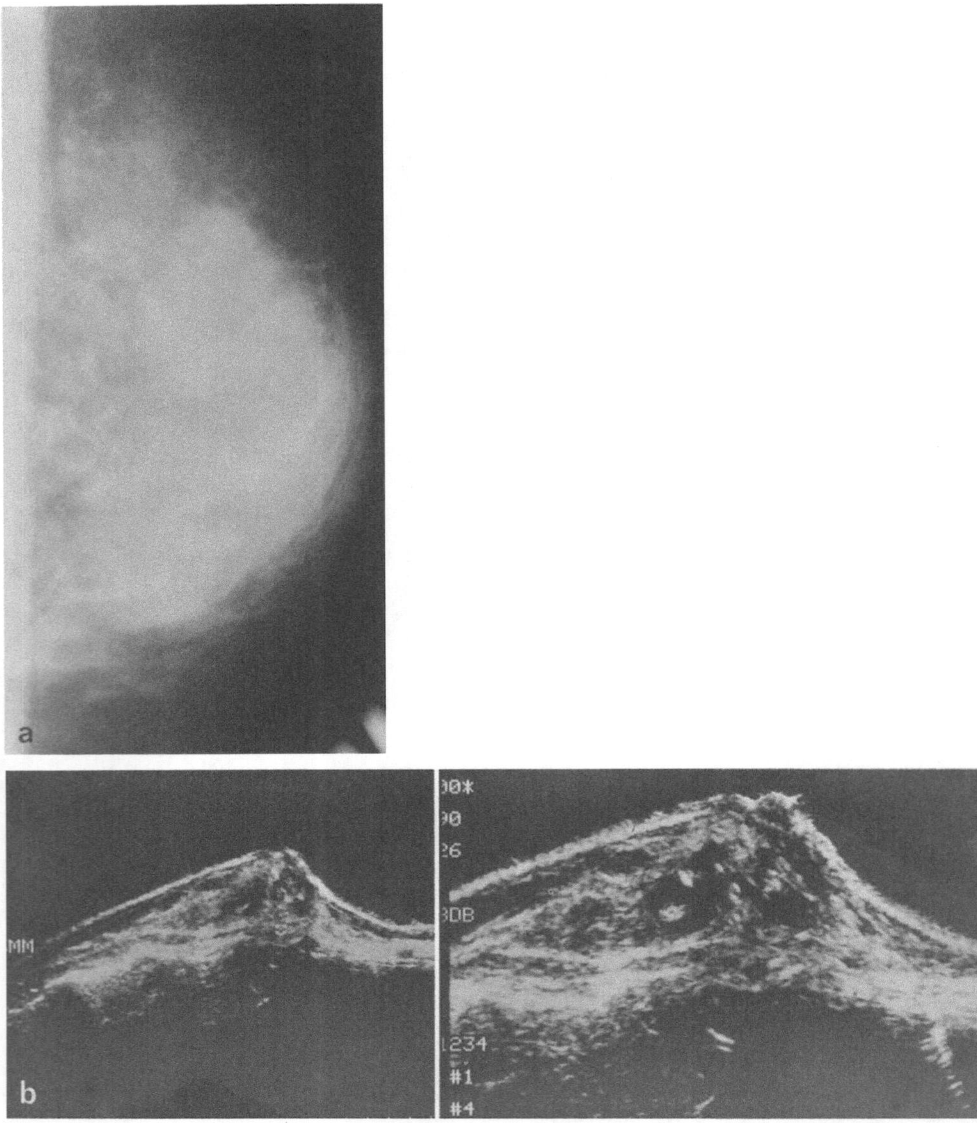

Fig. 3a, b. Right breast mass in 52-year-old female. **a** Mammogram demonstrates large area of increased density in central portion of breast. Multiple small foci of calcifications throughout upper half of breast. Impression – carcinoma. **b** Ultrasound visualization: Longitudinal section through midbreast showing central hypoechoic mass containing nonhomogeneous echoes. The mass attenuates the beam. Impression – carcinoma; the extent is better defined than on the mammograms. Pathologic findings: invasive duct carcinoma; multicentric comedo carcinoma

Fig. 4a, b. A 37-year-old female who had received augmentation prostheses 10 years prior to the present study. **a** Mammogram demonstrates irregular area in right upper outer quadrant of increased density adjacent to the prosthesis. **b** Ultrasound visualization shows hypoechoic solid mass compatible with carcinoma. Pathologic findings: infiltrating duct carcinoma

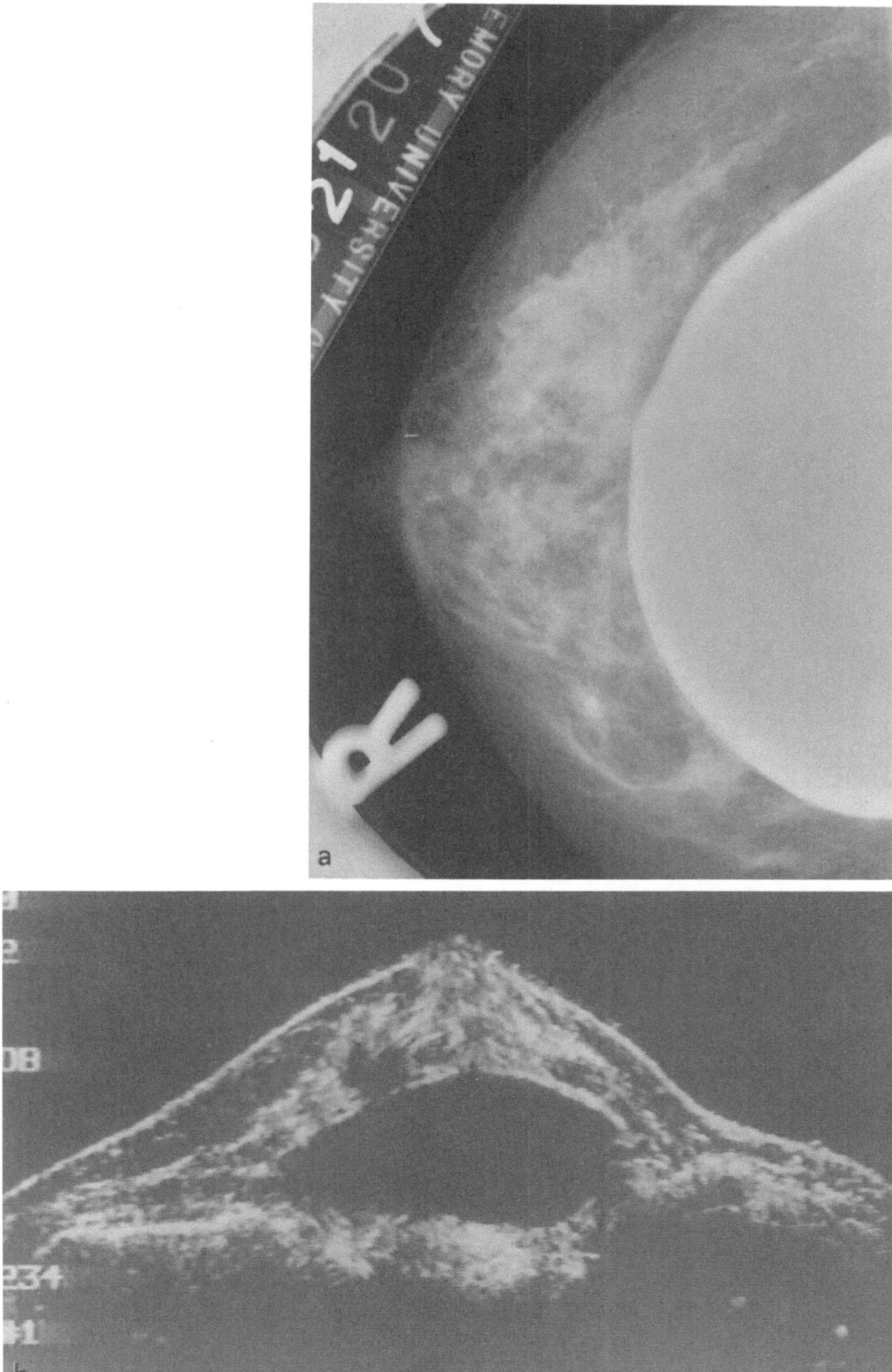
EMORY UNIVERSITY
a
b

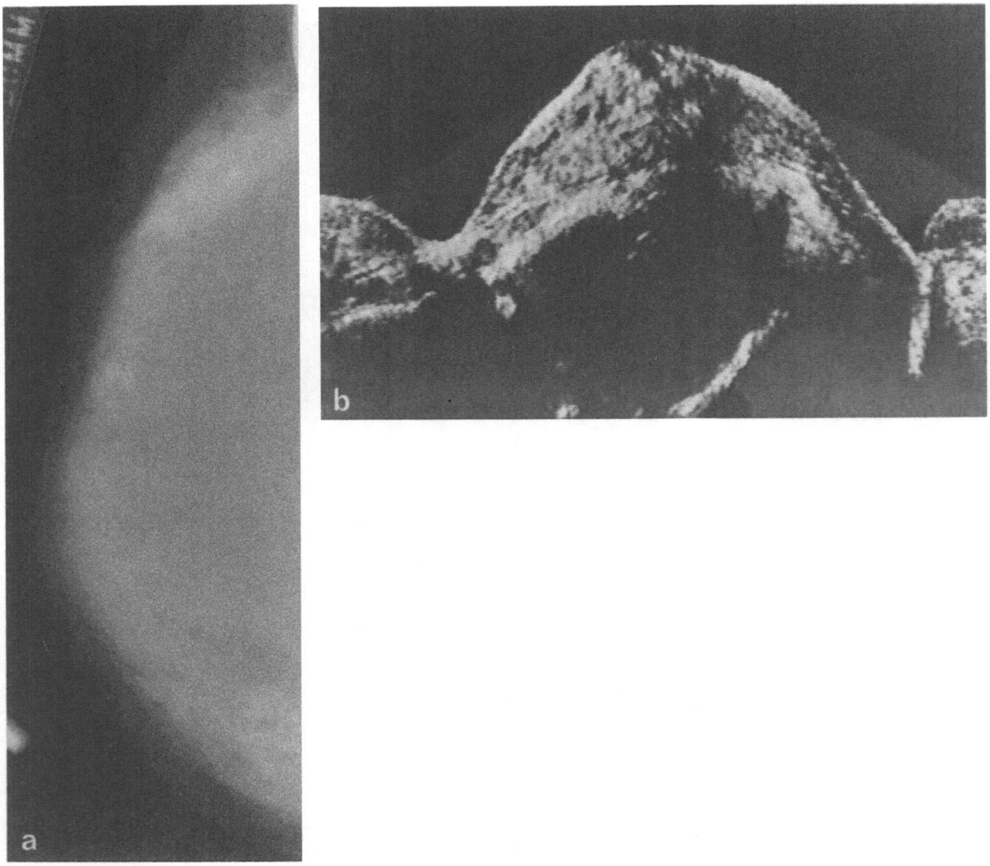

Fig. 5a, b. A 45-year-old female with painful breasts. Clinically, there was a thickening in the upper outer quadrant of the left breast (LUOQ). **a** Mammography demonstrates homogeneously dense left breast. **b** Ultrasound visualization: Hypoechoic LUOQ mass with bulging of skin. No abnormality in the LUOQ. Pathologic finding: LUOQ invasive lobular carcinoma

Discussion

From the onset, the lack of extended follow-up detracted from the protocol. The patients could not be randomized; with stratification the numbers became so small that only trends could be hoped for. Little age, or associated breast density, effect was noted. As usual, mammography and physical examination were less effective in the dense breast, Although cysts could be readily demonstrated in dense breasts when not clinically or mammographically apparent, the detection of carcinomas was not greater.

The inaccuracy of mammography in detecting carcinomas in these women was unusual. The study concentrated on young women. The cases were read without any clinical information, such as details of prior surgery, and prior studies were not available for protocol reading. Yet mammography had the highest accuracy in both benign and malignant lesions. On reviewing the cases with clinical information, only two carcinomas would have been overlooked and both in very dense breasts. In one of these latter cases, breast sonography was the only entity that led to the detection of the carcinoma. A palpable abnormality was present in a quadrant distant to the carcinoma but was not suspicious enough to warrant biopsy.

At times, it was difficult to assess the value of breast sonography in the clinical setting. Yet it was noted that even when there was no specific benefit, there was an increased sense of confidence when these studies corroborated those of X-ray and physical examination. Needle aspiration can establish the presence of a cyst if fluid is obtained but cannot exclude a cyst if no fluid is obtained (Fig. 2). Inpalpable cysts are of little clinical interest but may become significant if the mammographic appearance is not typical of a cyst. In these instances, ultrasound proved to be of benefit (Fig. 3).

There is an overlapping of the ultrasonic criteria for such benign lesions as fibroadenomas and such malignant lesions as medullary carcinomas. The recognition of small carcinomas and stippled calcifications not associated with a mass is not possible with ultrasound unless there is enough periductal fibrotic reaction to the in situ tumor to produce a pseudomass on the sonogram. The lack of demonstration of altered architecture or other abnormalities by breast sonography in the presence of calcifications detected by mammography has no clinical value since these borderline lesions must be localized and removed for specimen radiography.

Usually, the pectoral muscles and deep breast tissues are readily demonstrated by breast sonography. This may complement the screen-film mammography technique, where the breast tissues along the chest wall are not well demonstrated. In dense, very large breasts, even with high-power settings, attenuation of the beam may be so great that the retromammary area cannot be evaluated without compression.

This first protocol, designed only to evaluate the efficacy of breast sonography in a clinical setting, has produced a definite trend for the incorporation of sonography in the imaging of breast diseases (Figs. 1, 4, 5). Previous workers have suggested sonography as a complement to clinical examination and mammography (Kroll et al. 1982; Cole-Beuglet 1982; Fry and Harper 1979). The relative accuracy in demonstrating breast carcinoma approaches that of clinical examination with fewer false-positives and the detection of more cysts, but sonography cannot replace mammography.

The intention of this study was not to compare breast sonography units. However, the two instruments used did not produce equal results in our hands. It follows that for the individual radiologist, the selection of a breast sonography unit may be critical.

The study population may be compared with the 1,000 women referred from Winship Clinic annually with 350 biopsies and 100 breast carcinomas. In the present study, 40% of biopsies were for carcinoma, and indicator of selection. The low rate of biopsy, 10%, also suggests a different patient population. Since we encouraged referrals from outside the Emory University Clinic this now perhaps is a more representative study population similar to that of other breast imaging centers. This low biopsy rate but with a high yield of carcinoma was no doubt related to some degree of patient selection after prior mammography. The desire to study younger women also produced an element of bias.

One of us (RLE) has been involved with ultrasound of the breast since 1963 and has witnessed a clinically positive development in breast sonography over the past 2 years.

Conclusions

1. Breast sonography is a method of breast examination that does not utilize ionizing radiation.
2. Breast sonography is a time-consuming and expensive procedure compared with mammography.
3. At present, there are technologic limitations of breast sonography that make consistent diagnosis of small carcinomas, stippled calcifications, or small areas of altered architecture less reliable than mammography.
4. Corroboration of physical or X-ray findings by breast sonography in both benign and malignant diseases enhances confidence.
5. Sonographic diagnostic criteria for solid lesions must be refined.
6. There are overlapping changes in benign and malignant lesions for all modalities, as well as fatty deposits in breast sonography, making complementary roles imperative.
7. Breast sonography can differentiate cysts and solid lesions and demonstrate cysts, fibroadenomas, and an occasional carcinoma not found by X-ray or physical examination.
8. Despite its many limitations, breast sonography should be included in many breast imaging centers for its present contributions in the improvement of diagnostic accuracy and for continued evaluation of any technologic improvements.
9. At present, breast sonography can only be considered complementary to X-ray and clinical examination of the breast. In younger women, it may be the initial method of breast examination.

References

1. Cole-Beuglet C (1982) Sonographic manifestations of malignant breast disease. Semin Ultrasound 3:51–57
2. Fry EK, Harper P (1979) Examination of the female breast by means of mammography automated B-mode and rapid real-time ultrasound scanning. Proceeding of the Annual AIUM Meeting, p 89
3. Howry DH, Scott DA, Bliss WR (1954) The ultrasonic visualization of carcinoma of the breast and other soft tissue structures. Cancer 7:354–358
4. Jellins J, Kosoff G, Buddee FW, Reeve TS (1971) Ultrasonic visualization of the breast. Med J Aust 1:305–307
5. Kobayashi T (1975) Review: Ultrasonic diagnosis of breast cancer. Ultrasound Med Biol 1:383–391
6. Kroll J, Kotwich J, Tabrett M (1982) The diagnosis of benign disease and the exclusion of malignancy in patients with breast symptoms. Semin Ultrasound 3:38–50
7. Schneck CD, Lehman DA (1982) Sonographic anatomy of the breast. Semin Ultrasound 3:13–33
8. Wild JJ, Reid JM (1952) Further pilot echographic studies on the histologic structure of the living intact breast. Am J Pathol 28:839–861

Breast Cancer Screening: Expected and Observed Incidence and Stages of Female Breast Cancer in Gävleborg County, Sweden, and Implications for Mortality

B. Lundgren

Mammography Section, Gävle Hospital, 801 17 Gävle, Sweden

Breast cancer screening by single oblique-view mammography was introduced in Gävleborg county, Sweden in 1974. The total population of the county is 300,000, of which the 74,000 people 40 years old and over were invited to take part in screening. The optimal screening interval for this method should probably be on average 2 years. For various practical reasons, it was not possible to adhere to this interval. In two boroughs, the interval was nearly 5 years between the first and the second screening. For this reason, in the present study, an upper time limit for follow-up cases was set at 3 years.
The aim of the present study was to estimate the impact of this screening project on breast cancer mortality.

Materials and Methods

A study was made of all breast cancer cases diagnosed from the time of the first screening in all boroughs of the county up to 31 December 1981. Cases detected at first screening, prevalence cases, were excluded from this study, which only concerns *incidence cases,* i.e., those detected on repeated screening, in intervals between screenings, and among women who had not participated in the screenings. These *observed incidence cases* were clinically staged according to the TNM-system (UICC 1974).
To calculate the *expected incidence,* all breast cancer cases registered in the Staffan parish from 1961 to 1975 and in the Sandviken parish from 1969 to 1973 were used. These were checked against the National Cancer Registry. The cases from the Staffan parish were previously clinically staged and were used as a basis for comparison.

Results

Observed Incidence and Staging

The study population comprised 73,600 females, observed for periods of varying length depending on the date when they were first screened. The total number of person-years at risk was 356,200. During this observation period, 467 cases of breast cancer were diagnosed, corresponding to an incidence rate of 1.31/1,000/year. The stages of the observed cases are given in Table 1.

Recent Results in Cancer Research. Vol. 90

Table 1. Stages of breast cancer in subjects studied

Stage	I	II	III	IV	II–IV	Total
Observed no. cases	244	137	63	23	223	467
Percent	52	29	14	5	48	100

Table 2. Expected age-adjusted incidence for Gävleborg county

Parish	Population 31. 12. 74	Years at risk	Person-years	Cancer cases	Average incidence rate/ 1,000/year
Staffan	5,240	15	78,600	114.9	1.46
Sandviken	6,017	5	30,085	35.4	1.18
Total			108,685	150.3	1.38

Table 3. Cancer stages (Staffan parish 1961–1975)

Stage	I	II	III	IV	II–IV	Total
Observed no. cases	13	64	27	9	100	113
Percent	11	57	24	8	89	100

Expected Incidence and Staging

The expected incidence was calculated from the breast cancer material of the two control parishes. The age distribution was defined on 31 December 1974, and age adjustments were made against the distribution for Gävleborg county at the same point in time (Table 2).

Expected Incidence in Study Population. The observed study population comprised 356,200 person-years at risk and the expected incidence was 1.38/1,000/year, the number of expected cases, therefore, in the study population was:

$$\frac{1.38 \times 356{,}200}{1{,}000} = 492$$

which should be compared with the observed number of 467 cases.
The cancer stages of the observed cases in Staffan parish are given in Table 3.
The rates of cancer by stage given in Table 3 will be referred to as the *expected stages*.

Expected Stages in Study Population. The expected stages of the observed 467 cases (Tables 1, 3) would be as given in Table 4, and these may be compared with the observed stages as given in Table 5.

Table 4. Expected stages in study population

Stage	I	II	III	IV	II–IV	Total
Expected no. cases	51	266	112	38	416	467
Percent	11	57	24	8	89	100

Table 5. Expected and observed numbers and stages of breast cancer cases

Stage	I	II	III	IV	II–IV	Total
Expected no. cases	51	266	112	38	416	467
Observed no. cases	244	137	63	23	223	467
Difference	+ 193	– 129	– 49	– 15	– 193	

Table 6. Expected mortality-incidence rate

Stage	I	II–IV	Total
Expected incidence, no. cases	51	416	467
MIR (%)	10	40	37
Mortality, no. cases	5	168	173

Table 7. Observed mortality-incidence rate

Stage	I	II–IV	Total
Observed incidence, no. cases	244	223	467
MIR (%)	10	40	24
Mortality, no. cases	24	89	113

Implications for Breast Cancer Mortality

In Sweden, the cumulative mortality-incidence rate (MIR) for the years 1975–1977 was 37%. This means that 37% of females who were diagnosed as having breast cancer also died from this disease (Lundgren, to be published). It is not known exactly how the mortality is distributed according to the stage of disease. It seems, however, realistic to assume that the MIR in stage I is 10%. With this premise, the mortality of the observed material (Table 1) would be as given in Table 6 if the stages were the expected (Table 4).

The MIR in stages II–IV thus would be 40%. In the next table (Table 7), these MIRs are applied to the observed stages.

The difference in the estimated mortality between the expected and the observed stages would thus be 173 – 113, i.e., 60 cases, which would be the net mortality gain of screening, as performed in the study population. The MIR would decrease from 37% to 24%.

Discussion

The average survival time for breast cancer patients is about 15 years. Thus, it takes a very long time to observe the effects of screening on mortality even though randomized control groups are available. It is, therefore, important to collect as much supporting data as possible until incontrovertible evidence becomes available. This study represent such an effort.

The difference between the expected and observed numbers of cases of breast cancer was insignificant, whereas there was a considerable reduction in observed late-stage (II–IV) cases. The majority of the fatal cancers are to be found in these stages. Thus, a reduction in the mortality could be expected. So far, very little seems to be known about the mortality according to stage of breast cancer, though the total mortality in Sweden is known (MIR = 37%). Estimates can only be derived from the known MIR and from long-term survival in different stages, on which the premises of mortality by stage in this study are based (Henderson and Canellos 1980).

The mortality in stage I was assumed to be 10%, which might be at the lower limit. The reason for choosing this rate was the shift to smaller tumor sizes, which has occurred within this stage with the advent of mammography. Stage I tumors today are on average much smaller than before the introduction of mammography and also include nearly 10% in situ cancers, which were very uncommon. In the observed population, the rate of invasive carcinoma ≤ 10 mm and in situ cancer was 46%. In the control material (Staffan) this rate was 5%. The main point ist, however, the observed reduction in the actual number of cancers in stages II to IV, which in this material might mean a mortality reduction of 35%.

Conclusion

A study of the incidence and stages of breast cancer cases detected in screening was made with reference to the expected incidence and stages. There was no significant difference between observed and expected incidence, but there was a substantial reduction in the expected number of late-stage (II–IV) cancer cases, in spite of the screening not being carried out with optimum intervals. Based on the known total mortality-incidence rate (MIR) for breast cancer in Sweden (37%), the expected mortality reduction was calculated. Of 467 cancer cases detected, 173 patients would be expected to die from this disease if screening were not carried out, whereas as a consequence of screening and the reduced number of stage II to IV cancers, the number of deaths would be 113, i.e., about 60 lives saved, corresponding to a mortality reduction of 35%.

References

Henderson IC, Canellos GP (1980) Cancer of the breast. N Engl J Med 302: 17–30

Lundgren B (to be published) Cancer incidence and cancer mortality in Sweden 1960–1977. Real or apparent changes?

Union International Contra le Cancrum (1974) The TNM breast classification. UICC, Geneva

Five-Year Experience with Single-View Mammography Randomized Controlled Screening in Sweden

L. Tabár, E. Åkerlund, and A. Gad

Department of Mammography, Falun Central Hospital, 791 82 Falun, Sweden

A randomized, controlled, population-based breast cancer screening trial has been underway in two counties of Sweden since 1977 (Kopparberg county) and since 1978 (Östergötland county). The main goal of this study is to answer the question: What is the effect of mammography screening on mortality caused by breast cancer when using the single, mediolateral oblique view as the only screening method? The preliminary results gained in the first 5 years of screening in Kopparberg county are described here.

Materials and Methods

The Kopparberg-Östergötland projects involve a total of 161,000 females above 39 years of age, with no upper age limit. Of these 94,000 comprise the study population (47,000 in Kopparberg county and 47,000 in Östergötland county) invited to the screening (Tabár et al. 1979). The control group includes 67,000 age-matched females (45,000 in Östergötland and 22,000 in Kopparberg).

The screening trial is population-based, the females, being recruited by computer from the Swedish National Population Registry. The manner of randomization has been described in detail elsewhere (Tabár and Gad 1981). The interval time between two consecutive screenings in Kopparberg county is on average 20 months in the age-group 40–49 years and 35 months on average in females ≥ 50 years of age. Two screening rounds have been completed so far in women aged 40–49 years and the third round is underway; the second round of screening in females aged ≥ 50 years will be finished in the near future. Low-dose film-screen mammography is the only screening method employed. It is important to note that the single mediolateral oblique view is used primarily (Tabár et al. 1979).

Results

The attendance rate in the first and second round of screening is shown in Table 1. In the age-group 40–69 years, 92.5% of those invited attended the first screening. The second round of screening is not yet completed. The corresponding figure is at present 89.1%. Between October 1977, the start of screening, and July 1982, altogether 737 breast cancer cases were diagnosed in the combined total study population and control group. Of these, 176 were cases in the control population and 561 were carcinomas in the total study population. This latter includes all screening-detected cancers up to July 1982, all interval carcinomas, cancers detected among those who did not attend screening, as well as those cases that were diagnosed before the start of screening but after population registration. By

Recent Results in Cancer Research. Vol. 90

Table. 1 Attendance rate in the two rounds of screening

Age-group (years)	Attendance rate (%)	
	First round	Second round[a]
40–49	93.7	90.6
50–59	93.2	90.5
60–69	90.6	85.7
40–69	92.5	89.1
⩾ 70	62.7	50.4

[a] Data concerning the second screening are not yet complete

	First screening	Second screening
Examined	100	100
	↓	↓
Suspicion of abnormal finding	5 (4.9%)	3.3%
	↓	↓
Abnormal lesion(s) in the breast	2 (1.8%)	0.9%
	↓	↓
Referred to surgery	1 (1.1%)	0.6%
Number of surgical biopsies	65.3%	75.2%
Number of cancers	2/3	3/4

Fig. 1. Comparative work scheme of prevalent and incident screenings

July 1982, the control population had been at risk for 3.4 years due to the lack of screening and the incidence of breast cancer in the control group was 2.2/1,000/year. The national breast cancer incidence for those aged over 40 years was 2.1/1,000/year in 1976, the year before screening started.

Figure 1 illustrates the comparative work scheme of the prevalent and incident screenings. Of 100 females examined, 4.9% were recalled for further examination during the first screening because of the suspicion of an abnormal finding on the single oblique-view mammogram. The corresponding figure in the second round of screening was 3.3%. After complete mammographic and physical examination, 1.8% of all examined females proved to have abnormal lesion(s) in the breast(s) in the prevalent screening and 0.9% had such lesions in the incident screening. Two of three biopsied patients (65.3%) had cancer upon histologic examination at the time of the first screening, while this figure in the second screening was about three of four patients (75.2%).

Table 2 shows the distribution of screening-detected cancers (prevalent and incident) in all ages over 40 years, according to tumor size. In the first screening, 39,713 women were examined; because the second round is not yet completed, the figures are based on the examination of 24,509 females. Table 3 illustrates the results of histologic examination of those cancers detected in the prevalent and incident screenings. Tables 2 and 3 and Tables 4 and 5 make it possible to compare the screening results with the distribution of tumors and lymph node status in the age-matched control group.

Among those 39,713 females examined in the first round of screening, 278 breast carcinomas were diagnosed (prevalence 7.0/1,000 examined) (Tabár et al., to be published). Figure 2 shows the number of interval cancers detected in the period between

Table 2. Distribution of screening-detected cancers (prevalent and incident) according to tumor size, in subjects ≥ 40 years of age

	First round screening (prevalent) (39,713 examined)		Second round screening (incident) (24,509 examined)	
Cancer	No.	Percent	No.	Percent
TIS	21	7.6	11	10.1
≤ 5 mm	10	3.6	9	8.2
6–10 mm	78	28.4	22	20.2
Minimal cancer	109	39.6	42	38.5
11–20 mm	103	37.5	52	47.7
≥ 21 mm	63	22.9	15	13.8
Total	275[a]	100.0	109	100.0

[a] Additional three cancers diagnosed by cytology only

Table 3. Distribution of cancers according to the result of histologic examination of axillary lymph nodes in females over 40 years of age

	First screening		Second screening	
	No.	Percent	No.	Percent
No metastasis	181	65.8	64	58.7
Metastasis	52	18.9	27	24.8
Not examined	42	15.3	18	16.5
Total	275	100.0	109	100.0

Table 4. Distribution of cancers in the control group, according to tumor size in subjects over 40 years of age

Size	No.	Percent
TIS	4	2.3
≤ 5 mm	8	4.5
6–10 mm	16	9.1
"Minimal cancer"	28	15.9
11–20 mm	60	34.1
≥ 21 mm	88	50.0
Total	176	100.0

Table 5. Distribution of cancers in the control group in subjects over 40 years of age according to histologic examination of the axillary lymph nodes

	No.	Percent
No metastasis	87	49.4
Metastasis	56	31.8
Not examined	33	18.8
	176	100.0

the first and second screenings. One interval carcinoma was diagnosed among these females within the first 6 months after negative screening; a further 12 cases were detected in the 7–12-months period, 32 cases between 13–24 months, and 32 cases after 25 months. Altogether, 72 interval cancers have been diagnosed so far in the age-group 40–69 years in the interval period between the first and second as well as in the interval time between the second and third screenings. Histopathologic staging of these cases reveals that 61.2% of the interval cancers were either stage I or tumor in situ (TIS) (Fig. 3). In the age-group 40–49 years, altogether, 21 interval cancer cases have been diagnosed to date (Fig. 4). Five

Prevalent		I.–II. Interval months detected cancers			
Examined women	Detected cancers	0–6	7–12	13–24	≥ 25
39,713	278	1	12	32	32

Control incidence: 2.2/1,000/year
First year interval incidence: 0.3/1,000/year

Fig. 2. Interval cancers detected between first and second screenings

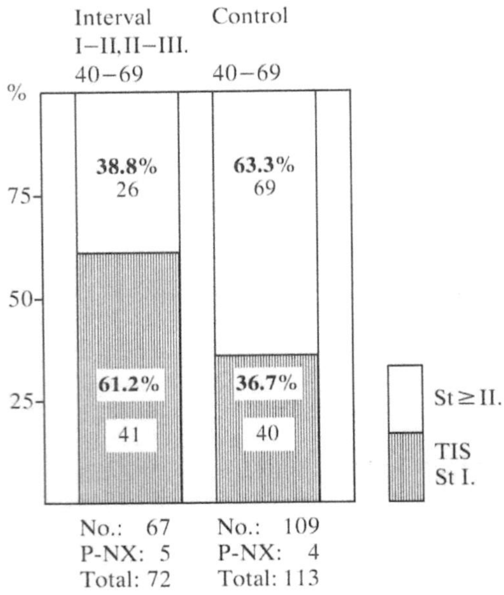

Fig. 3. Distribution of all interval cancers diagnosed in females aged 40–69 years according to stage, compared with cancers diagnosed in females aged 40–69 years in the control population

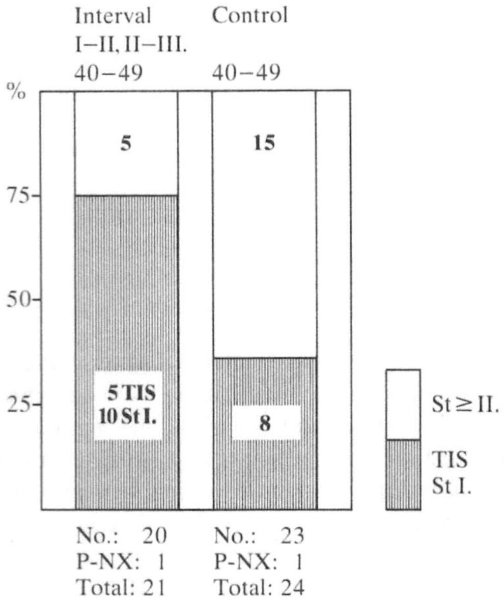

Fig. 4. Comparative stage distribution of cancers diagnosed in the control group (aged 40–49 years) and interval cancers (40–49 years) diagnosed between the first and second and second and third screenings

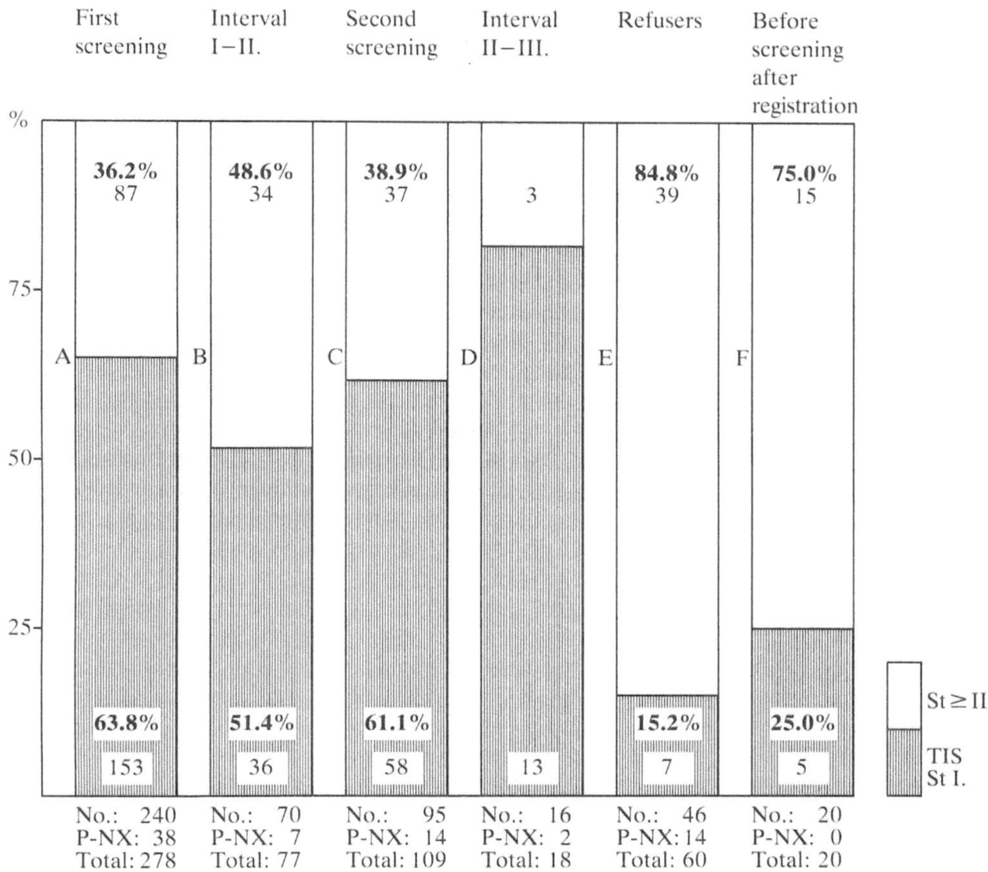

Fig. 5. Distribution of cancer in the study population according to stage (UICC 1978). All subjects ⩾ 40 years of age. *Column A* illustrates those cancer diagnosed in the first screening. *Column B:* interval carcinomas diagnosed between the first and second screenings. *Column C:* cancer cases diagnosed in the second round of screening. *Column D:* interval carcinomas discovered so far between the second and third screenings. *Column E:* cancers detected among those who refused to be screened. *Column F:* carcinomas diagnosed in the study population before start of screenings but after registration of population

of these were TIS, ten were stage I cancers, and five cases were stage ≥ II. The tumor size was ≤ 20 mm in one case but the axillary lymph nodes were not examined histologically [nodes pathologically not examined (p-NX)].

All breast cancers diagnosed in the total study population between October 1977 and July 1982 can be seen distributed according to stage in Fig. 5. The stage distribution of cancers in the different subgroups of the study population (Fig. 5) and in the total study population (Fig. 6) can be compared with the stage distribution of cancers diagnosed in the control population of those aged over 40 years (Fig. 6). Figure 7 shows the stage distribution of breast cancers detected in the total study population, aged 40–69 years, as compared with the age-matched control group, 40–69 years. Of the 337 cancers diagnosed in the total study group, age 40–69 years, 193 were either stage I or TIS, 116 were stage ≥ II cancers, while in 28 cases the tumors were ≤ 20 mm in diameter, but the axillary lymph nodes were not examined histologically (p-NX).

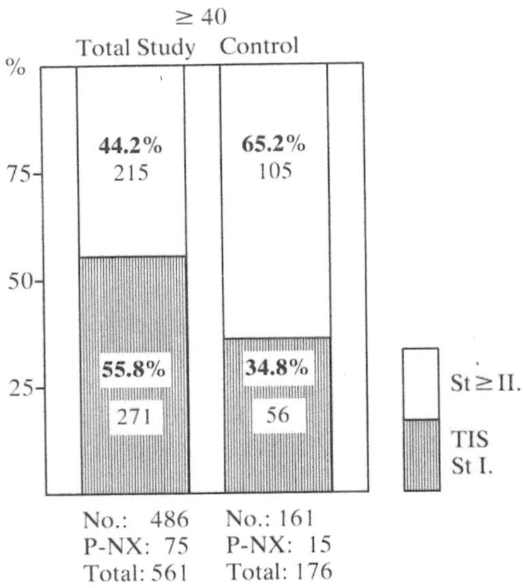

Fig. 6. Comparative stage distribution of cancers diagnosed in the control group (all ages ≥ 40 years) and in the total study population (all ages ≥ 40 years)

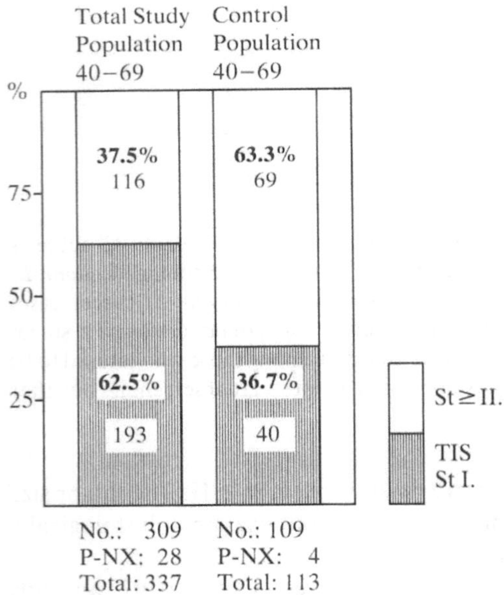

Fig. 7. Distribution of cancers according to stage (UICC 1978)

In the control population, which includes about half as many females in Kopparberg county as the total study population, the number of stage I and TIS cases was 40, while 69 cases were stage ≥ II. In four cases (p-NX), no histologic examination of the lymph nodes was performed. Figure 8 compares the control group incidence with the prevalent (per 1,000 examined) and incident figures (second screening and interval cancers/1,000/year) in different age-groups.

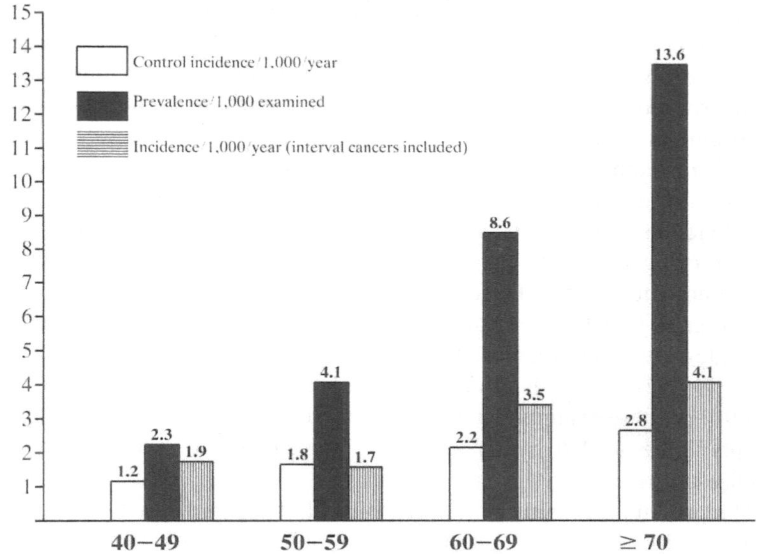

Fig. 8. Comparison of control group incidence with prevalent and incident figures

Discussion

Can breast carcinoma be controlled, i.e., can one achieve significantly decreased mortality from breast cancer by performing mammography screening at regular intervals? What is the magnitude of benefit and net benefit/risk when using the single mediolateral oblique view alone as a screening method? What is the ideal, most beneficial interval time between two consecutive screenings? These are the main questions that the ongoing Swedish breast cancer screening projects intend to answer.

During the first screening (October 1977 and May 1982), about 47,389 females were invited to a mammographic examination. The attendance rate in the age-group 40–69 years was 92.5%, in females aged 70–74 years it was 81.0%, and among females ≥ 75 years it was 50.8%. Altogether, 39,713 females participated in the first screening (83.8%). The attendance rate in the second round of screening was also high, 89.1% in the age-group 40–69 years and 50.4% in females over 70 years of age. This indicates that the screening method is acceptable for females. The low rate of nonresponders makes statistical evaluation easier and more reliable. Furthermore, breast cancer incidence in the control group (2.2/1,000/year) and the expected national breast cancer incidence (2.1/1,000/year) were practically equal, which shows that there is no considerable "contamination effect" in the control group.

The prevalence of breast cancer (7/1,000 examined) was more than three times the incidence in the control group (2.2/1,000/year) in all subjects ≥ 40 years of age. However, it should be noted that the prevalence/control incidence ratio varies among the different age-groups: 2.3/1.1 = 2.1 in females aged 40–49 years and 13.6/2.8 = 4.8 in females ≥ 70 years. These observations are important because they give a basis for the calculation of the duration of the preclinical existence of breast cancer and for calculation of the lead time. In practical terms, these are the key issues in determining the ideal interval time between two consecutive screenings. Because the calculated mean detection lead time in premenopausal females is shorter than in postmenopausal females, one can conclude that before menopause females should be screened with a 1–(max.) 1.5-year interval, and the time between two consecutive screenings of postmenopausal females should be 1.5–2.0 years and should definitely not exceed 2 years. Further studies are needed to confirm these preliminary observations.

It is important to analyze the potential risks in every population-based screening program, e.g., if the specificity of the primary screening procedure is low, too many healthy individuals will be suspected of having the disease, i.e., the rate of false-positive cases will be too high. This results in too many unnecessary recalls for further examinations and psychological harm. During the prevalent screening in Kopparberg county, 4.9% of all examined females (1947 of 39,713) were recalled because of suspected abnormality on the single-view mammogram. In the second round of screening, the corresponding figure is 3.3% (809 of 24,509). Since 1.8% (721 females) of those examined in the first screening and 0.9% of those examined in the second screening had in fact pathologic lesions in the breast, only 3.1% (1,226 cases) and 2.4% (588 cases) of those screened can be considered false-positives.

The primary screening procedure must have high sensitivity, i.e., there should be very few or ideally no false-negative cases at all. To reach this goal, uniformly high-quality examinations are necessary and the mammographer should be highly skilled in the perception and analysis of mammographic abnormalities. Accurate preoperative diagnosis can prevent many unnecessary operations and their harmful effects without lowering sensitivity. The diagnostic workup of the lesions detected in our prevalent and incident screening seemed to be efficient since in, respectively, two of three and in three of four surgical biopsies the histologic diagnosis was cancer. In addition, only 13 cancers were diagnosed among 39,435 females within 1 year after their negative screening, i.e., the cancer incidence was significantly lower (0.3/1,000/year) in the screened population in the year after the first screening examination, compared with the incidence in the control population (2.2/1,000/year).

The efficacy of breast cancer screening can be measured by quantitative and qualitative analysis of those cancers diagnosed between two consecutive examinations (interval carcinomas). We believe that the screening has a positive educational effect upon the population, resulting in more awareness of the breast cancer problem. This and the efficient application of breast self-examination in the interval period, taught by a simple personal letter, can explain the diminished patient delay and the fact that more than 61% of our so-called interval cancers in the age group 40–69 years were diagnosed as stage I tumors.

Eventually, two factors can result in a significant change in the stage distribution of breast cancers in the study population as compared with the control group – efficient mammography screening and increased patient awareness. In different screening centers with properly carried out mammography techniques, about 40% of the discovered breast carcinomas are ≤ 10 mm in size and the rate of cancers with axillary metastases is low. As Figs. 5–7 show, significantly more stage I/TIS cancers were diagnosed in our study during the first and second screening and in the interval periods than among those in whom mammography did not play a role in the detection of cancer (control group, nonparticipants, females in whom the carcinoma was diagnosed after population registration but before the start of screening). While roughly two-thirds of all detected breast cancers in the total study population (40–69 years age-group) consisted of stage I/TIS cases, the situation was reversed in the control group: about two-thirds of all cancers were diagnosed as advanced stage ≥ II carcinomas. Most of the nonparticipants in our study were over 70 years of age and nearly all of the cancers diagnosed among nonparticipants were discovered in this age-group. This explains the difference between the data shown in Figs. 6 and 7.

When the tops of the prevalent columns are connected by a line (Fig. 8) and the same is done with the tops of the incident columns, it is interesting to observe that the two curves differ considerably. The "refill" happens slowest in the age-group 50–59 years, where the incident figure reaches the level of the control incidence as early as after one screening.

Although it is very important to analyze the preliminary data gained in different phases of a screening project, one should not predict whether the preliminary benefit, the significant change in stage distribution of cancers, will eventually result in decreased mortality from breast cancer in the study population. The main question can be answered only by a long-term thorough follow-up of the total study and control populations.

References

1. Andersson I, Andren L, Hildell J et al. (1979) Breast cancer screening with mammography. Radiology 132: 273–276
2. Lundgren B (1979) Population screening for breast cancer by single view mammography in a geographic region in Sweden. J Natl Cancer Inst 62: 1373–1379
3. Tabár L, Dean PB (to be published) Risks and benefits of mammography in population screening for breast cancer. In: Bonadonna G (ed) Breast cancer. Recent advances in diagnosis and treatment. Wiley, New York
4. Tabár L, Gad A (1981) Screening for breast cancer. The Swedish trial. Radiology 138: 219–222
5. Tabár L, Gad A, Åkerlund E et al. (1979) Screening for breast cancer. A randomized controlled trial. In: Logan WW, Muntz EP (eds) Reduced dose mammography. Masson, New York, pp 407–414
6. Tabár L, Gad A, Åkerlund E, Holmberg L (1983) Screening for breast cancer in Sweden. Results of the first round of screening. In: Feig SA (ed) Breast carcinoma. Current diagnosis and treatment. Masson, New York, pp 315–326

Breast Cancer Screening in Malmö

I. Andersson

Department of Diagnostic Radiology, Allmänna Sjukhuset, 214 01 Malmö, Sweden

In January 1977, a breast cancer screening program was started in Malmö, which is a city in Sweden with about 235,000 inhabitants. The study was designed as a randomized trial and all females born from 1908 to 1932 were allocated to either a study group or a control group. The randomization was done on an individual basis. Each group consisted of about 21,000 women. The main aim of the study is to demonstrate the effect of mammographic screening on the mortality of breast carcinoma. Mammography is the only screening modality employed. In the first and second screening rounds, two views – the oblique and the craniocaudal – were obtained. All patients were classified according to the system of Wolfe (1976). In the third round, females with an N 1 or P 1 pattern underwent only the oblique-view screening and females with the P 2 or DY pattern underwent screening with both views.

Malmö is a city suitable for epidemiologic studies. For instance, all patients with breast carcinoma are investigated and treated at one hospital by a team consisting of radiologists, cytologists, surgeons, oncologists, and pathologists. Thus, patients with breast cancer are easily traced. Clinical mammography is available at the hospital and in one private practice. Females belonging to the control group who are left to their usual medical care can undergo a mammographic examination even without symptoms.

Three screening rounds have been completed. It should be pointed out that data for the third round and control group given in the following are preliminary. The first screening round was attended by 15,748 females, which corresponds to an attendance rate of 74%. The screening rounds were offered to all the females, i.e., even to those who did not attend the preceding screening. The attendance rate at the second and third screenings was 70%.

Between 3% and 4% of the screened women were selected for complete mammography on the basis of the screening mammograms (Table 1). The purpose of the complete mammography was to increase the specificity of the screening, i.e., to reduce the number of false-positives. After complete mammography, less than half of those originally selected were referred for further investigation. In the first two rounds, 1.2% of those screened

Table 1. Proportion of females selected, referred, and operated upon (percentage of those screened)

	Selected	Referred	Operated upon
First screening	3.4	1.6	1.2
Second screening	3.8	1.5	1.3
Third screening	3.1	0.9	0.6

Recent Results in Cancer Research. Vol. 90

were operated upon but only 0.6% of those screened in the third round underwent operation.

From the date of entry through the third screening, carcinoma was found in 222 women in the screening (Table 2). Fifty females who were negative in screening appeared with carcinoma between screenings (interval carcinomas). The interval between the screenings was on average 22 and 20 months, respectively. Forty-six females who had been invited but did not participate in the screening also appeared with breast carcinoma. This makes a total of 318 females with carcinoma in the invited half of the population. During the same period, 204 females in the control group had a diagnosis of breast carcinoma.

In the control group, 11% of the carcinomas were noninvasive and 16% were invasive with a diameter of at most 10 mm, making a total of 27% of what could be called small carcinomas (Table 3). Among screening-detected cases, the proportion of small carcino-

Table 2. Number of females with carcinoma from date of entry through third screening

	No. subjects
First screening	118
Second screening	58
Third screening	46
Subtotal	222
Interval	50
Nonparticipants	46
Subtotal invited group	318
Control group	204
Total	522

Table 3. Proportion of patients with "small" carcinomas

	Noninvasive (%)	Invasive (≤ 10 mm)	Total (%)
First screening	16	43	59
Second screening	21	48	69
Third screening	15	46	61
Intervals	14	14	28
Nonparticipants	2	9	11
Control group	11	16	27

Table 4. Proportion of patients with advanced disease

	Axillary metastasis (%)	Stages II–IV (%)
First screening	18	20
Second screening	18	26
Third screening	17	17
Interval	30	42
Nonparticipants	61	65
Control group	38	52

mas was significantly higher, over 60%, which was mainly due to a much larger proportion of small invasive carcinomas. Among interval carcinomas, the proportion of small carcinomas was almost the same as in the control group, while among nonparticipants it was smaller, 11%.

In the control group, 52% of the patients were in stages II–IV (Table 4). Among screening-detected cases, approximately 20% were in the corresponding stages. There was an overrepresentation of advanced disease among nonparticipants, 65%, as compared with the control group. Among interval carcinomas, the proportion of advanced disease was a little lower (42%) than in the control group.

Concerning the distribution of histologic types, the following deserves mention. The proportion of noninvasive carcinoma, the majority being intraductal carcinoma, was approximately the same in the first, second, and third screening rounds – 14%, 16%, and 13%, respectively. Also, highly differentiated tubular carcinoma, continued to be found. The proportion was 35%, 22%, and 26% in the first, second, and third screening rounds, respectively. Noninvasive carcinoma as well as highly differentiated tubular carcinoma are believed to be slowly progressive, rather benign types of carcinoma. However, the results indicate that the transition from a radiographically nondetectable to a detectable stage occurs within a rather short period of time.

In summary, a large proportion of the tumors detected by mammographic screening are small, without axillary metastasis. By prognostic parameters established in a clinical series of patients, this group should have a better than average prognosis. However, when evaluating the primary results, one should be cautious for several reasons, one of which is the length-biased sampling, which means that screening tends to pick up slowly growing carcinomas with a better than average prognosis. Thus, although the results so far indicate a favorable effect, firm conclusions cannot be drawn until mortality data are available.

Reference

Wolfe JN (1976) Breast patterns as an index of risk for developing breast cancer. AJR 126:1130–1139

Experience from Randomized Controlled Breast Screening with Mammography in Östergötland County, Sweden: A Preliminary Report

G. Fagerberg

Institution for Diagnostic Radiology, Mammographic Section, University of Linköping, Regionsjukhuset, 581 85 Linköping, Sweden

A randomized controlled study on breast cancer screening with mammography was started in Östergötland county, Sweden, in 1978. The basic question asked in this trial is: Can screening for breast carcinoma with single-view mammography as the only screening modality reduce mortality in the disease? A total of 93,000 females aged 40 years and older living in Östergötland county have been selected to the study. Randomization was carried out on the basis of municipalities and parishes. The control group includes 46,000 women and the study group offered examination with single-view mammography comprises 47,000 subjects. These females will be invited to two examinations with an interval of 2–3 years. The second screening is now underway and will be finished in 1983. The preliminary results are reported.
The overall participation rate in the first screening was 79%. A total of 294 cases of breast carcinoma were diagnosed as prevalent cases, which is about 8/1,000 females examined. In the control group, the incidence of breast carcinoma was 2.0/1,000/year. In the screened population, tumor in situ and invasive carcinoma up to 10 mm in diameter constituted 51% of the carcinomas diagnosed among females aged 40–69 years. The corresponding figure in the control group was 14%. The frequency of axillary lymph node metastases in screened carcinomas was 19%; in the control group it was 44%. In the screened group, 20% of the carcinomas were classified as p.TNM (postsurgical histopathologic classification) stage II carcinomas; in the control group the corresponding figure was 60%. One and a half years after finishing the first screening round, the total number of stage II carcinomas or higher stages was 80 in the study group, while in the control group so far 100 cases of breast carcinomas in these stages have been recorded.
Conclusive evidence of the effect of a cancer screening program upon mortality in cancer calls for randomized studies, and the only valid end point is an overall reduction in deaths from cancer in a population randomly selected and offered screening, compared with deaths in a comparable control group. From this study, comparable mortality data may be expected within the next 3–4 years.

Recent Results in Cancer Research. Vol. 90

*Breast Cancer Screening: Significance of Minimal Breast Cancers**

M. Moskowitz

Breast Cancer Detection Center, University of Cincinnati, Cincinnati, OH 45267, USA

Abstract

Analysis of cancers occurring during an aggressive screening program indicates: (1) In our study, during 3 years of active incidence screening of women under the age of 50 years, 24 cancers occurred, 14 of which were minimal. In the 3 years that there has been very limited screening, 23 cancers occurred, only five of which were minimal ($p = 0.02393$). (2) We projected that 110 breast cancers should have occurred in the incidence years of observation of this self-selected population of 10,531 women. In our screened population, 124 cancers occurred. This is not significantly different from the expected number. (3) In a similar period of observation of a similar sized screened population 112 cancers occurred in Louisville and 113 cases of cancer occurred in Seattle. There is no significant difference from the 124 cases reported in Cincinnati nor from the 110 cases expected. However, of all forms of cancer (prevalent, incident, interval) in Cincinnati, 67 cases were minimal, as against 35 in Louisville and 23 in Seattle ($p = < 0.0001$). All in all, these data supported the concept that screening for breast cancer does not in any significant way increase the number of cancer cases detected, it only advances the stage of detection. The data also suggest that, for an aggressive screen, length-biased sampling does not seem to be an insurmountable obstacle.

Introduction

Screening for neoplastic disease, by its very intent, is intended to detect subclinical, and presumably "earlier" stages of disease. Is the cancer found by screening real cancer? Implicit in this question is the assumption that screening an asymptomatic population may detect many cancers that would never have otherwise developed in the patient's lifetime. This further presumes that many "small" lesions are "precursor," or perhaps even reversible, cancers; that there are a large number of such lesions prevalent in the population, far in excess of the number expected to develop clinically; and, due to length-biased sampling, periodic screening will tend to detect primarily the slower growing of such cases.

We believe that the data we have accrued over the past 6 years allow us some check on the validity of these assumptions vis-a-vis breast cancer in our screened population.

---

* This paper was originally published in the American Journal of Roentgenology (vol. 136 pp. 735–738, 1981) and is republished here with kind permission; this work is supported in part by: The National Cancer Institute, N01 CN 55310, and The American Cancer Society, DPBC-11

Recent Results in Cancer Research. Vol. 90

Materials and Methods

The material to be reported is generated from a net total of 10,531 self-selected women who enrolled in a breast cancer screening program in two cohorts separated by 1 year, beginning in 1973. Annual screening with mammography and clinical breast examination was to be offered to these women for 5 years, and follow-up of the entire cohort was to be carried on for an added 5 years. In April, 1977, screening was sharply curtailed for women aged 35–49 years.

From August 1973 through 30 June 1979, we maintained a patient contact rate of 94%. This contact, plus our ongoing surveillance of breast biopsies performed in the metropolitan area, has yielded for the period indicated what we believe to be reliable incidence data for breast cancer for this total cohort for the above period. From 30 June, 1979 to the present, the data are not yet complete and, therefore, subject to increase. These data for the years 1979–1980 are used only in one context and are clearly indicated when used.

For this paper, the data are analyzed by age of patient at time of surgery for the neoplasm. The number of persons at risk in each age-group was calculated for each calendar year and corrected appropriately for aging of the population.

As can be seen in Table 1, 222 cancers (prevalent, incident, interval) occurred in this population from 1 August 1973 through 30 June 1979. Of these cancers, 40% were either 5 mm in size, wholly intraductal, in situ lobular, tubular cancer, cancers with less than 10% microinvasion, or Paget's disease with no other pathologic finding of cancer in the breast.

Since April 1977, only 18% of the females under the age of 50 years have undergone a full screening. From 1978 to 1979, only half of the population over the age of 50 years would have been eligible for full screening. The data presented in Table 1, however, include all cancers occurring in all patients, prevalent, incident, and interval until 30 June 1979. As indicated, data for 1980 are not yet complete. We are aware, however, of nine cancer cases proven since June 1979, but they are not included in Table 1 because the data for the calendar years 1979–1980 are not complete.

Table 1. Cancers occurring 1973–June 30, 1979 (includes interval, incident, and prevalent cancers)[a]

Cancer	No. cases
Stage I invasive cancer	78 (35.0%)
Stage II invasive cancer	59 (26.0%)
Microinvasive (< 10%)	12 (5.4%)
5-mm invasive cancer	13 (5.8%)
Intraductal cancer	40 (17.9%)
Paget's disease	1 (0.5%)
Lobular cancer in situ	12 (5.8%)
Tubular carcinoma	4 (1.8%)
Unknown stage	3 (1.3%)
Total	222 (100 %)

[a] Cases occuring since July 1, 1979, are not included in this tally

Expected Incidence Versus Observed Incident Cancers

Since such a large proportion of the breast cancers detected in our study are minimal breast cancers, if they were unreal (i.e., would never have developed into clinical cancers with a life-threatening potential), the total incidence rate should markedly exceed the expected incidence as approximated by the appropriate self-selection-adjusted and region-adjusted incidence rates. Unless the incidence rates seen in our population are in excess of what would reasonably be expected, it would be very likely that most of the cancers detected are biologically significant and would have otherwise presented clinical symptoms in the patient's lifetime.

Seidman's analysis (1977) of the demographic data provided by the Breast Cancer Detection Demonstration Projects (BCDDP) suggests that self-selection bias should increase the annual incidence of breast cancers expected by approximately 25%. Mortality rates for all ages for the Cincinnati region (Mason et al. 1975) are approximately 25% greater than national rates. Since regional bias was not included in Seidman's calculations,

Table 2. Expected and observed cases of cancer (incident cancers only, age adjusted)[a]

	Expected cancers				Observed cancers
	TNCS	SS bias	Regional bias	Total expected	
Age 35–49 years	23	25%	25%	35	44
Age > 50 years	51	25%	25%	75	80
All ages	74			110	124

TNCS, Third National Cancer Survey; *SS*, self-selection
[a] Data until June 1979

Table 3. Persons at risk during incidence years by age

Calendar year	Age (years)	No. persons at risk	Expected incidence/year/ 1,000 people TNCS[a]	No. cancers/ year/1,000 people expected[a]
1974–1975	35–49	2,763	1.04	2.9
	50 +	2,113	2.08	4.4
1975–1976	35–49	5,480	1.04	5.7
	50 +	5,051	2.08	10.5
1976–1977	35–49	5,114	1.04	5.3
	50 +	5,417	2.08	11.3
1977–1978	35–49	4,699	1.04	4.9
	50 +	5,832	2.08	12.1
1978–1979	35–49	4,289	1.04	4.5
	50 +	6,242	2.08	13.0

[a] *TNCS*, Third National Cancer Survey

this suggests that regional bias would increase the expected national incidence by another 25%. Thus in the age-group 35–49 years based upon national incidence data (Table 2) and adjusting appropriately for increasing age of the population (Table 3), we should have expected 23 cancers during the incidence years of screening 1974–1979. If 1979–1980 is included, 28 cases of cancer would be expected. Correction for self-selection and regional bias should increase the 1974–1979 expectation to 35 cases; if 1979–1980 is included, 42 cases would be expected. Over the age of 50 years, 51 cancers would have been expected at national levels for 1974–1979; self-selection and regional biases should increase that total to 75 cases. Thus, it would not be unreasonable to expect a total of 110 cases with appropriate self-selection and regional adjustments for 1974–1979.

In the age-group 35–49 years, we observed 44 cancers versus the 35 expected ($p = 0.37$), and in the age-group over 50 years, 80 cancers were observed versus the 75 expected ($p = 0.75$). The total observed was 124 cases versus the 110 expected. The observed totals include all incident and interval (nonscreen detected) cases of cancer for 1974–1979.

It might be argued that the estimates of self-selection bias and regional biases make too high an adjustment for expected incidence in this population. In fact, it is possible that the 44 cases observed in younger women versus the 23 expected by the Third National Cancer Survey (TNCS) is due to the inclusion of 19 "precancer" cases. However, in any 3-year period, on average 14 cancers would be expected by the TNCS (Table 3). Our model would predict that the corrected incidence should be 21 cases for this population for a 3-year period. In the 3 years (1977–1980) in which there was a *marked curtailment* of screening, 23 cancers occurred. During 3 *active* screening years in females aged 35–49 years, 24 cancers were found. This is direct supporting evidence that the approximation we made of the base incidence in this screened population is accurate. This simple model also seems to predict equally well the 5-year total *incidence* of cancer in all ages for Louisville, Seattle, and Cincinnati, all of which have a significantly different frequency of minimal cancer detection. These data will be expanded in subsequent sections.

Thus, there is no significant excess of the number of cancers detected over those expected. Perhaps some of the cancers detected in younger women would not have shown clinical symptoms in the patient's lifetime, but it is likely that the number of such cases is relatively small.

Change When Screening Stops

Due to certain events surrounding the breast cancer screening problem, as of 24 April 1977 a marked restriction in mammographic screening of younger women was introduced. Females under the age of 50 years were only to be offered mammographic screening if they had a personal history of breast cancer themselves, a maternal or sibling history of breast cancer, or a significant clinical abnormality on physical examination. As a result of this restriction, approximately 18% of females in this age-group received complete screening. The data for all females under the age of 50 years after 1977 when screening was seriously altered, therefore, can be looked at in comparison with the observations in all females under the age of 50 years that occurred prior to that time, i.e., the group can serve as its own control.

If screening is to be effective it should draw on future incidence to some extent. The time represented by this gain over usual clinical detection is the lead time. If the lead time to detection gained by screening is sufficiently long, i.e., approaching infinity, the number of cancers occurring in the observation period after screening is reduced will sharply drop off.

Table 4. Screen sensitivity in younger women (all cancers included)

	Total	Minimal	Stages I–II
1974–1977	24 (100%)	14 (58%)	10 (42%)
1977–1980[a]	23 (100%)	5 (22%)	18 (78%)

$p = 0.02393$, χ^2 test (Yates corrected)
[a] Data complete until 1979; the data are not complete for 1980 (three cases)

In the 3-year period 1974–1977, 24 cancers (including interval cancers) were found. When screening was sharply curtailed in 1977–1980 23 cancers occurred. Therefore, there is *no* evidence to indicate a drop in incidence. This observation is inconsistent with an infinitely long lead time, and is not supportive of a mean lead time significantly longer than 2 years. If the *mean* lead time is not longer than 2 years, it is unlikely that there are a significant number of cases with an infinitely long lead time.

Based on prevalence data, our model previously estimated (Fox et al. 1978) for younger females that the lead time gained over clinical detection was 2.1 ± 0.5 years. This model has accurately predicted the lead time gained by a controlled clinical trial now in progress in Falun, Sweden for each age-group screened (personal communication L. Tabar).

In the incidence years 1974–1977 for women aged 35–49 years, only three breast cancer cases were *not* detected by the screen; none were stage II. Two interval breast cancers occurred in one patient. In the years 1977–1979, when screening was markedly reduced, 11 breast cancers were detected in nonscreened women, two of which were minimal, four of which were stage I, and five of which were stage II. Since July 1979, three more cancers have been found, all of which were stage II. In the period 1974–1977, the average time to clinical detection after the last screening was only 6 months. In the 1977–1979 period, the average time to detection after the last full screening was 21 months, or 9 months after the date of what would have been their regularly scheduled full sensitivity screen. Although incomplete, the data up to 1980 average out to a lead time of 26 months. Thus, the apparent average lead time gained by clinical detection is 26 months, well within the variation predicted by our model for this age.

Of the 24 cases of cancer detected during active screening, 14 or 58% were minimal and 42% were invasive (Table 4). Of the 23 cancers in the next 3-year period, five (22%) were minimal, and 18 (78%) were invasive. Thus, the cancer incidence has remained at the same level over national incidence during this period when there was little screening, but the distribution has significantly shifted toward advanced invasive disease ($p = 0.02393$, χ^2 test, Yates corrected).

All of the cancers that occurred during screening and those that occurred after screening stopped seem to have equal biologic significance.

Incidence in Screens of Different Threshold Sensitivities

Another way to estimate the clinical significance of the minimal cancers is to compare the incidence years of screens of different threshold sensitivities. Once a screen has established its size threshold of detection sensitivity, the annual incidence rate developing within that screen should remain relatively stable. Thus, screens of different size threshold sensitivity should detect the same total number of incident cancers. The only difference between the screens should be in the stage at detection. If incidence is indeed equal and stage is significantly different, then all the cancers discovered by each screen should have the same biologic properties.

Let us examine screens of three different threshold sensitivities in what are supposedly similar metropolitan areas. For Cincinnati and Louisville (Heuser et al. 1979; Moskowitz 1980), the data are available for 3 and 5 years after the prevalence year. In Cincinnati, 70 incident (including interval) cancers occurred in the 3 years after the prevalence year. During a similar period in Louisville, 76 cancers were reported. The number of breast cancers reported in Louisville (Heuser et al. 1979) as stage II were twice as high as the stage II cancers found in Cincinnati during the same period. The rate of detection of these advanced cancers is statistically significantly different at the $p = < 0.045$ level (Moskowitz 1980).

In Seattle, the total incidence of cancers over a 5-year period is 113 (personal communication from Dr. Thomas Carlile) as compared with the Cincinnati rate of 124. For Louisville, after 5 years there were 112 cancers (personal communication, Dr. Jerry Buchanan). The total number of cancers found after 5 years in Cincinnati, Louisville, and Seattle, are not statistically significantly different ($p = 0.47$, χ^2 test). In Cincinnati, of all the cancers detected, 67 were either ductal in situ, lobular in situ, Paget's disease, or less than 5 mm in size. (For this comparison microinvasive and tubular cancers are omitted.) In Seattle, of all cancers found (prevalent, incident, and interval), the preliminary data to date indicate that 23 cancers fall into a similar category ($p = < 0.0001$), and for Louisville 35 such cancers were found.

Therefore, these data suggest: (1) aggressive screening does not significantly increase the total number of cancers found, it only advances the stage of detection; (2) aggressive screening significantly alters the natural history of the disease such that the rate of advanced disease per 1,000 patients examined is significantly reduced.

Length-Biased Sampling

It has been theorized that due to length-biased sampling (Zelen 1976), screens will tend to detect primarily slower growing cancers. No doubt, due to the intermittent nature of screening this is to some extent correct. However, in a tumor population with a heavy component of intermediate and slow growth rate tumors, one would expect the effect of length-biased sampling to be maximal in the prevalence year (Zelen 1976; Henderson and Canellos 1980). That is to say that many indolent tumors of varying size and stage will be uncovered in the 1st year. Thereafter, those tumors that reach detection threshold at the intervals of the screening, or between screenings, will be more aggressive in their growth rates. Inefficient screening with high miss rates will lead to an excess interval cancer load, and faulty conclusions concerning tumor biology will be drawn.

The aggressive screening we performed was associated with an interval, or miss, rate. From 1973–1979, in all age-groups, 35 cancers were detected outside the screening 17 of these occurred, in patients who had not received a mammogram in the preceding 12 months. One of these occurred 13 months after the last full screening, two occurred after 15 months, the remainder at intervals from 20 to 69 months for an average of 27 months.

Eighteen cases (19 cancers) can reasonably be considered true interval cancers for a false-negative rate of 9%. Interestingly, 10 of 18 of the true interval cancers had a family history of breast cancer and only two of 17 of the patients with no previous mammograms had such a history.

At this point, it would do well to recall that during the period of active screening of younger women, 58% of all cancers (including interval cancers) were minimal.
One might argue that aggressive screening is not necessary because the slow-growing tumors will survive for long periods, no matter when detected. However, if nonaggressive screening is performed, the more rapidly growing tumors are not detected until they reach clinical threshold, and they appear often as interval cancer, usually more advanced disease (Heuser et al. 1979; Moskowitz 1980).
Taken as whole, these data suggest that while length-biased sampling somewhat affects early detection and, therefore, probable outcome, for breast cancer screening it is simply not an insurmountable problem.

Acknowledgements. We thank Drs. Thomas Carlile and Jerry Buchanan, for providing the data from the Seattle and Louisville projects, and Dr. Laszlo Tabar for data from the screening project in Falun, Sweden.
The author is deeply indebted to Dr. Stanley Fox for his stimulating and provocative role in the crystallization of many of the concepts presented here.
The analyses of statistical significance were performed by Dr. Peter Gartside of the University of Cincinnati, Department of Environmental Health.

References

1. Fox SH, Moskowitz M, Saenger EL, Kereiakes JG, Milbrath J, Goodman MW (1978) Benefit/risk analysis of aggressive mammographic screening. Radiology 128: 359–365
2. Henderson IC, Canellos GP (1980) Cancer of the breast: the past decade. N Engl J Med 302: 17–30
3. Heuser L, Spratt JS, Polk HC, Buchanan JB (1979) Relation between mammary growth kinetics and the intervals between screenings. Cancer 43: 857–862
4. Mason TJ, McKay FW, Hoover R, Blat WJ, Fraumeni JF Jr (1975) Atlas of cancer mortality for U.S. Counties: 1950–1969 (DHEW publication no. (NIH)75-780). U.S. Department of Health Education & Welfare, Public Health Service – National Institutes of Health
5. Moskowitz M (1979) Screening is not diagnosis. Radiology 133: 265–268 [addendum: Restructured data comparing screening approaches. Radiology 134: 262 (1980)]
6. Seidman H (1977) Screening for breast cancer in younger women: Life expectancy gains and losses. An analysis according to risk indicator groups. CA 27: 66–87
7. Zelen M (1976) Theory of early detection of breast cancer in the general population. In: Heuson JC, Mattheim WA, Rozencweig M (eds) Breast cancer: trends in research and treatment. Raven, New York, pp 287–304

Localization and Significance of Clinically Occult Breast Lesions: Experience with 469 Needle-Guided Biopsies

G. F. Schwartz, S. A. Feig, A. L. Rosenberg, A. S. Patchefsky, and G. S. Shaber

Department of Surgery, Jefferson Medical College,
1015 Chestnut Street, Suite 510, Philadelphia, PA 19107, USA

Introduction

As the use of mammography has become ubiquitous in medical practice, radiographic findings in the absence of a palpable mass have been recognized as valid indications for a breast biopsy. When the radiologist's observations provoke the recommendation for biopsy, the surgeon's objectives must be to insure the removal of the entire suspicious area for precise histologic examination while removing the minimum volume of contiguous normal breast tissue.

It is incumbent upon physicians to understand and explain the possible significance of these impalpable findings in order to convince their patients of the need for biopsy when they are encountered. Unless this "earlier" detection leads to greater survival or less radical therapy, there is little stimulus to patients or their physicians to embark upon screening programs to uncover asymptomatic breast cancer.

In the past several years, 469 clinically occult breast lesions have been treated at Thomas Jefferson University Hospital. This report describes the technique of "needle-guided biopsy," which has been used to localize these tiny suspicious areas precisely and guarantee their removal and presents the microscopic diagnoses encountered and their significance.

Methods and Materials

General recommendations for biopsy of the breast based upon suspicious radiographic observations include the following: (1) Calcifications indicative of malignancy because of size (less than 2 mm), shape (punctate, microlinear, or branching), and distribution (clustered or grouped along ducts or more than $5/mm^2$); (2) stellate masses; (3) breast masses with ill-defined borders or nodular contours; (4) dominant, well-circumscribed smooth masses that are significantly larger than any other mass in either breast; and (5) areas of increased tissue density or distorted breast architecture.

The insertion of needles into the breast to localize clinically occult breast lesions was described originally by Dodd et al. (1965). Only in the past several years has the procedure gained popularity, with some investigators advocating the use of special needles with hooks or barbs to avoid their being dislodged during transport of the patient between radiology suite and operating room, to avoid pneumothorax as a complication, etc. (Homer 1979; Homer et al. 1980; Kopans and DeLuca 1980; Meyer and Kopand 1982). However, we have found these devices to be unnecessary if care is taken with needle placement and preparation for the subsequent operative procedure.

Recent Results in Cancer Research. Vol. 90

The area in question is identified on the mammograms and its distance from the nipple is measured on both craniocaudal and lateral films. These measurements are used to select a topographic site in the same horizontal and vertical planes. Following the aseptic preparation of the skin and the infiltration of a few milliters of local anesthetic, a standard, disposable, 25-gauge, $1\frac{1}{2}$-in. needle is inserted into the breast, directed toward the lesion and taped in place. Mammograms are repeated in both projections to determine the proximity of the needle tip to the suspicious area, and if the needle is "on target," the patient is sent to the operating room. Our own earlier experience also determined that the use of vital or radiopaque dyes injected through the needle to mark the tissue more precisely was unnecessary and, in fact, interfered with the interpretation of the specimen radiograph or obscured the operative field (Schwartz et al. 1978). Although the current trend is for breast biopsies to be performed under local anesthesia, these needle-guided biopsies, for the most part, were performed under general anesthesia, especially when the radiographic finding was a group of clustered microcalcifications. Looking for this "needle in the haystack" occasionally requires considerable tugging and pulling, especially since the incisions are usually small ones, and this is more uncomfortable than the usual biopsy for a palpable lesion. Moreover, we have been loathe to disturb the architecture of the suspicious area by the infiltration of a bolus of anesthetic solution, possibly creating a difference between the specimen radiograph and the preoperative mammogram.

A circumareolar incision centered in line with the needle is used whenever possible, but when the suspicious area is judged too far from the center of the breast for this incision, one that is parallel to the areolar margin in the skin lines is used instead, directly over the expected site. There is no need to excise any skin whatever. By tunneling through the breast using appropriately sized hooks and retractors, the suspicious area is approached.

A volume of tissue only slightly larger than the radiographic abnormality is exised, and specimen radiology is performed. The tabletop X-ray machine used for specimen radiography is kept in the pathology department near the operating room. This radiograph indicates whether the suspicious lesion has been excised; if necessary, additional tissue is removed until the mass, calcifications, or other abnormality has been unequivocally removed. While most specimens are fixed and embedded in their entirety for serial sectioning, especially those containing calcifications, occasionally a frozen section may be possible if a large-enough mass has been encountered. When the mammograms show a mass that is impalpable because of its small size or deep location, but which might be amenable to frozen section when visualized directly, it is possible to prepare the patient so that a definitive procedure may be performed under the same anesthesia if the mass proves to be malignant and the patient concurs.

Most patients are discharged the evening after surgery or the next morning with the assurance that they will be apprised of the final diagnosis as soon as possible. By insuring that the suspicious area is within the initial specimen excised and keeping this volume of tissue as small as possible, about a 1-cm diameter greater than the mammographic abnormality, those patients who prove to have benign disease show no deformity or loss of breast contour as a result of the procedure. If malignancy is encountered, appropriate workup and options of therapy may be discussed with the patient.

Results

Between early 1974 and 1 May 1982, 430 females underwent needle-guided biopsy in the manner described above at Thomas Jefferson University Hospital. Of these, 39 required

Table 1. Age distribution of clinically occult breast lesions

Age (years)	No.	Percent
Under 30	3	0.7
30–39	38	8.8
40–49	120	27.9
50–59	168	39.1
60–69	81	18.8
70 or older	20	4.6
Total	430	

Table 2. Radiographic findings in clinically occult breast lesions

	No.	Percent
Calcifications (size, shape, distribution)	268	57.1
Stellate masses	8	1.8
Other masses (ill-defined or well circumscribed)	153	32.6
Masses with associated calcifications	21	4.5
Abnormal density or parenchymal distortion	19	4.1
Total	469	

bilateral biopsy, so the total number of biopsy specimens was 469. Those radiologic findings that necessitated biopsy and the ages of the patients encountered are summarized in Tables 1 and 2.

Of the entire group of 469 needle-guided biopsies, 318, or 67.8%, proved to be for benign disease, and malignancy was demonstrated in 151 (32.2%). "Fibrocystic disease," implying a melange of benign conditions, constituted 81.7% (260 of 318) of these benign biopsies. We have attempted to subdivide this imprecise category, "fibrocystic disease," according to the degree of epithelial proliferation observed microscopically. In this regard, diagnoses of cystic disease, apocrine metaplasia, adenosis, fibrous mastopathy, and mammary duct ectasia were considered "without" epithelial proliferation, and the diagnoses of papillomatosis, ductal or lobular hyperplasia, and florid adenosis, or the proliferative phase of sclerosing adenosis, were considered "with" epithelial proliferation. The entire distribution of these benign lesions is summarized in Table 4.

The histology of the 151 cancers detected by needle-guided biopsy is summarized in Table 5. Microinvasive ductal cancer is defined as one that is predominantly intraductal but with up to 10% of the histologic sections showing stromal invasion (Patchefsky et al. 1977). A single malignant carcinoid tumor of the breast was encountered, documented by electron microscopy and histochemical staining techniques. Lobular carcinoma in situ (lobular neoplasia) (Haagensen et al. 1972) is presented as a separate entity, listed under malignant diagnoses, recognizing the controversy that surrounds this lesion. It should not be listed along with in situ ductal carcinoma because of the different implications of these two diagnoses in terms of patient management recommendations.

Axillary contents were available for review for 82 women with Frankly invasive carcinomas (82 of 89 = 92%), including the patient with a carcinoid tumor. Three females had

Table 3. Histologic findings in clinically occult breast lesions

Diagnosis	No.	Percent
Benign	318	67.8
Malignant	151	32.2
Invasive carcinoma	89	19.0
Microinvasive duct	9	1.9
In situ duct	40	8.5
In situ lobular (lobular neoplasia)	13	2.8
Total	469	

Table 4. Histology of 318 benign biopsies

Diagnosis	No.	Percent
Fibrocystic disease without epithelial proliferation	193	60.7
Fibrocystic disease with epithelial proliferation	67	21.1
Fibroadenoma	43	13.5
Intramammary lymph node	3	0.9
Normal breast tissue or fat necrosis	12	3.8
Total	318	

Table 5. Histologic findings in 151 cancers

Histology	No.	Percent
Invasive duct cancer	83	55.0
Invasive lobular cancer	5	3.3
Malignant carcinoid	1	0.7
Microinvasive duct cancer	9	6.0
In situ duct cancer	40	26.4
In situ lobular cancer (lobular neoplasia)	13	8.6
Total	151	

symptoms of disseminated disease at the time of diagnosis, and thus did not undergo mastectomy with axillary dissection. Four other females either underwent radiation therapy without axillary node dissection, or their records were unvailable. The status of the axillary nodes in those females for whom the data are available is shown in Table 6. Of the nine women with microinvasive duct carcinomas, all of them underwent mastectomy with axillary dissection, either radical or modified radical, and the axillary nodes were negative for metastases in every patient. Each of these patients had undergone biopsy because of the mammographic finding of clustered calcifications. Within this small group of nine patients, histologic examination of the entire breast detected the presence of multifocal cancer in four of them (44%), multifocal being defined as the presence of in situ or invasive cancer, ductal or lobular, in a quadrant of the breast other than the one in which the primary carcinoma had been found (Schwartz et al. 1980).

Table 6. Axillary node status in 82 invasive cancers

	No.	Percent
All nodes negative	49	59.8
Level 1		
Only one positive node	8	9.8
2 or 3 positive nodes	9	10.9
4 or more positive nodes	1	1.2
Multiple levels		
Less than 4 positive nodes	1	1.2
4 or more positive nodes	11	13.4
Distant metastases	3	3.7
Total	82	

Table 7. Multifocal carcinoma

Primary diagnosis (no. of cases in brackets)	Other foci of carcinoma (no. of cases in brackets)
Invasive ductal or lobular (97)	Invasive ductal or lobular (5)
	Noninvasive ductal (20)
	Noninvasive lobular (10)
	Total 35/97 = 36.1%
Minimally invasive ductal (9)	Minimally invasive ductal (1)
	Noninvasive ductal (3)
	Total 4/9 = 44.4%
Carcinoid, primary (1)	Total 0/1 = 0%
Noninvasive ductal carcinoma (31)	Noninvasive ductal (10)
	Noninvasive lobular (4)
	Total 14/31 = 45%
Lobular in situ carcinoma (4)	Noninvasive lobular (1)
	Noninvasive ductal (1)
	Total 2/4 = 50%
	Total 54/142 = 38%

In situ ductal carcinomas were found in 40 biopsies, of which 35 were detected as areas of clustered calcifications within the breast. In each of these biopsies, the area of in situ carcinoma was found in the area of the calcifications. One patient had a impalpable mass with calcifications; although the mass was benign, the area of calcifications demonstrated foci of intraductal cancer. Four patients underwent biopsies for impalpable masses, which proved to be either fibroadenomas or cysts, and the areas of intraductal cancer were incidental findings.

None of the 16 females who underwent axillary dissection as part of the treatment for intraductal carcinoma had axillary metastases. However, it was noteworthy that 14 of 31 patients who underwent mastectomy for intraductal carcinoma had areas of multifocal cancer.

Of the 13 patients with lobular carcinoma in situ (lobular neoplasia), seven underwent biopsy because of clustered calcifications and six because of a impalpable mass. In each patient with a mass, the mass was benign and the lobular carcinoma in situ was an incidental finding. Four of these females with lobular carcinoma in situ underwent mastectomy, whereas the others chose careful follow-up when the controversial nature of the disease was discussed with them. The observed incidence of multifocal cancer in this group was 50% (two of four). Table 7 notes the overall incidence of multifocal cancer encountered within the 142 breasts removed subsequent to a needle-guided biopsy disclosing malignancy.

Discussion

This report documents the success of needle-guided biopsy in the precise localization of radiographic abnormalities in the breast without accompanying clinical findings. Close cooperation between surgeon, radiologist, and pathologist insures that the suspicious area(s) are removed in their entirety with the sacrifice of the minimal amount of contiguous normal breast tissue. Such excision need not be accompanied by loss of breast contour or conspicuous scars. Our experience, moreover, refutes the need for any specialized needles or injected dyes to accomplish the biopsy. A standard, readily available, disposable 25-gauge needle suffices; in patients with deep-seated lesions or very large breasts, a longer, fine-gauge spinal needle may be preferred.

The age distribution of these patients may not be representative of the actual incidence of clinically occult breast lesions. Many of the females had been enrolled in a screening program at the Thomas Jefferson University Hospital, which was directed at females between the ages of 45 and 65 years. Their lesions were disclosed as a direct result of their participation in this program rather than having been referred for mammography as part of routine health care or because of a complaint related to the breast.

Clustered calcifications alone prompted more than half of the biopsies, but some of the cancers detected were visualized as actual masses on the mammogram. They were not palpable because of their small size in most cases, but there were several patients whose cancers might have been considered big enough to be felt had they been located elsewhere in the breast, or if the breast had been smaller. For example, one obese, large-breasted patient had a 3-cm (T-2) cancer, which was located almost against the chest wall. Only by accident of patient size and tumor geography was this an impalpable lesion. In several other cases, the initial breast examination was considered "normal," but a subsequent mammogram demonstrated the presence of a significant finding, usually a mass or parenchymal distortion. Armed with the mammograms, the examiner could feel a questionable area on physical examination, which corresponded to the suspicious site on the mammogram.

It is imperative in similar cases that needle-guided biopsy be used to prove that the X-ray findings and the clinical findings are identical. For example, one patient in this series had a clinically palpable mass, which was thought, on the basis of its characteristics, to be a fibroadenoma. The patient's mammogram suggested the presence of a stellate mass in the same general location of the breast. Without needle-guided biopsy, it would have been possible to remove the palpable mass, which was a fibroadenoma, and miss the carcinoma, the stellate mass, situated in the same area of the breast, but deeper within the same quadrant.

These examples raise the question of the definition of clinically occult. Certainly, those cancers evident only as clustered calcifications within the breast are occult by any definition. However, are masses in the breast that are not palpable because of location or because of the large size of the breast still to be considered clinically occult? The notation T-0 has been used to describe those cancers that are not palpable because there is no evidence of primary tumor on physical examination. We suggest that only if there is no mass in the breast should this be used. Let T-0 stand for those cancers detected by mammography alone as clustered calcifications or areas of parenchymal distortion, but if a cancer is seen as a mass, stellate or circumscribed, on the mammogram, the same criteria for staging should apply whether it is palpable or not. In other words, if less than 2.0 cm, it is T-1, if 2–5 cm, T-2, etc. Most of these cancers will be T-1 lesions, but, as we have noted, there may be an occasional larger one missed because of its deep location or the patient's large breast. An additional notation might be made, if desired, in staging that the cancer was not detected on physical examination but only on mammography, such as T-1_m, or in the case of clustered calcifications that prove to be malignant the lesion might be considered T-0_m. Thus, our patient with an impalpable 3-cm carcinoma and clinically negative axilla would still be considered stage II (T-2_m, N-0, M-0) and recorded appropriately for follow-up.

Our observation that several of the in situ ductal carcinomas and the lobular carcinomas in situ were detected only as incidental findings in specimens removed for other reasons should not imply that biopsy includes a large segment of contiguous normal-appearing breast surrounding the radiographic abnormality. Although the entire area seen on the mammogram should be identified and excised, using specimen radiography when necessary to prove its excision, this should not be an excuse for a wide excision of normal-appearing breast tissue, just because something else might be found in the neighborhood (Roses et al. 1980).

Although it might be considered presumptuous to draw conclusions from the histologic findings, which might influence the treatment of other early lesions, or with regard to the effect of detecting impalpable cancers on ultimate survival, several observations are appropriate. The high proportion of microinvasive or noninvasive cancers should be noted. None of these patients had axillary metastases, so these data do substantiate the consideration of less drastic procedures as possible treatment, such as total mastectomy without axillary dissection, or at most, level I dissection rather than a complete axillary dissection. This high proportion of noninvasive or microinvasive cancers also suggests a higher long-term survival for this entire group of patients as compared with patients with palpable masses found to be cancers. Even among the invasive cancers, the incidence of axillary metastases is approximately half of what might be expected for clinically apparent lesions (Haagensen 1971a). This in turn suggests a better prognosis for these patients, since it is not unreasonable to make the extrapolation of survival from axillary node metastasis (Haagensen et al. 1972). The high incidence of multifocal cancer in this and earlier studies, close to 40%, must be considered when offering therapeutic recommendations (Schwartz et al. 1980).

Any treatment that does not include the entire breast, even for in situ ductal carcinoma or microinvasive carcinoma, may leave other areas of cancer behind within that breast. Even if one excludes those patients with multifocal areas of lobular carcinoma in situ, the multicentricity of ductal carcinoma remains significant. For invasive carcinomas, the same treatment should be recommended as if the lesion were palpable. Small does not imply inconsequential! Additionally, attention to the axillary nodes is demanded, since these small cancers have a significant likelihood of involving these nodes. If radiotherapy is chosen in lieu of mastectomy for any of these patients with invasive carcinoma, a preliminary level I axillary dissection is recommended to determine the extent of radiotherapy needed and the need for subsequent adjuvant chemotherapy. If mastectomy is chosen, then total mastectomy with complete axillary dissection should be considered. Whether the underlying pectoralis major muscle is removed with the specimen should depend upon the location and size of the lesion. If the mass is located in proximity to the fascia of this muscle, it does not seem reasonable to leave the muscle behind.

Lobular carcinoma in situ (lobular neoplasia) continues to be a challenge and a dilemma. Currently, our patients undergo no further treatment. Instead, they are apprised of the controversy surrounding this disease, and if they concur, they are followed-up at quarterly intervals by clinical examination and by periodic, usually annual, mammography, rather than undergoing any prophylactic surgical procedure.

Summary

Experience with 469 clinically occult breast lesions is presented. The overall incidence of malignancy observed was 32%, just about one in three. The technique of needle-guided biopsy is described, insuring precise localization and excision of minute radiographic findings, yet without leaving a conspicuous scar to remind the patient of her experience. Although it is too early to speculate about a possible increase in survival of these "earliest" breast cancers, the observed decreased incidence of axillary node metastasis implies a lowered death rate from breast cancer in these patients. It is not unreasonable to extrapolate the extent of patient salvage from axillary node status. Many of these cancers were uncovered in the course of screening asymptomatic patients, and this further implies the efficacy of such screening programs in the early detection of breast cancer. The surprisingly high incidence of multicentricity in these tiny cancers must not be ignored when recommending adequate and appropriate therapy for these impalpable malignancies.

References

Dodd DG, Greening RR, Wallace W (1965) In: Nealon TF Jr (ed) The management of the patient with cancer. Saunders, Philadelphia, p 88

Haagensen CD (1971a) Diseases of the breast, 2nd edn. Saunders, Philadelphia, pp 396–410

Haagensen CD (1971b) Diseases of the breast, 2nd edn. Saunders, Philadelphia, p 706

Haagensen CD, Lane N, Lattes R (1972) Neoplastic proliferation of the epithelium of the mammary lobules. Surg Clin North Am 52: 497–524

Homer MJ (1979) Percutaneous localization of breast lesions: Experience with the Frank Breast Biopsy Guide. J Assoc Can Radiol 30: 238–241

Homer MJ, Rangel DM, Miller HH (1980) Pre- and transoperative localization of nonpalpable breast lesions. Am J Surg 139: 889–891

Kopans DB, DeLuca S (1980) A modified needle-hookwire technique to simplify preoperative localization of occult breast lesions. Radiology 134: 781

Meyer JE, Kopand DB (1982) Preoperative roentgenographically guided percutaneous localization of occult breast lesions. Arch Surg 17: 65–68

Patchefsky AS, Schwartz GF, Shaber GS, Feig SA, Nerlinger (1977) The pathology of breast cancers detected by mass population screening. Cancer 40: 1659–1670

Roses DF, Harris MN, Gorstein F, Gumport SL (1980) Biopsy for microcalcification detected by mammography. Surgery 87: 248–252

Schwartz GF, Feig SA, Patchefsky AS (1978) Clinicopathologic correlations and significance of clinically occult mammary lesions. Cancer 41: 1147–1153

Schwartz GF, Patchefsky AS, Feig SA, Shaber GS, Schwartz AB (1980) Clinically occult breast cancer. Ann Surg 191: 8–12

The Selective Treatment of "Early" Carcinoma of the Breast by Lumpectomy, Level I Axillary Dissection, and Radiation Therapy

G. F. Schwartz, B. F. Danoff, S. A. Feig, H. M. Rosenblum, J. D. Bloss, and J. R. Gall

Department of Surgery, Jefferson Medical College,
1015 Chestnut Street, Suite 510, Philadelphia, PA 19107, USA

Considering the choice of treatment for "early" breast cancer controversial might be likened to calling a monsoon a small rainfall. Enthusiastic and vocal advocates of widely disparate forms of therapy resemble carnival barkers hawking their games, promising a prize with each toss. At one extreme are those who believe that no one any longer must submit to mastectomy, and at the other end are those who refuse to consider anything but mastectomy. In the middle of this maelstrom of rhetoric stands the all-but forgotten patient, who, quite understandably, feels that half of her is being pulled inexorably toward the linear accelerator while the other half is being drawn into the operating room. Not only is this decision between mastectomy and radiation therapy thrust upon the patient when she is most vulnerable, but the patient is all too often made to feel that the decision must be made immediately, any delay between biopsy and therapy jeopardizing the ultimate chances of survival.

Patients confronted with the diagnosis of breast cancer are not interested in listening to shibboleths about the need for randomized trials and the alleged lack of definitive proof that any one therapy is better than another. Their breast, if not their life, depends upon the careful collection, collation, and comparison of the available data related to various forms of treatment and the enumeration of the advantages and disadvantages of each. For some females, it may be inconceivable that anyone would sacrifice her breast if radiation therapy had a reasonable chance of accomplishing the same goal. For other females, irradiation is comparable to carrying a firecracker in a back pocket, waiting for someone to light the fuse. The decision must be made today, without the luxury of waiting for someone's 10-year clinical trials to be completed and analyzed.

What information can we, as concerned physicians, communicate to our patients, to help them along this difficult path to a decision, assuming that there is more than one way of handling the situation? This report outlines our own manner of managing this problem, offering what we believe to be reasonable bases for difficult decisions. We shall also present our own approach to the selective use of radiation therapy for "early" breast cancer, combining lumpectomy and level I axillary dissection as a preliminary step to determine the extent of radiation therapy necessary and the need for adjuvant chemotherapy.

In the USA, the term "informed consent," at least in terms of breast cancer treatment, has come to mean not only a discussion of all possible complications of the intended procedure but also a pretreatment dialog, which includes mention of all of the so-called options of treatment. Implicit in this concept of informed consent is the temporal separation of biopsy to establish the diagnosis and the subsequent definitive therapy. Otherwise, every patient undergoing breast biopsy would need to know all of the possibilities beforehand and undergo metastatic workup before biopsy, even if the lesion were likely to be benign. We, therefore, perform biopsy of the breast under local anesthesia whenever possible in a

Recent Results in Cancer Research. Vol. 90

hospital operating room, but as an outpatient procedure. Frozen section is used when appropriate so that the patient can be told whether the lesion is malignant before she leaves the hospital, and a portion of the tumor is sent for the determination of estrogen and progesterone receptors.

Benign lesions are generally excised in toto; incisional biopsy is used for clinically obvious cancers, unless the diagnosis is in doubt on frozen section or if the cancer is so small that excisional versus incisional biopsy is only an exercise in semantics. Although a core-needle biopsy (Tru-Cut) may secure the diagnosis of cancer, it does not excise enough tissue for receptors and may not reveal enough about the architecture and morphology of the entire mass to allow discrimination between various treatment alternatives. Although a portion of tumor may be sent for the determination of hormone receptors at the time of subsequent therapy, since we have the opportunity to do so and because these analyses are so difficult we prefer to send portions of tumor both at biopsy and later, at the time of therapy.

Following the documentation of a malignant diagnosis, the patient is so apprised and the next steps in management are outlined. We recommend chest X-ray, bone scan, and liver function studies in every patient, recognizing the negligible yield from these tests, especially in patients with stage I cancers. Patients are somewhat reassured when they are told these tests are negative, and these studies serve as comparisons for later ones. Patients are told that these are only crude assessments but the best available currently.

Many patients express concern about the reliability of the frozen-section diagnosis of breast cancer, although they are told that a mistake almost never occurs. Nevertheless, almost all feel more comfortable that no treatment will be advocated until after the paraffin sections have been reviewed. The patient is scheduled for a conference appointment upon completion of the metastatic workup and review of the histologic sections, assured that all of her many questions will be addressed at that time. It is at the time of this conference that the various options of therapy are discussed with the patient. Each patient must feel that her own problem will be considered on an individual basis, her treatment custom-tailored, not as though she is just one among many, all patients being treated alike because they have the same disease.

This concept of the selective treatment of breast cancer is presented, reinforcing this sense of individualized treatment. Most females are not aware of variations in histology, clinical stage, degrees of invasion, etc., among breast cancers, which require differences in treatment recommendations. Most of them expect to be told that they must have mastectomy, and many come prepared to challenge this recommendation even before its is made.

The other great concern shared by patients is the implied urgency with which a decision must be made. Again, most have been led to believe, either by their family physician or by what they may have read in magazines, that any delay is dangerous and may jeopardize the likelihood of being "cured." This fear is the first one covered in the discussion, and each patient, within the limits of her perceived ability to understand it, is apprised of the concept of tumor doubling time and growth, specifically mentioning that a cancer of the breast may be present within the breast, undetected, for up to 8 years from the time of its inception until it becomes large enough to be felt. This protracted period is then compared with the relatively short time between biopsy and treatment in the natural history of the disease.

Patients are universally relieved to learn that they need not feel so pressed for time that a decision must be made on the spot, without being able to consider the alternatives of treatment in a reasonable, careful manner. If a "second opinion" is desired, there is enough time to proceed, and each patient is assured that her slides and records will be made available to her personally or any physician of her choice. The admonition is offered that, although a reasonable delay is not dangerous, one should not procrastinate for the sake of delay itself. Three to four weeks are suggested as the maximum time between the biopsy that proves the diagnosis of cancer and the definitive treatment. This allows sufficient time for the patient to make whatever plans she feels necessary for her subsequent care as well as obtain any other consultations she desires. Obviously, once the therapeutic decision has been made, treatment should be instituted as soon thereafter as feasible.

The individual factors that lead to different recommendations among the various surgical procedures for breast cancer are not germane to this discussion, except to emphasize that the reasons for the recommendations are made clear to the patient. For example, if the cancer is entirely intraductal (in situ), total mastectomy may be suggested, whereas if the patient has an invasive cancer situated in the inner half of the breast, lying on the pectoralis major muscle, classic radical mastectomy is required. Radiation therapy as an alternative to mastectomy is mentioned to every patient with stage I and II (Columbia clinical stage A and B) carcinoma of the breast. The manner in which it is approached varies, however, in relation to our own opinions of this option.

Preceding this discussion about radiation therapy is the statement that although there may be a controversy about the selective use of radiation therapy for "early" breast cancer, no treatment has been shown to exceed radical mastectomy in terms of the proportion of treated patients alive and free from disease 10 years later. The Haagensen data are quoted to support this opinion (Haagensen 1971). What has changed in recent years has been the traditional approach that every patient with breast cancer needs this operation to achieve such a likelihood of long-term survival (Findlay and Goodman 1981). We have begun to recognize that at least for some if not many patients, radical mastectomy is not necessary, and the current controversy relates to the process of selection for lesser treatment. "Overkill" is better than "underkill" although neither is desirable!

At this time, the unique features of each patient's cancer are mentioned, indicating what surgical recommendation would be traditional. Radiation therapy is then offered as an alternative. Initially, irradiation as a form of therapy is discussed only in generalities, mentioning that it may be a reasonable option to consider. There are some patients who have an inherent distrust of radiation therapy, regardless of the manner in which it is presented, and they wish to hear nothing further. (In recent years, this number has diminished.) For those patients who wish to continue this dialog, a brief description of what they may expect to undergo is outlined, including reexcision of the biopsy site, the application of metal markers (clips) to the margins of this wound, and complete level I axillary dissection in preparation for the radiation therapy. The patients are reminded that irradiation is a protracted procedure, lasting 2 months from the time of the preliminary surgical step to the completion of the "boost" to the primary site and involving a commitment of 5 days each week. If the patient remains receptive, she is referred to the radiation therapist (B.F.D.) for a more complete discussion of the technique, the results, and complications, etc. Patients are advised that involvement of axillary nodes by metastases implies adjuvant chemotherapy for 6–12 cycles whether treatment is by mastectomy or irradiation, so this subsequent reommendation has no bearing on the immediate decision.

Before leaving, the patient is given a final recommendation by the surgeon member of the team (G.F.S.), since it is not fair for patients to be forced to make decisions without the advice of their physicians. It is not strictly a matter of patient preference, although often it is the patient's own choice that finally determines the course she will follow, after she has had opportunity to assimilate all of the available information. Every patient is told that the data extant about the long-term results of irradiation are not as voluminous as those for mastectomy, but that for selected patients the results *may* be as good. Precise use of language is essential, and we never say that irradiation has been proved unequivocally to be as good as mastectomy.

There are situations when both surgeon and radiation therapist agree that either mastectomy or irradiation is inappropriate for the individual patient. If the mammogram reveals multifocal cancer, or if the tumor is large in relation to the size of the breast so that lumpectomy would be tantamount to simple mastectomy, irradiation is interdicted. Conversely, if the tumor is located so eccentrically in the breast that adequate skin margins cannot be excised around it at the time of mastectomy, or if the cancer is of relatively favorable histology, e.g., tubular or papillary carcinoma, but located medially in the breast in close proximity to the underlying pectoralis major fascia so that this accident of location mandates radical mastectomy, radiation therapy is preferable to mastectomy.

This, then, constitutes what may be called truly informed consent when considering the options of therapy for breast cancer. Both avenues, irradiation and mastectomy, are explained fully to the patient, and a recommendation is made for one or the other based upon individual considerations, recognizing that these recommendations are prejudiced by our own interpretations of the available data and our own experience. The amount of individual patient input into the final decision is obviously variable, most patients asking only for a recommendation which they then accept with complacence, and at the other extreme some patients insisting upon one form of treatment (usually irradiation) despite contrary advice from both the surgeon and radiation therapist. In the few instances of the latter, we have been torn between acquiescence, respecting the patient's right to decide her own fate, and courteously suggesting that she seek care elsewhere, offering to help her find another physician who agrees with her point of view and who, in good conscience, might treat her as she wishes.

If irradiation is chosen, it has been our practice, regardless of how the initial biopsy had been performed, incisional or excisional, to reexcise the site of the primary tumor. Among our first patients treated by irradiation were two females who underwent what had been called excisional biopsy prior to our seeing them. Both of these patients were treated by irradiation without reexcision of the site, on the assumption that the operative report had been correct. Both of them developed recurrence at this primary site less than 1 year after completion of radiation therapy. Therefore, we have become unwilling to accept anyone else's criteria of "lumpectomy," and we reexcise the primary site, removing all gross evidence of disease with a small, 1–2-cm margin of contiguous normal breast tissue. Small metal clips are fixed to the margins of the wound and at the base of the wound for subsequent radiographic localization of this area. If the tumor is deep within the breast and not extending superficially to the skin or subcutaneous tissue, a clip is also placed on the most superficial aspect of the tumor site, truly localizing the lumpectomy wound in three dimensions. This is especially valuable when the original biopsy had been performed through a circumareolar incision for a mass located at some distance from the areolar margin. The breast is then reconstituted in as cosmetically acceptable a manner as possible.

A complete level I axillary dissection is performed, the lateral limit of the dissection being the point at which the axillary vein crosses the white tendon of the latissimus dorsi muscle. The axillary vein defines the superior margin of the dissection, and the medial boundary is the edge of the pectoralis minor muscle. The dissection is carried in a caudad direction until the fifth rib is reached, at the lowermost origin of the pectoralis minor muscle. The thoracodorsal nerve is cut intentionally in this dissection, being transected where it emerges from beneath the axillary vein, because of its course through the level I lymphatics and lymph nodes. (We have never been impressed by any limitation of motion or other difficulties resulting from this nerve section and the resultant atrophy of the lastissimus dorsi muscle. We routinely cut this nerve in all mastectomies that involve axillary dissection.) This block of axillary fat and areolar tissue with the nodes it contains is delivered to the surgical pathology laboratory for meticulous dissection, looking for every node. A portion of the primary tumor, if there is residual cancer present, is sent for the determination of estrogen and progesterone receptors, even if this had been done at the time of the original biopsy.

Patients are in the hospital for 3–6 days following this procedure, the drainage from the axillary wound being the limiting factor influencing the time of discharge. Some patients require more drainage than others from the small lymphatics transected at the time of dissection, which are too small to visualize and clip, but which continue to weep postoperatively.

Uusally, radiation therapy begins about 2 weeks following this procedure. The entire involved breast is treated with tangential fields using 4- or 6-MV photons. Wedges are employed for dose homogeneity, and no (skin) bolus is used. A minimum tumor dose of 4,600–5,000 rads is delivered over $4^1/_2$–$5^1/_2$ weeks. For outer quadrant lesions with negative axillary nodes, only the breast is treated. For inner quadrant or central lesions, the internal mammary nodes are treated either with the tangential fields or by a separate direct 12- or 15-MeV electron beam field. When the axillary nodes are involved by metastatic disease, axillary and supraclavicular nodes are treated with a single anterior photon field (4 or 6 MV). A tumor dose of 4,500 rads is delivered to the regional nodes. An additional 1,500–2,000 rads is then delivered to the site of the primary cancer either by an iridium-192 interstitial implant or an electron beam. This boost volume is delineated by the metal clips placed at the time of lumpectomy and includes a 1–2-cm margin around the clips in all dimensions. The precise localization of the clips within the breast is determined by computed tomographic (CT) scan of the breast.

Justification for our choice of the preliminary surgical procedure in preparation for irradiation is warranted. We have been satisfied that radiation therapy is capable of "sterilizing" microscopic cancer, but that it is less effective treatment for gross, macroscopic cancer. For this reason, we advocate lumpectomy only without excising a large margin of normal-appearing breast. To excise a full quadrant of breast in preparation for irradiation seems to be unsound reasoning. The only current justification for radiation therapy in preference to mastectomy is cosmetic; to create an unpleasant aesthetic appearance of the breast by the excision of the primary disease seem to vitiate this concept altogether.

Some radiation therapists have suggested the excision of some axillary nodes as what has been called loosely and inaccurately a node-sampling procedure. We feel that the information which this type of incomplete operation provides is inadequate. Our own data indicate the number and status of the lymph nodes contained within the complete level I dissections we have performed. In the 54 patients thus far treated in this manner (Table 1) the mean node count has been 27 (median – 25 nodes; mode – 24 nodes; range ∸ 10–47 nodes). Most of the patients had stage I clinical disease, but seven patients treated by irradiation did have clinically involved axillary nodes. All of these seven patients proved to have microscopic metastases as well. Of the entire group of 54 patients, exactly one-third had axillary metastases (Table 2). Perhaps of greater significance in justifying complete level I dissection instead of a "sampling" procedure, whatever that means, is that 23.4% of

Table 1. Clinical stage

Stage	No.	Percent
T1–N0	33	61.1
T1–N1	2	3.7
T2–N0	14	25.9
T2–N1	5	9.3

Table 2. Incidence of node metastases

Clinical stage	Involved nodes	No.	Percent
T1–N0	None	25	46.3
	1	1	1.9
	2	3	5.5
	3	0	0
	4 or more	4	7.4
T1–N1	None	0	0
	1	1	1.9
	2	1	1.9
	3	0	0
	4 or more	0	0
T2–N0	None	11	20.4
	1	1	1.9
	2	0	0
	3	1	1.9
	4 or more	1	1.9
T2–N1	None	0	0
	1	0	0
	2	1	1.9
	3	2	3.7
	4 or more	2	3.7
Overall incidence of metastases		18 of 54	33.3

the patients with clinically negative axillae were found to have positive axillary nodes, and 44.4% of these patients had only one or two involved nodes out of as many as 41 nodes recovered from the axillary contents. If the entire lymph node package had not been removed, it is likely that positive nodes would have been missed in some of these patients, and the subsequent treatment would have been inappropriate. Irradiation to the regional nodes would not have been implemented nor would these patients have received adjuvant chemotherapy.

We do not dissect the entire axilla, i.e., all three levels. This would require a somewhat longer and more conspicuous incision than the very small one currently employed for the level I dissection, but this is a minor consideration. We are more concerned that removal of the entire axillary node package, as performed in Patey modified radical mastectomy or radical mastectomy, would be more likely to be accompanied by permanent and significant edema of the breast following radiation therapy.

What are the chances of leaving behind involved lymph nodes at levels II and III if all of the nodes at level I are negative? This is a reasonable question which we have tried to answer by a retrospective analysis of patients undergoing mastectomy who had positive nodes. We reviewed 50 randomly chosen pathology reports of patients with clinical stage I and II invasive ductal or lobular breast cancers who underwent classic radical mastectomy or Patey modified radical mastectomy. All were patients of the senior author, and their mean node count was 35 for all three levels. Only three of these patients had any involved nodes at level II or III without concomitant involvement of at least one node at level I. Thus, 94% of these women with positive nodes had involvement of level I if they also had positive nodes at levels II or III. Based upon these observations, we continue to advocate level I dissection in preparation for irradiation. We are currently subdividing the level I nodes into their respective anatomic groups, according to the Haagensen grouping, i.e., central group, scapular group, and (partially) the axillary vein group, to see if there are any more subtle patterns of nodal metastases we can discern.

Naturally, it is much too early to try to assess the results of this approach, and another decade must pass before we can extract meaningful data from this experience. However, in the past 3 years, with about half of our 54 patients undergoing therapy within the past year, we have been able to make some observations. Three patients have developed local recurrence at the site of the primary tumor. Two of these have been mentioned previously as not having undergone reexcision of the primary site because the entire cancer had been allegedly excised at the time of biopsy. These recurrences were noted after 10 and 18 months, respectively, and both patients had simultaneous recurrence/metastases in sites beyond the breast so that mastectomy was not feasible. Both of these women had multiple positive nodes (13 of 23, 5 of 32) although both were initially clinical stage I, T-1, N-0 tumors. A third patient was advised to undergo mastectomy rather than irradiation because of widespread calcifications within the entire upper half of the breast on mammography, presumably indicating multifocal disease. She refused mastectomy and also refused lumpectomy, declaring herself in favor of irradiation only, although she permitted level I dissection. All 30 level I nodes were negative for metastases. Nine months later, the patient was noted to have recurrence at the primary site at the time of a quarterly routine examination. She then acquiesced to mastectomy, which was performed, but no further axillary dissection was added. Approximately 10 months later, fundoscopic examination revealed bilateral retinal metastases and chest X-ray showed a pulmonary nodule.

A fourth patient initially underwent irradiation for two very small, less than 0.5-cm diameter contiguous cancers. She had previously had bilateral augmentation mammoplasty and these tiny tumors were quite easy to palpate. Twenty-five axillary nodes were negative. About 3 years later, she found another, less than 0.5-cm mass in another quadrant of the same breast, which proved to be a tubular carcinoma. Total mastectomy was performed, and she continues to do well. This is the first patient of our group who has developed a new primary cancer of the same breast following radiation therapy.

One patient died suddenly of systemic pneumocystis infection 3 months after completion of radiation therapy, without prior knowledge of this disease. Autopsy failed to demonstrate evidence of residual breast cancer, but she must be counted as dead from cancer for any statistical analysis of these data henceforth.

Thus, with a follow-up of 2 months to 3 years, obviously inadequate for anything but speculation, 49 of the 54 patients are well and free from disease. The cosmetic results of the combined surgical and radiotherapeutic approach have been excellent, and all of the patients except one are glad they chose radiation therapy. The one patient who is less than happy had undergone modified radical mastectomy 2 years previously for carcinoma of the opposite breast. At the time of her annual mammogram 2 years later, an area of parenchymal distortion was noted in the remaining breast, close to the chest wall. When this was biopsied using the needle-guided technique we have described, a tiny invasive cancer was discovered. Because of its location on the pectoral fascia, almost at the inframammary fold, a radical mastectomy requiring the excision of an unusually large amount of skin would have been the surgical treatment, and radiation therapy was advised as an alternative. Although the radiated breast looks excellent, she has continued to compare the protracted course of therapy with the rapid recovery she made after her mastectomy.

In summary, radiation therapy will continue to be an alternative to mastectomy that is recommended by physicians and/or chosen by patients at least until there are enough data accumulated to indicate that it is not appropriate. Even if this does come to pass, it will be at least another 10 years before this is apparent. Until such time as we know the answer without equivocation, it is our duty to inform our patients of the dilemma we face, and allow them to participate in the decision-making process. If radiation therapy is chosen, it is also incumbent upon us to see that it is used in an optimal fashion for the patient's benefit. We believe that the combination of lumpectomy and level I axillary dissection in preparation for radiation therapy accomplishes this aim. Our limited experience with this technique seems to support this conclusion.

References

Findlay PA, Goodman RL (1981) Lumpectomy and irradiation as an alternative to mastectomy in early carcinoma of the breast. In: Schwartz GF, Marchant DJ (eds) Breast disease: Diagnosis and treatment. Elsevier/North Holland, New York, pp 237–250

Haagensen CD (1971) Diseases of the breast, 2nd edn. Saunders, Philadelphia, p 706

Breast Conserving Treatment in Breast Cancer: Clinical and Psychological Aspects

M. Blichert-Toft

Surgical Department, Division of Endocrine Surgery, Odense University Hospital, 5000 Odense C, Denmark

Introduction

When dealing with operable breast cancer, the treatments of choice are either Halsted's radical mastectomy or a less radical form of mastectomy associated with loco-regional radiotherapy, the so-called McWhirter variant. The aim is total loco-regional demolition of cancer tissue. However, distant treatment failures and survival rates have in recent times led to the conviction that breast cancer in a high proportion of cases is a systemic disease at the time of diagnosis, especially when clinical series are considered.

The altered perception of biologic behavior may justify the idea that less comprehensive surgery than that associated with the Halstedian and McWhirter ways of treatment can be introduced without affecting the outcome provided that irradiation to residual breast tissue is given. Breast-saving therapy has, therefore, been contemplated. In fact, the procedure has already gained ground in several centers in Europe as well as in the USA.

Breast Conservation: A Matter of Dispute

By a careful study of the literature supported by own experience, the Danish Breast Cancer Group (DBCG) agrees with the statement put forward by Wolmark and Fisher (1981) that necessary data from well-conducted randomized trials proving the efficacy of breast-saving procedures are lacking. We also favor the attitude that breast resection as the only surgical intervention should be regarded as experimental and ought not to be conducted outside the framework of randomized trials.

Two English randomized trials by Atkins et al. (1972) and Hayward (1981) as well as one from the Milan group led by Veronesi (Veronesi et al. 1981) are highly regarded. In these studies, radical mastectomy with (Atkins et al. 1972; Hayward 1981) or without (Veronesi et al. 1981) adjuvant radiotherapy was compared with segmental resection of the breast followed by radiation therapy of residual breast tissue. In the English studies, local control of the disease in the resection groups was found to be significantly inferior to that achieved by mastectomy. As for survival, Hayward (1981) demonstrated significantly lower figures for stage I patients treated by resection. The reasons for these disappointing findings are claimed to be associated with the use of insufficient radiation doses (Table 1). In the study carried out by Veronesi et al. (1981), no significant difference was found between the resection and mastectomy groups in local control of the disease, distant failure, or survival. However, the observation time was short; the median time was 4 years. In their study, high-voltage radiation was used in doses considered adequate according to present

Table 1. Loco-regional recurrences and survival rates are given for three randomized clinical trials, in which mastectomy is weighted against breast conservation

Randomized clinical trials	Clinical stage	Therapeutic principles	Radiation dose	Duration of radiation in weeks	Number of patients	Loco-regional recurrence (5 years)	Survival (5 years)
Atkins et al. (1972)	I	RM + X-ray	25–27 Gy	2	108	4%	80%
		T + X-ray	35–38 Gy	3	112	13%	80%
	II	RM + X-ray	25–27 Gy	2	80	11%	72%
		T + X-ray	35–38 Gy	3	70	43%	58%
Hayward (1981)	I	RM + X-ray	25–27	2	132	approx. 6%	82%
		T + X-ray	35–38 Gy	3	121	approx. 32%	62%
Veronesi et al. (1981)	I	RM			349	1%	90%
		T + X-ray	50 Gy + 10 Gy	5	352	0.3%	90%

RM, radical mastectomy; *T,* tumorectomy

knowledge. Further, in patients with metastatic lymph nodes in the axilla, systemic therapy was given (Table 1).

In all three studies, the cosmetic results were far from perfect in many patients. The use of wide excisions, including a zone of 3 cm of normal tissue around the tumor (Atkins et al. 1972; Hayward 1981) and quadrantectomy technique (Veronesi et al. 1981), were the cause. Several other studies have been performed, but based on highly selected patient groups. A review is given by Leis (1981). The therapeutic and cosmetic results were satisfactory, but from a scientific point of view the relevance of such studies is limited as far as conclusive evidence is concerned.

Obviously, we cannot advocate breast-saving procedures to be performed outside the context of randomized clinical trials.

Demands on Breast Conservation

To assess the efficacy of breast-conserving therapy it is necessary to prove that the procedure will maintain both local control and distant control of the disease at least equally as well as to mastectomy. To reach such a verdict it is necessary randomly to assign a calculated sample of eligible patients to receive either mastectomy or breast resection within the context of a consecutive trial. At least 5–10 years of observation is needed. This has not yet been done using modern adjuvants. The reason why so few trials of conservative surgery have been organized is associated with very difficult ethical considerations with regard to the randomization procedure and ensuring truly informed consent from the participants.

Benefits from Breast Conservation

As mentioned, mastectomy is a highly traumatizing experience to any female (Polivy 1977; Maguire et al. 1978; Morris 1979; Stehlin et al. 1979). According to our own investigations dealing with young mastectomy patients (Christensen et al. 1981), it was found that body image and femininity were severely damaged in about 60% of patients. About 35% had serious sexual difficulties, and the vast majority complained about various affective disorders. Finally, the phantom breast syndrome was present in approximately 30%, predominating in the group of young females working as employees outside the home.

Comparative studies between psychosocial sequelae after mastectomy and breast conservation disclosed in general a much better adjustment to the conservative therapy with respect to body acceptance, femininity, and sexual function (Sanger and Reznikoff 1981; Beckmann et al., to be published). Anxiety was not differentially affected by the two surgical procedures, indicating a certain concern of having had cancer. The marital status was more stable and satisfying in the conservative group (Beckmann et al., to be published).

This experience may indicate that the following benefits can be accomplished by breast-saving strategies:

1. The psychological strain of breast cancer management may be relieved.
2. Emotional well-being may be improved.
3. Preserved body acceptance and femininity may be achieved.
4. Sexual difficulties may be diminished.
5. Breast cosmesis may be more satisfying.

With regard to breast cosmesis, the results have varied considerably. The surgical techniques used in the three randomized trials (Atkins et al. 1972; Hayward 1981; Veronesi et al. 1981) lend support to the assumption that the amount of tissue removed was too large. It remains to be clarified whether smaller resections will suffice. Apparently, some women delay their visit to the doctor due to fear of the surgical consequences if cancer is confirmed. It is hoped that limited surgery may lead to a change so that unnecessary delay is avoided.

Emotional well-being may be of some importance to survival. Greer et al. (1979) made the observation that the psychological response to breast cancer apparently had an effect on the outcome defined as recurrence-free survival 5 years after surgery. If this assumption is correct, it would seem appropriate to try and diminish affective disorders as far as possible. Breast-saving procedures may be a valuable means for that purpose (Beckmann et al., to be published).

Danish Trials Concerning Breast Conservation

In Denmark, today, the basic primary treatment of operable breast cancer is mastectomy. Approximately 95% of all eligible patients are mastectomized according to the procedure described by Cady (1973), slightly modified with regard to axillary node dissection. A radical dissection of the axillary nodes is not intended. On the contrary, the aim is to remove approximately five to ten lymph nodes for staging purposes. Node-positive patients are considered a high-risk group and receive adjuvant radiotherapy as well as systemic treatment.

Since 1977, breast cancer treatment in Denmark has been undertaken within the context of nationwide randomized trials in an attempt to evaluate the efficacy of different adjuvant regimens to mastectomy (Andersen et al. 1981). Since October 1982, new protocols have been adapted with the main object of investigating the efficacy of breast-conserving treatment. Before the start of the new protocols, a pilot study was conducted at Odense University Hospital during the previous 2 years. The object was to assess the feasibility of the program and to achieve some experience with regard to operative conduct, technique, and interplay between surgery, high-voltage irradiation, and combination systemic therapy.

Operative Technique for Breast Conservation

According to the pilot study and the forthcoming protocol (DBCG-82TM) for breast-saving procedures, a small segmental resection of the tumor bearing part of the breast is undertaken (Fig. 1). The deep fascia is removed as well as the overlying skin. Around the tumor, only a narrow zone of up to 1 cm of normal tissue is included. Radial

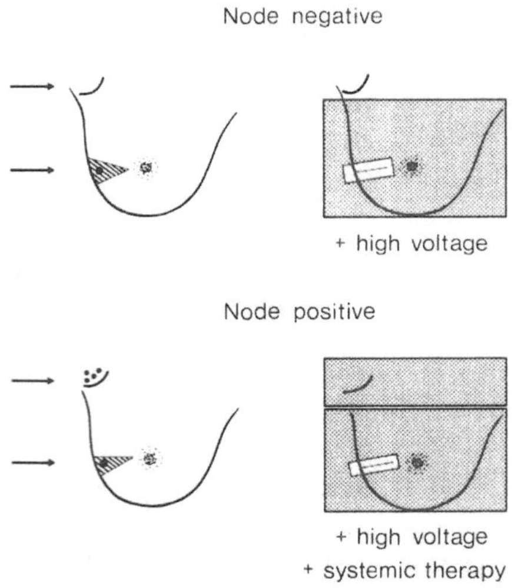

Fig. 1. Therapeutic principles for breast conservation. *Arrows* indicate the axillary incision and the wedge resection of the breast

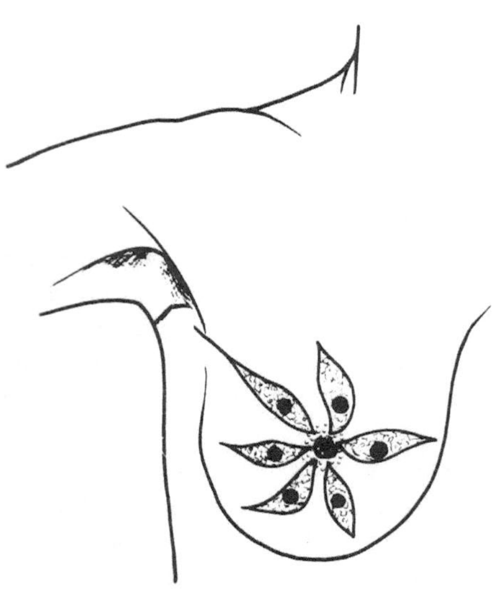

Fig. 2. Principles for skin incision and axillary incision in breast conservation

incisions are preferred (Fig. 2). Both peripherally and centrally located tumors are dealt with. If the tumor is within a proximity of less than 1 cm from the papilla, the papilla region is resected together with the tumor-bearing part (Fig. 3). To improve cosmesis, only the most superficial part of the resection line is sutured leaving a submammary cavity for drainage (Fig. 4). Using this technique, a smaller reduction in the size of the breast than that anticipated is accomplished.
For staging of the disease, axillary node sampling is carried out by a separate incision (Fig. 1). The central axillary fat pad is removed together with five to ten lymph nodes for the histologic examination to determine the degree of spreading.

Adjuvants

Node-negative patients receive high-voltage irradiation given to residual breast tissue (Fig. 1). The dose approximates 50 Gy + 10 Gy as a boost to the tumor bed. Radiation is administered as daily fractions 5 days each week for 6 weeks.
Node-positive patients receive high-voltage irradiation given to residual breast tissue as well as to regional lymph nodes (Fig. 1). The strategy and dose size is the same as for node-negative patients. Additionally, combination systemic therapy is applied.

Criteria for Inclusion

The following criteria for eligibility to breast-saving therapy are used:
1. Females 70 years or younger.

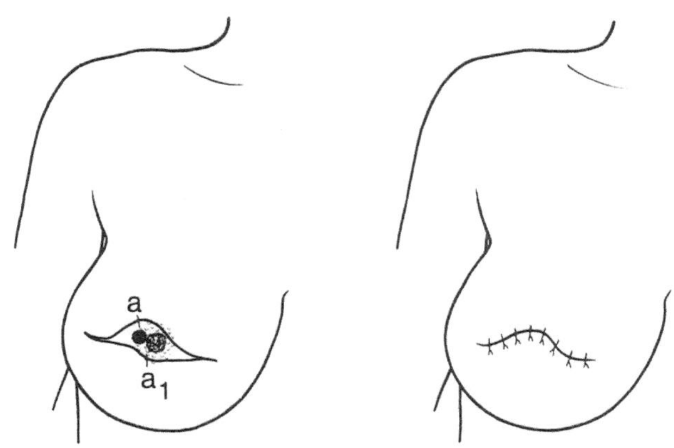

Fig. 3. Principle for breast resection in cases with the malignant tumor close to the papilla

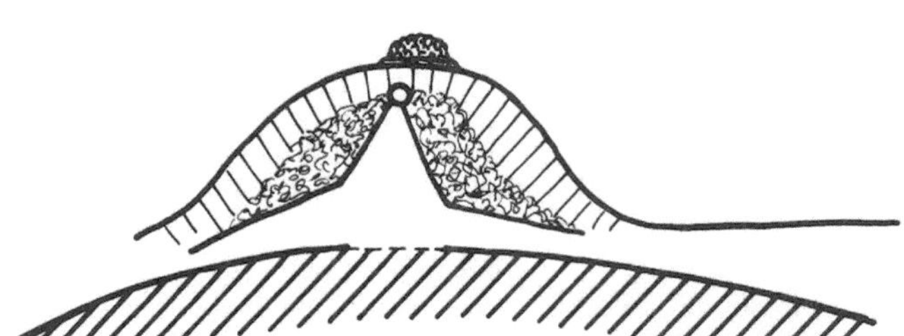

Fig. 4. Principle for closure of the mammary resection line leaving a submammary cavity for drainage

2. Tumor of any size leaving at least two-thirds of the breast tissue after resection.
3. Invasive ductal carcinoma.
4. Mammography is preferred and should be performed before decision-making with regard to eligibility.

Protocol Design

Eligible patients are asked for a surgical preference. If they do not want to make the choice themselves, they are randomly assigned to receive either breast-conserving therapy or mastectomy. It has been stressed very firmly by the ethical committees that a choice of surgery be offered before a random assignment is done. Of course, such considerations weaken the scientific quality of the trial but, regrettably, these difficulties and drawbacks have to be faced when dealing with biomedical research involving human subjects.

Results of Pilot Study

These are very promising and encourage us to proceed with the planned DBCG-82TM protocol, in which the results of breast-saving therapy are weighted against those of mastectomy on a random basis. During the period of pilot study, about 30 patients underwent limited surgery for breast cancer in accordance with the protocol design. Surgical complications were few – one instance of hematoma developed in the submammary cavity. Two patients temporarily experienced moderate breast edema during the period of irradiation. The low frequency of breast edema appears to be related to the limited axillary dissection (Clarke et al. 1982).

Breast cosmesis was excellent to good according to a four-point scale described by Harris et al. (1978). The observation period was up to 2.5 years. Local recurrence of the breast cancer did not occur during follow-up. One case of regional failure with spread to the axillary lymph nodes verified by biopsy was recorded. No instance of distant failure was observed.

References

Andersen KW, Mouridsen HT, Castberg T et al. (1981) Organisation of the Danish adjuvant trials in breast cancer. Dan Med Bull 28: 102–106

Atkins H, Hayward JL, Klugman DJ, Wayte AB (1972) Treatment of early breast cancer: A report after ten years of clinical trial. Br Med J 2: 423–429

Beckmann J, Johansen L, Richardt C, Blichert-Toft M (to be published) Psychological reactions in younger women operated on for breast cancer: Amputation versus resection of the breast with special reference to body-image, sexual identity and sexual function. Dan Med Bull [Suppl]

Cady B (1973) Total mastectomy and partial axillary dissection. Surg Clin North Am 53: 313–318

Christensen K, Blichert-Toft M, Giersing U, Richardt C, Beckmann J (1981) Postmastectomy problems in young women after operation for cancer of the breast. Ugeskr Laeger 143: 1641–1643

Clarke D, Martinez A, Cox RS, Goffinet DR (1982) Breast edema following staging axillary node dissection in patients with breast carcinoma treated by radical radiotherapy. Cancer 49: 2295–2299

Greer S, Morris T, Pettingale KW (1979) Psychological response to breast cancer: Effect on outcome. Lancet 2: 785–787
Harris JR, Levene MB, Hellman S (1978) Results of treating stage I and II carcinoma of the breast with primary radiation therapy. Cancer Treat Rep 62: 985–991
Hayward J (1981) The surgeon's role in primary breast cancer. Breast Cancer Res Treat 1: 27–32
Leis HP (1981) The surgeon's role in breast cancer: changing concepts. Breast Cancer Res Treat 1: 5–15
Maguire GP, Lee EG, Bevington DJ, Küchemann CS, Crabtree RJ, Cornell CE (1978) Psychiatric problems in the first year after mastectomy. Br Med J 1: 963–965
Morris T (1979) Psychological adjustment to mastectomy. Cancer Treat Rev 6: 41–61
Polivy J (1977) Psychological effects of mastectomy on a woman's feminine self-concept. J Nerv Ment Dis 164: 77–87
Sanger CK, Reznikoff M (1981) A comparison of the psychological effects of breast-saving procedures with the modified radical mastectomy. Cancer 48: 2341–2346
Stehlin JS, Evans RA, Gutierrez AE, Cowles J, Ipolyi PD, Greff PJ (1979) Treatment of carcinoma of the breast. Surg Gynecol Obstet 149: 911–922
Veronesi U, Saccozzi R, Vecchio M et al. (1981) Comparing radical mastectomy with quadrantectomy, axillary dissection and radiotherapy in patients with small cancers of the breast. N Engl J Med 305: 6–11
Wolmark N, Fisher B (1981) Surgery in the primary treatment of breast cancer. Breast Cancer Res Treat 1: 339–348

Prognostic Pathologic Factors Among Breast Cancers Detected on Screening by Mammography

S. A. Feig and G. F. Schwartz*

Department of Radiology, Thomas Jefferson University Hospital,
Philadelphia, PA 19107, USA

Since screening by both mammography and physical examination have been advocated as means of reducing breast cancer mortality, it is crucial to understand the relative contribution of each modality toward this goal. One means of dealing with this problem is through the use of pathologic parameters related to patient survival. These are lesion size, ratio of infiltrating to intraductal growth, histologic type, histologic grade, extent of tubule formation, lymphatic vessel invasion, and axillary lymph node metastasis. This paper analyzes results of a breast cancer screening project in terms of these pathologic factors. Most cancers classified as minimal or included in other favorable prognostic categories were seen on mammography but were occult to physical examination.

Of extreme importance was the finding that most impalpable cancers did possess the potential for metastatic spread, which probably would have occurred had they not been discovered by mammography at an early curable stage. If mammography had been omitted and the cancers detected at a relatively later stage by physical examination, it is likely that they would have already progressed to threaten patient life.

Although decreased breast cancer mortality can be proven only through a randomized clinical trial, analysis of prognostic pathologic factors indicates that substantially improved survival through mammographic screening is a reasonable expectation. This will be shown for all patients studied between 45 and 64 years of age.

Materials and Methods

The material for this investigation consists of 183 breast cancers detected on screening 17,000 self-selected women, 45–64 years of age, by xeromammography and physical examination. These studies were evaluated, respectively, by radiologists and clinical physicians specializing in breast diseases. Both were interpreted independently without knowledge of findings from the other modality. Biopsies were performed at our institution and other hospitals. All biopsies, regardless of initial pathologic diagnosis of benign or malignant disease, were reviewed by a single pathologist. The current study represents a more complete biopsy case follow-up than previously reported (Feig et al. 1977a, b; Patchefsky et al. 1977).

* The authors wish to express their appreciation to Arthur S. Patchefsky, M.D., Dept. of Pathology, Jefferson University Hospital, for having reviewed the original histologic slides

Recent Results in Cancer Research. Vol. 90

Results

Histologic Types

One important determinant of survival is histologic type. All of our 183 breast cancers were classified by histologic type according to the method of McDivitt et al. (1968). Of these, 79% (145 of 183) were detected by mammography and 54% (98 of 183) by physical examination (Fig. 1). Most breast cancers, 113 in our series, were of the invasive ductal variety but the highest survival rates have been reported in other types with more specific histologic designations such as in situ ductal (Ashikari et al. 1977; Cancer Surveillance Epidemiology, and End Results 1980; Gillis et al. 1960; Millis and Thynne 1975), microinvasive ductal (less than 10% invasive growth) (Silverberg and Chitale 1973), and tubular carcinoma (Carstens et al. 1972; Contesso et al. 1977). These were associated with 5-year survival rates of 96%–100% and accounted for 51 cancers in our study. Among them, physical examination detection rates were by far the lowest, ranging from 13% to 25%, whereas mammographic detection rates were from 85% to 93%.

We found ten in situ lobular carcinomas, only four of which were palpable on physical examination. At this stage, lobular carcinoma always can be cured by appropriate surgical therapy (Ashikari et al. 1973). If untreated, a minority of these may develop into infiltrating lobular carcinoma, where survival is not as good as in infiltrating ductal carcinoma (Adair et al. 1974; Ashikari et al. 1973; McDivitt et al. 1967, 1968). Infiltrating lobular carcinoma was among the largest of all cancers detected and formed the only group in which detection by physical examination exceeded mammography.

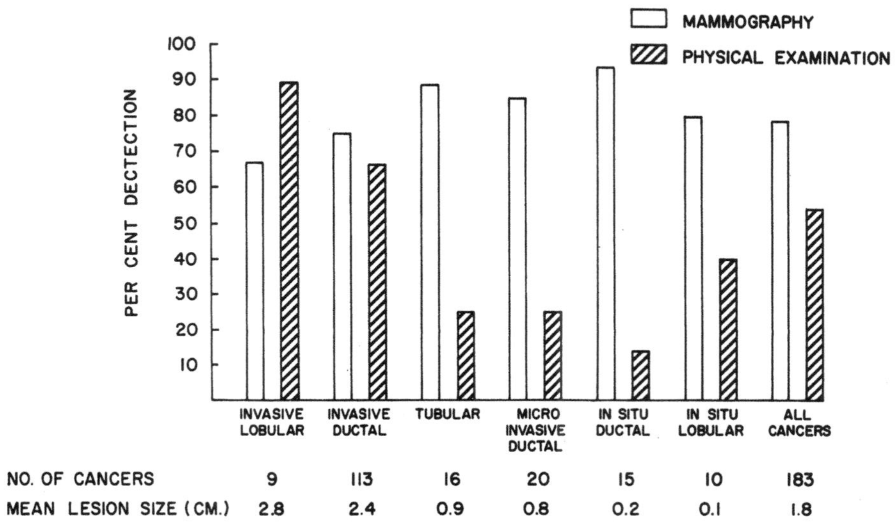

Fig. 1. Relationship of tumor histology to detection of 183 breast cancers by mammography and physical examination. Cancers included in more favorable prognostic groups such as tubular, microinvasive ductal, in situ ductal, and in situ lobular were considerably less likely to be found on physical examination and more likely to be evident on mammography than were all cancers in general

Stage of Cancer Development

Lesion Size. The correlation between breast cancer size and prognosis has been repeatedly demonstrated in numerous clinical studies (Adair et al. 1974; Alderson et al. 1971; Bloom 1950a, b; Bloom and Richardson 1957; Contesso et al. 1977; Cutler et al. 1969; Fisher et al. 1969; McDivitt et al. 1968; Wallgren et al. 1976). Smaller lesions have a much greater likelihood of long-term survival. In the current investigation, mean tumor diameter, as measured on pathologic examination, was taken as the lesion size. For all 183 cancers, the mean size was 1.6 cm. Figure 2 illustrates that physical examination becomes a decreasingly sensitive modality in the smaller ranges of lesion size. For example, among 41 cancers from 0.5 cm down to microscopic diameter, 93% (38 of 41) were found on mammography but only 20% (8 of 41) were palpated on physical examination.

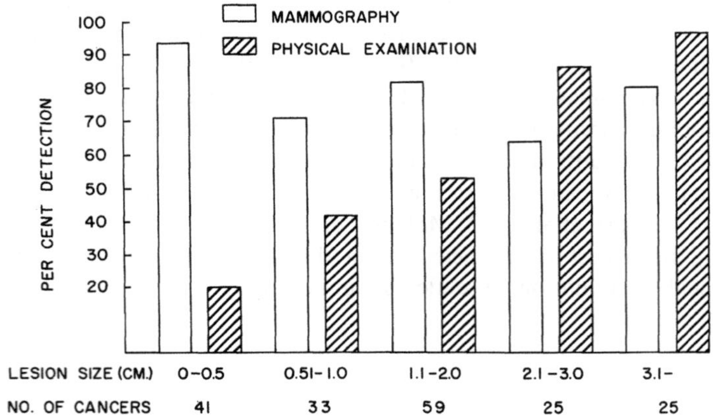

Fig. 2. Relationship of lesion size to detection for 183 breast cancers. The performance of physical examination declines as smaller lesions are considered while detection rates for mammography remain high

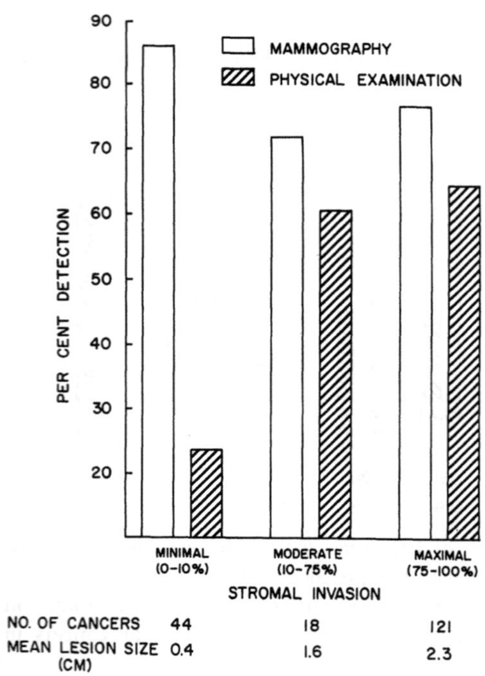

Fig. 3. Relationship of stromal invasion to detection of 183 breast cancers. Accuracy of physical examination shows little change between moderate and maximal invasion but drops considerably for minimally invasive lesions. Mammographic accuracy remains high for all three categories

Proportion of Infiltrating to Intraductal Growth. Nearly all breast cancers arise in the ducts and lobules but later may break through the basement membrane to invade the breast stroma (Gallager and Martin 1969b). Another means of relating prognosis to stage of breast cancer development is based on the work of Silverberg and Chitale (1973) who found increasing mortality as progressive proportions of infiltrating to intraductal growth were attained. Accordingly, invasion of ductal and lobular tumors in our series was classified as minimal (0–10%), moderate (10%–75%), and maximal (75%–100%). For each of these three categories, physical examination was less effective than mammography (Fig. 3). The disparity between the two detection modalities was greatest for minimally invasive lesions, became less for moderately invasive lesions, but showed little additional change with further increase in stromal invasion.

Lymphatic Vessel and Lymph Node Involvement. Following stromal invasion, breast cancer may infiltrate the breast lymphatics that drain to the regional nodes. Observation of tumor cells in breast lymphatic vessels has been associated with an increased chance of

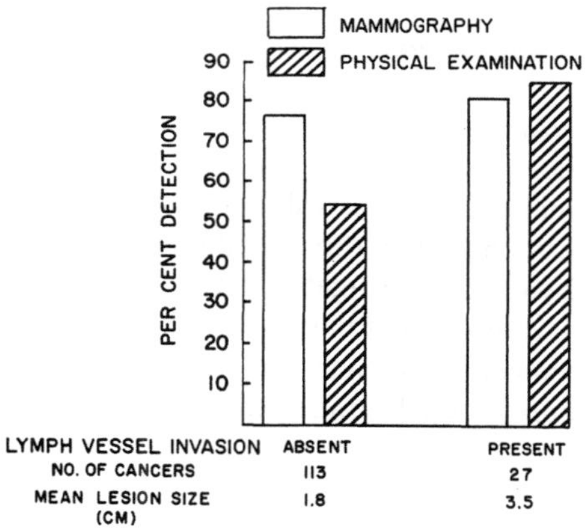

Fig. 4. Relationship of lymphatic vessel invasion to breast cancer detection. Mammography and physical examination detected similar numbers of cancers associated with lymphatic vessel invasion. For lesions with no demonstrable lymphatic vessel involvement, only detection by physical examination diminished significantly

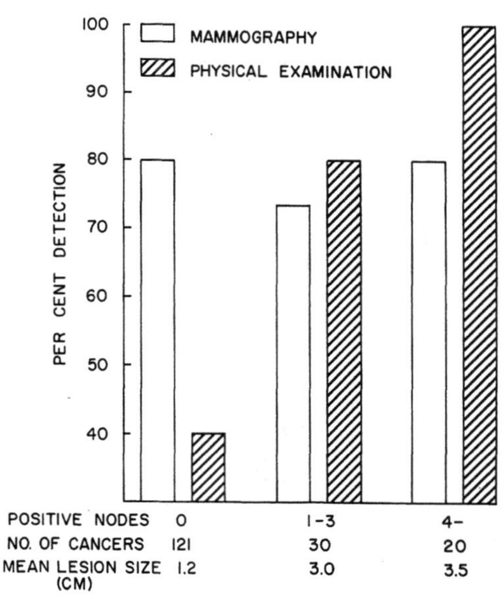

Fig. 5. Relationship of axillary lymph node metastases to method of detection for 171 breast cancers. Physical examination did least well for 121 lesions without nodal involvement. In this favorable prognostic category, mammography found 80% (97 of 121) of tumors but only 40% (48 of 121) were evident on physical examination

treatment failure (Fisher and Fisher 1977). Since lymph flow is continuous, histologic examination can detect the presence of intravascular tumor cells only at a particular moment. This finding was demonstrated on biopsy specimens in 27 of 140 patients for whom sufficient histologic material was available. Of these, mammography detected 81% (22 of 27) and physical examination 85% (23 of 27) (Fig. 4). Among 113 patients in whom lymphatic vessel invasion could not be found, 77% (87 of 113) were detected by mammography and 54% (61 of 113) by physical examination.

Previous investigators have found prognosis to be best in patients without axillary lymph node metastases, intermediate in those with one to three involved nodes, and worst when four or more nodes were involved (Fisher et al. 1969). When our patients were grouped according to these designations (Fig. 5), physical examination performed slightly better than mammography in the latter two categories, probably because nodal involvement is more readily assessed by palpation than by mammographic visualization. Among 121 cancers without axillary metastases, 80% (97 of 121) were seen on mammography but only 40% (48 of 121) could be palpated.

Intrinsic Tumor Factors

Histologic Grade. Based on nuclear size, shape, staining, mitoses, and tubule formation, ductal carcinomas may be classified as grade I (low), II (moderate), and III (high) malignancy. The validity of such a histologic grading system as a prognostic indicator was established by Bloom (1950a, b; Bloom and Richardson 1957) and subsequently confirmed by other investigators (Alderson et al. 1971; Fisher and Fisher 1977; Tough et al. 1969). Histologic grading is believed to reflect intrinsic tumor aggressiveness. Among early cancers of similar size, grade I lesions have the least immediate potential for metastatic spread. Of 27 grade I cancers in our study, 89% (24 of 27) were apparent on mammography

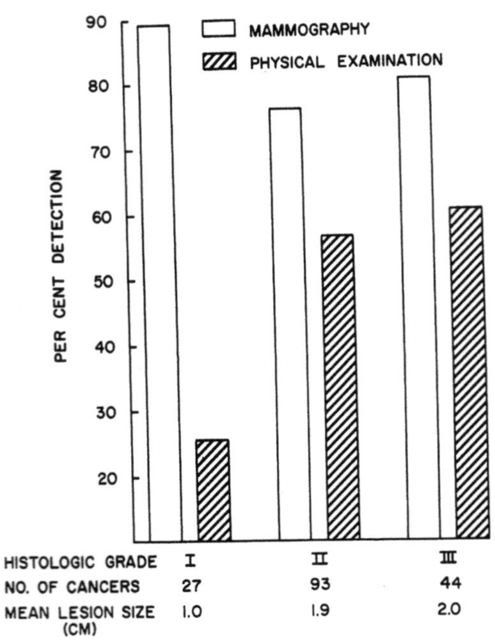

Fig. 6. Relationship of histologic grade in 164 ductal carcinomas to detection by mammography and physical examination. Mean size of grade I lesions was approximately half that of those in grades II or III. Because of their smaller size, grade I lesions were most likely to be occult to physical examination

and 26% (7 of 27) on physical examination (Fig. 6). Physical examination detection rates for grade II and III lesions were higher than those for grade I but still less than those obtained by mammography.

Tubule Formation. Most invasive ductal carcinomas are characterized by a loss of normal ductal morphology. A minority show ductal structures (tubules) that are well preserved. Tubular carcinoma can be defined as a histologic grade I invasive ductal carcinoma composed of 90% or greater tubule formation. There were 16 such lesions in our study (Fig. 1), and in these cases excellent long-term survival can be expected. Improved survival has also been seen in lesions containing lesser degrees of tubule formation even though they may not conform to the definition of pure tubular carcinoma. Several studies indicate that survival may be proportional to the degree of tubule formation (Bloom 1950a; Fisher and Fisher 1977; Wallgren et al. 1976). Data from our study indicate that the accuracy of physical examination decreases with increasing tubular formation. This was most apparent for pure tubular carcinoma (90%–100% tubule formation) where 88% (14 of 16) were found by mammography but only 25% (4 of 16) by physical examination (Fig. 7).

Tumor Margins. Although several investigators have suggested that cancers possessing a well-delimited border on gross pathologic examination have a more favorable survival than those with stellate borders (Lane et al. 1961; Wallgren and Silfersward 1976), others have found no such difference (Alderson et al. 1971; Silverberg et al. 1971). In our study, the gross nature of tumor margins did not significantly influence the detection rates of mammography or physical examination. Mammography detected 77% (58 of 75) of tumors with irregular borders and 67% (20 of 30) of those with circumscribed borders. Physical examination detected 65% (49 of 75) and 67% (20 of 30) of these groups, respectively.

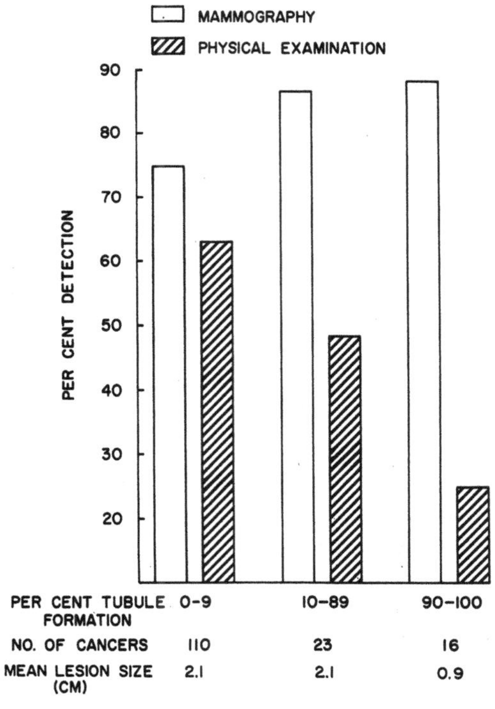

Fig. 7. Relationship of tubule formation to detection of 149 minimally invasive and invasive ductal and tubular carcinomas. Accuracy of physical examination is inversely proportional to the percent age extent of tubule formation

Prognostic Categories

Several of the prognostic factors considered thus far have been incorporated into favorable prognostic categories such as minimal carcinoma. For patients with lesions conforming to these categories, excellent long-term survival has been demonstrated by previous investigators. To assess the expected survival of patients with cancers detected by mammography and/or physical examination in our own project, these lesions were placed into one or more of these categories where appropriate (Fig. 8).

One such favorable prognostic category is comprised of cancers less than 2 cm with negative axillary lymph nodes. These have been associated with 5-year survival rates of 85%–95% (Adair et al. 1974; Cutler et al. 1969; Fisher et al. 1969; Wallgren et al. 1976). There were 105 such lesions in our study. Of these, mammography found 84% (88 of 105) and physical examination 31% (33 of 105).

One definition of minimal carcinoma is that defined by Wanebo et al. It includes all in situ ductal and lobular cancers, all invasive carcinomas measuring 1.0 cm or less arising in the outer breast with no clinical evidence of axillary lymph node metastases, and all low-grade infiltrating carcinomas such as tubular carcinoma (Wanebo et al. 1974). For these lesions, they have reported a 98% 5-year survival rate. There were 59 cases in our series fitting this definition. Of these, 88% (52 of 59) were detected on mammography and 31% (18 of 59) on physical examination.

Gallager and Martin (1971) defined minimal carcinoma as all noninvasive ductal and lobular carcinomas and all invasive carcinomas of 0.5 cm or less. Among patients with cancers conforming to this definition, a 20-year survival rate of 93% has been reported (Frazier et al. 1977). In our study, there were 42 cancers fulfilling the Gallager and Martin criteria. Of these, 93% (39 of 42) were evident on mammography and 17% (7 of 42) on physical examination.

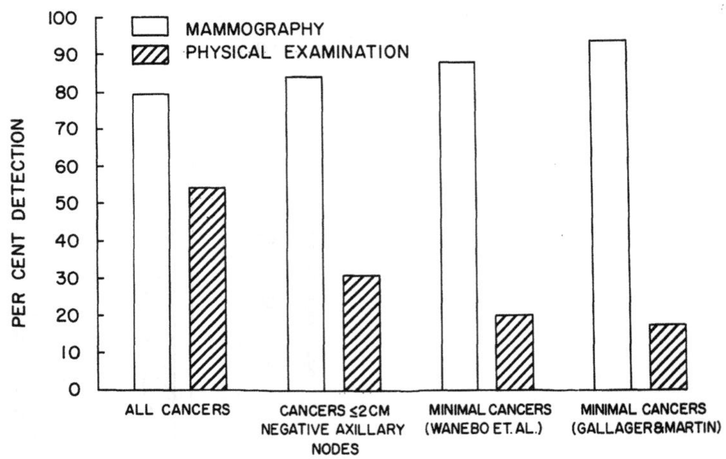

TOTAL NO. OF CANCERS	183	105	59	42
MEAN LESION SIZE (CM)	1.7	0.9	0.5	0.2

Fig. 8. Detection of breast cancers in various prognostic categories. When these are arranged according to increasing long-term survival – all cancers, cancers measuring 2 cm or less with negative axillary nodes, and minimal cancers – relative contribution of mammography increases whereas that of physical examination decreases

Discussion

Significance of Early Detection

There can be only two basic reasons for placing a breast cancer in a favorable prognostic category. Either: (1) It is an early cancer as determined by its size, high proportion of in situ growth, or negative axillary nodes; or (2) the lesion has less inherent metastatic potential because of tubule formation or low histologic grade. The relationship of detection by mammography and physical examination to each of these pathologic factors has been presented in Figs. 1–7. For each prognostic factor, lesions included in the most favorable division were much more likely to have been positive on mammography but negative on physical examination than those in less advantageous divisions. The reason for this becomes apparent when, in any given figure, one compares mean lesion size for each division. Since cancers included in the more favorable divisions are smaller, they are more likely to be occult on physical examination.

Most early cancers appear to be relatively aggressive since factors suggesting less metastatic potential were seldom present. For example, only 20% of all tubular and ductal cancers 2.0 cm or less were of histologic grade I (Fig. 9). Similarly, only 15% of all tubular, minimally invasive and invasive ductal lesions 2.0 cm or less were comprised of 90%–100% tubule

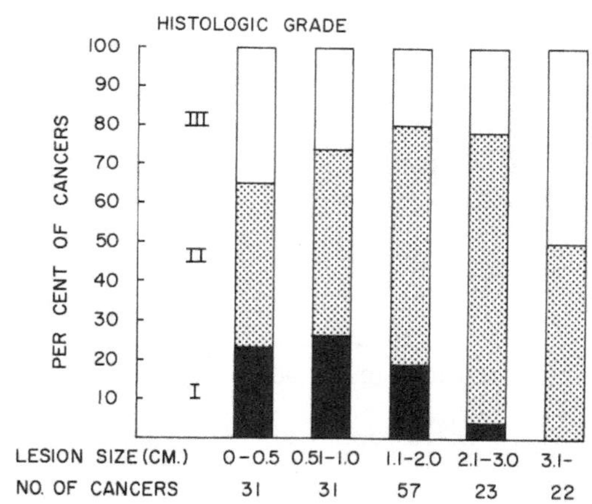

Fig. 9. Proportion of cancers in each size-group according to histologic grade. Each of the 164 ductal and tubular cancers was given a single grade based on its dominant histology. Most grade I cancers were seen in the lower size ranges, but even there represented a relatively small percentage of cases

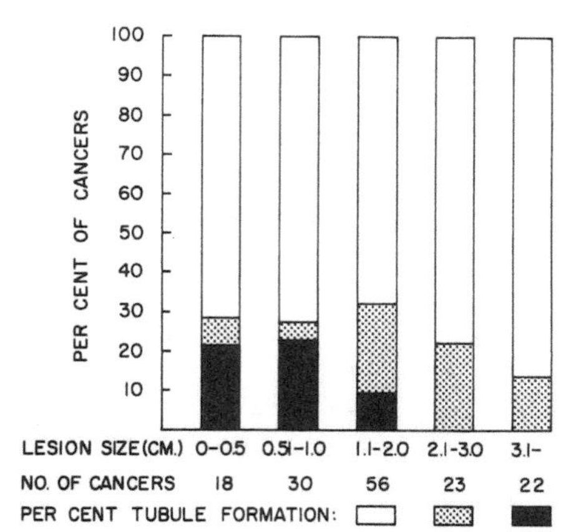

Fig. 10. Proportion of cancers in each size-group according to percentage extent of tubule formation; 149 minimally invasive and invasive ductal and tubular lesions were analyzed. Although tubule formation was more commonly seen in the smaller size-ranges, even there it was observed only in a minority of cases

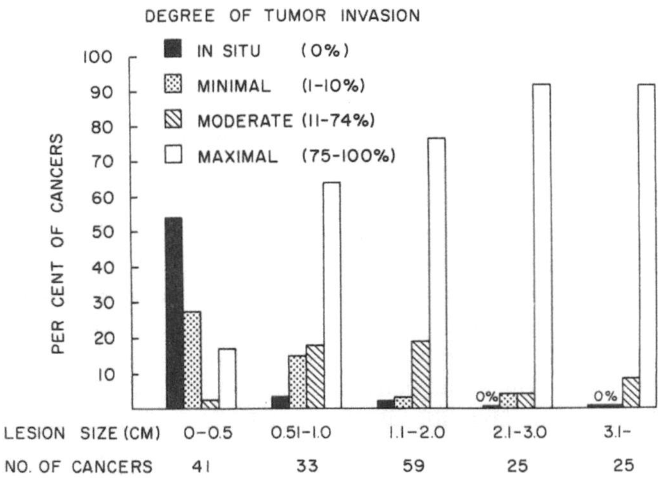

Fig. 11. Proportion of cancers in each size-group according to degree of tumor invasion. All 183 cancers in our study were analyzed. Transition from in situ to invasive growth occurs rapidly around 0.5 cm

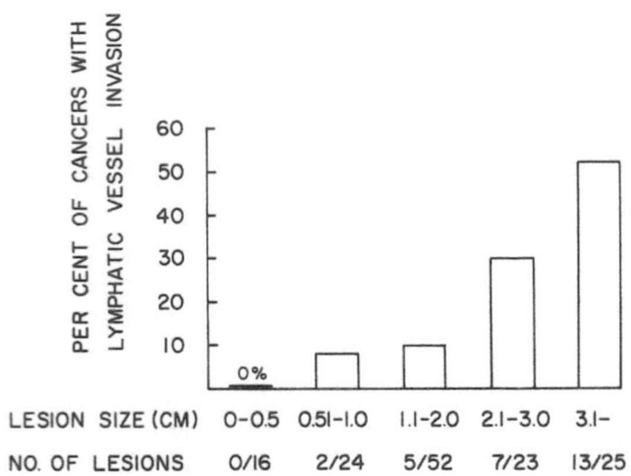

Fig. 12. Frequency of observed lymphatic vessel invasion according to lesion size in 140 invasive breast cancers

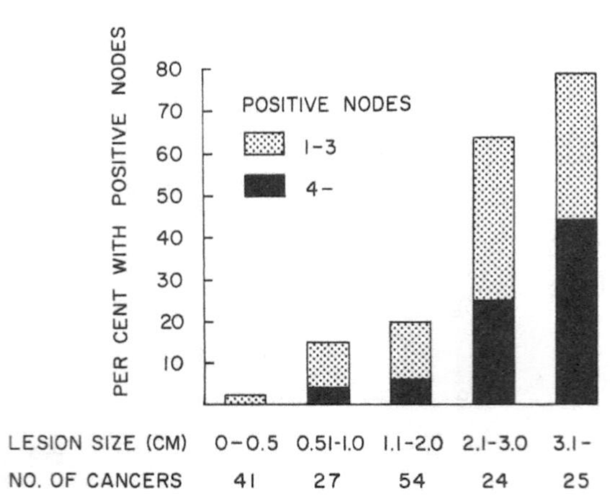

Fig. 13. Frequency of axillary lymph node metastasis according to lesion size in 171 breast cancers. Sharp increase in metastasis occurs above 2.0 cm

formation (Fig. 10). Nearly all of these preponderantly tubular lesions were included in histologic grade I.

Virtually all breast cancers began to manifest their aggressive behavior at an early stage (Fig. 11). Though in situ lesions accounted for half of all cancers 0.5 cm or less, this proportion decreased rapidly with even a slight increase in size. They represented only 3% of cancers between 0.51 and 1.0 cm.

After this change from in situ to invasive growth, lymphatic vessel invasion and axillary lymph node metastases can occur. Figures 12 and 13 relate the appearance of these two phenomena to lesion size. This occurs slowly at first, but beyond 2.0 cm, the slope steepens. Apparently, 2.0 cm represents a critical size above which axillary metastases are much more likely to occur. Above this size, axillary metastases were seen in 71% (35 of 49) of lesions. At or below 2.0 cm, axillary metastases were present in only 13% (16 of 122) of lesions. For all cancers in the latter more favorable size range, 82% were found by mammography but only 40% by physical examination.

These observations strongly support the relationship of in situ carcinoma to invasive disease indicated by Gallager and Martin (1969a, b, 1971). Our data suggest that most breast cancers possess metastatic potential from a relatively early stage in their development. Most small lesions have the capacity for further growth and spread but this may not eventuate if they are detected at an early, impalpable stage by mammography while still confined to the breast.

Significance of Multiple Prognostic Factors

Favorable prognostic factors tend to occur in association. For example, smaller lesions are more likely to be associated with negative axillary nodes. Nevertheless, in most cases, for any given factor or set of factors, prognosis is usually improved by the presence of any additional favorable factor. It has been shown by multiple regression analysis that each factor has an independent effect on the chance of survival (Alderson et al. 1971; Wallgren and Silfersward 1976; Wallgren et al. 1976). Therefore, analysis of multiple prognostic factors strengthens the contention that mammographic screening will lead to improved survival.

Early Detection and Patient Age

Since our study population consisted of females between 45 and 64 years of age, this enabled us to compare early detection in females both above and below 50 years of age. The proportion of cancers with favorable prognostic indices was similar in both groups. Two indices were measured: (1) Cancers 2 cm or less with negative axillary nodes (Fig. 14); and (2) minimal cancers as defined by Gallager and Martin (1971) (Fig. 15). Among lesions 2 cm or less with negative axillary nodes, the proportion detected by physical examination was low for females in all age-groups (Fig. 16). The same conclusion was also reached for minimal cancers (Fig. 17).

Most investigators have concluded that breast cancer survival is unrelated to patient age (Stoll 1976). In our study, among females 45–49 years of age, 43 cancers were detected. Of these, 44% (19 of 43) could not be palpated, which is not significantly different from the 47% (66 of 140) of cancers that were impalpable in females over 50 years of age. This being the case, mammographic screening should lead to improved survival in females 45–49 years of age as well as in older age-groups.

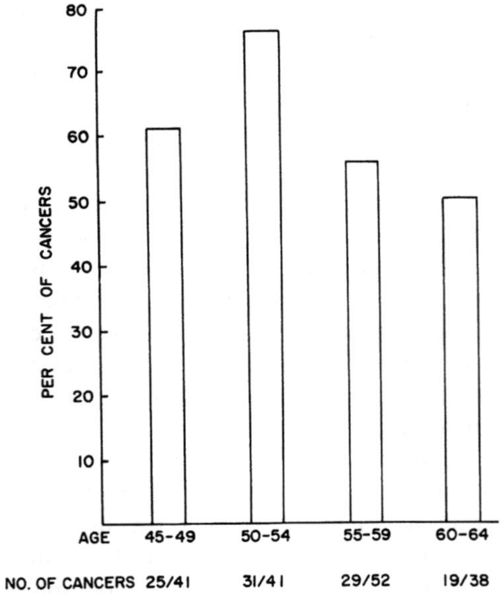

Fig. 14. Percent, in each age-group, of cancers that measure 2.0 cm or less and have negative axillary nodes

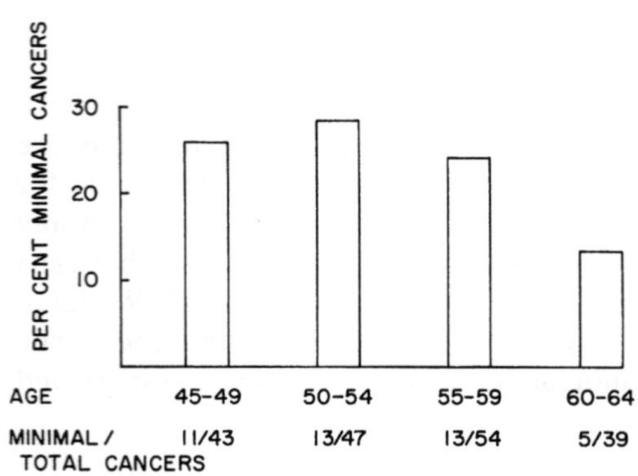

Fig. 15. Percent, in each age-group, of cancers that represent minimal cancer as defined by Gallager and Martin (1971)

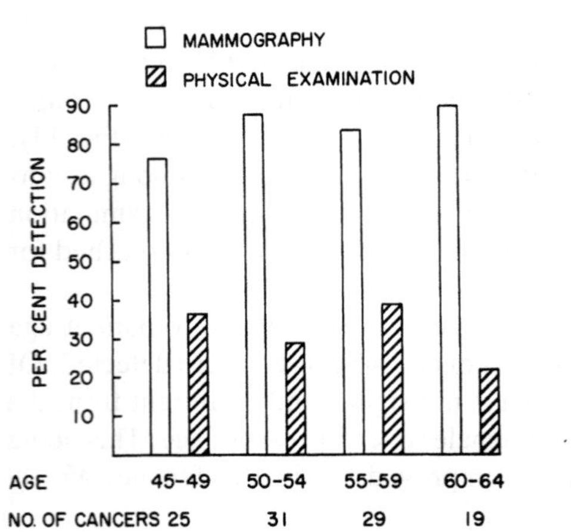

Fig. 16. Detection of cancers, 2.0 cm or less and with negative axillary nodes, by mammography and physical examination, according to patient age

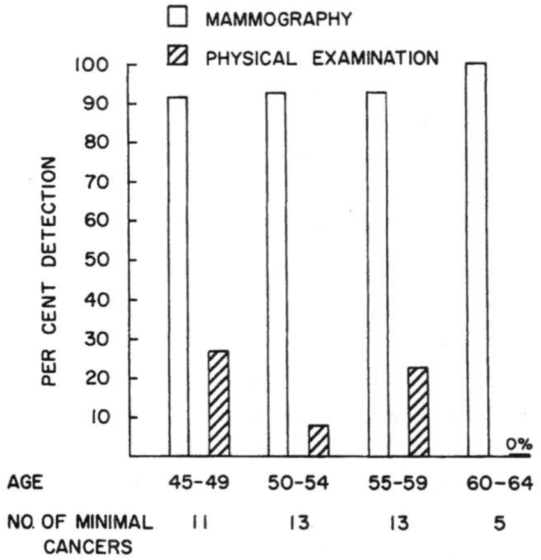

Fig. 17. Detection of minimal breast cancers (definition of Gallager and Martin), by mammography and physical examination, according to patient age

Conclusion

Breast cancers detected on screening by mammography and physical examination were analyzed by multiple prognostic parameters, such as lesion size, histologic type, histologic grade, tubule formation, proportion of intraductal to infiltrating growth, lymphatic vessel invasion, and axillary lymph node metastasis. Based on this analysis, excellent long-term survival can be anticipated for the large group of females, both above and below 50 years of age, whose cancers were detected by mammography but were impalpable on physical examination.

One observation of vital consequence was that most impalpable cancers possessed significant metastatic capacity as evidenced by their moderate to high histologic grade, low percentage of tubule formation, and early invasive growth. Fortunately, these cancers were detected by mammography before metastases had occurred.

Another important finding was that metastatic activity began to accelerate when most cancers reached a size of 2 cm. Substantial metastases had occurred before most cancers reached sufficient size to be palpable on physical examination. Thus, combined screening by mammography and physical examination should lead to a reduction in breast cancer mortality far beyond that which might be achieved using physical examination alone.

References

Adair F, Berg J, Joubert L, Robbins G (1974) Long term followup of breast cancer patients. The 30-year report. Cancer 33: 1145–1150

Alderson MR, Hamlin I, Staunton MD (1971) The relative significance of prognostic factors in breast carcinoma. Br J Cancer 25: 646–656

Ashikari R, Huvos AG, Urban JA, Robbins G (1973) Infiltrating lobular carcinoma of the breast. Cancer 31: 110–116

Ashikari R, Huvos AG, Snyder R (1977) Prospective study of noninfiltrating carcinoma of the breast. Cancer 39: 435–439

Bloom HJG (1950a) Prognosis in carcinoma of the breast. Br J Cancer 4: 259–288

Bloom HJG (1950b) Further studies on prognosis of breast carcinoma. Br J Cancer 4: 347–367

Bloom HJG, Richardson WW (1957) Histological grading and prognosis in breast cancer. Br J Cancer 11: 359–374

Carstens PHB, Huvos AG, Foote FW Jr, Ashikari R (1972) Tubular carcinoma of the breast. A clinicopathologic study. Am J Clin Pathol 58:231–238

Contesso G, Rouesse J, Pettit J-Y, Mouriesse H (1977) Les facteurs anatamopathologiques du prognostic des cancers du sein. Bull Cancer (Paris) 64:525–536

Cutler SJ, Black MM, Torbjorn M, Harvei S, Freeman C (1969) Further observations on prognostic factors in cancer of the female breast. Cancer 24:653–667

Feig SA, Shaber GS, Patchefsky AS, Schwartz GF, Edeiken J, Libshitz HI, Nerlinger R, Curley RF, Wallace JD (1977a) Analysis of clinically occult and mammographically occult breast tumors. AJR 128:403–408

Feig SA, Shaber GS, Schwartz GF, Patchefsky A, Libshitz HI, Edeiken J, Nerlinger R, Curley RF, Wallace JD (1977b) Thermography, mammography, and clinical examination in breast cancer screening. Review of 16,000 studies. Radiology 122:123–127

Fisher ER, Fisher B (1977) Relationship of pathologic and some clinical discriminants to the spread of breast cancer. Int J Radiat Oncol Biol Phys 2:747–750

Fisher B, Slack NH, Bross IDJ (1969) Cancer of the breast. Size of neoplasm and prognosis. Cancer 24:1071–1080

Frazier TG, Copeland EM, Gallager HS, Paulus DD, White EC (1977) Prognosis and treatment in minimal breast cancer. Am J Surg 133:697–701

Gallager HS, Martin JE (1969a) The study of mammary carcinoma by mammography and whole organ sectioning. Cancer 23:855–873

Gallager HS, Martin JE (1969b) Early phases in the development of breast cancer. Cancer 24:1170–1178

Gallager HS, Martin JE (1971) An orientation to the concept of minimal breast cancer. Cancer 23:1505–1507

Gillis DA, Dockerty MB, Clagett OT (1960) Preinvasive intraductal carcinoma of the breast. Surg Gynecol Obstet 110:555–562

Lane N, Husnu G, Salerno RA, Haagensen CD (1961) Clinico-pathologic analysis of the surgical curability of breast cancers. Ann Surg 153:483–498

McDivitt RW, Hutter RVP, Foote FW, Stewart FW Jr (1967) In-situ lobular carcinoma. A prospective follow up study indicating cumulative patient risk. JAMA 201:81–86

McDivitt RW, Stewart FW, Berg JW (1968) Tumors of the breast. Atlas of tumor pathology, 2nd ser, fasc 2. American Forces Institute of Pathology, Washington, p 86

Millis RR, Thynne GSJ (1975) In situ intraductal carcinoma of the breast. A long term follow-up study. Br J Surg 62:957–962

Patchefsky AS, Shaber GS, Schwartz GF, Feig SA, Nerlinger R (1977) The pathology of breast cancer detected by mass population screening. Cancer 40:1659–1670

Silverberg SG, Chitale AR (1973) Assessment of significance of proportions of intraductal and infiltrating tumor growth in ductal carcinoma of the breast. Cancer 32:830–837

Silverberg SG, Chitale AR, Levitt SH (1971) Prognostic significance of tumor margins in mammary carcinoma. Arch Surg 102:450–454

Stoll BA (1976) Effect of age on growth pattern. In: Stoll BA (ed) Risk factors in breast cancer. Year Book Medical Publishes, Chicago, pp 129–148 (New aspects of breast cancer vol 2)

Tough ICK, Carter EC, Fraser J, Bruce J (1969) Histological grading in breast cancer. Br J Cancer 23:294–301

Wallgren A, Silfersward C (1976) Clinical and histological factors of prognostic importance in breast cancer. Int J Radiat Oncol Biol Phys 8:611–617

Wallgren A, Silfersward C, Eklund G (1976) Prognostic factors in mammary carcinoma. Acta Radiol (Stockh) 15:1–16

Wanebo HJ, Huvos AG, Urban JA (1974) Treatment of minimal breast cancer. Cancer 33:349–357

Young JL Jr, Percy CL, Asire AJ (eds) (1981) Surveillance, epidemiology, and end results: Incidence and mortality data 1973–1977. National Cancer Institute Monograph 57. National Cancer Institute, NIH Publication No. 81–2330

What Can We Learn from Interval Carcinomas?

I. Andersson

Department of Diagnostic Radiology, Allmänna Sjukhuset, 214 01 Malmö, Sweden

Malignant tumors appearing in the interval between screenings are often referred to as "interval carcinomas". It is to be anticipated that some of these tumors were detectable on the preceding screening mammograms although overlooked for some reason, while others surfaced because they were rapidly growing. It is also reasonable to assume that rapidly growing tumors with a worse than average prognosis should be overrepresented due to the effect of length-biased sampling at screening.

Since the beginning of 1977 a breast screening project has been running in the city of Malmö, Sweden. A 50% random sample of all females aged 45–69 years, approximately 21,000, was invited to screening with mammography while the remaining 50% constitute a control group. Three screening rounds have been completed, with an average interval of 22 and 20 months, respectively, between the first and second and second and third screenings. Of those invited, 15,748 females participated in the first screening round and 14,300 in the second.

Thirty-three females who were considered normal at the first screening appeared with carcinoma before the second screening, i.e., in the first interval (Table 1). The corresponding figure for the second interval was 17, making a total of 50 interval carcinomas up to the third screening. Of these, 43 were invasive and seven noninvasive. The age-specific rate of interval carcinoma decreased with increasing age, opposite to the increasing detection rate at screening.

Of 43 invasive carcinomas, 18 appeared within 12 months of the previous screening, while 25, or 58%, appeared more than 12 months after the previous screening, although the latter period, i.e., up to the next screening was somewhat shorter. Five of seven noninvasive carcinomas were diagnosed more than 12 months after the preceding screening. Of the 50 females with interval carcinoma, 41 sought advice for symptoms from the breasts while nine had no symptoms. In the groups with and without symptoms, five and four carcinomas, respectively, were demonstrated only by mammography, i.e., 18% of all cases.

The screening mammograms were reviewed for any signs of carcinoma (Table 2). In 24 of the 50 cases nothing abnormal could be seen. In nine cases some abnormality could be seen

Table 1. Carcinomas detected at screening and in the intervals between screenings

	At screening	Between screenings
First screening	118	
		33
Second screening	58	
		17
Third screening	46	

Recent Results in Cancer Research. Vol. 90

Table 2. Review of preceding screening mammograms

Findings at review	No.	Percent
Nil	24	48
Slight abnormality	9	18
Clear abnormality		
Typical/highly suspected	8	16
Not typical but suspected	9	18

Table 3. Prognostic variables

	Carcinoma detected		
	Between screenings (%)	At screenings (%)	In controls (%)
Invasive growth	86	83	92
Axillary metastasis	30	17	38
Stage II–IV	42	20	52

retrospectively, which was, however, considered too slight to warrant a suspicion of malignancy. On the other hand, 17 cases or one-third were considered to be diagnostic errors, 12 of which belonged to the first and five to the second interval. In 8 of the 17 cases there was an evident abnormality that was considered clearly indicative of carcinoma, some of which were probably overlooked at screening. In nine cases the abnormalities, although evident, were atypical of carcinoma. Most abnormalities in this group were reasonably identified at screening but misinterpreted. Faulty image quality was not an important factor. In four cases it might have been a contributing factor.

The proportion of invasive carcinomas among interval carcinomas was 86%, which is only slightly different from that among carcinomas detected at screening and among carcinomas appearing in the control group (Table 3). The proportion with axillary metastasis was 30%, which is clearly more than among carcinomas detected at screening but a little less than among controls. Accordingly, the proportion of patients with stage II–IV disease was smaller than among controls but double that of patients with carcinoma detected at screening. Only one, or 8%, of the patients in the two oldest 5-year cohorts had axillary metastasis compared with 45% of the three younger cohorts.

An attempt was made to assess the growth rate of invasive interval carcinomas. Tumors with a doubling time of 100 days or less may be considered rapidly growing. Of 43 invasive carcinomas, 20, or 47%, were in this category. As we do not know the distribution of growth rates among cases detected at screening or in the control group we cannot state that the proportion is larger among interval carcinomas. However, it is our firm impression that there is a subgroup of very rapidly growing tumors among the interval carcinomas. Of the 20 rapidly growing tumors, only three had an abnormality on the preceding screening mammogram that should have been possible to detect. Furthermore, nine, or almost half of them appeared within 12 months of the preceding screening.

Table 4. Follow-up of patients with invasive carcinoma

	No. patients	No. patients with tumor volume doubling time ≤ 100 days
Dead from breast carcinoma	7	6
Alive with „recurrence“	7	6
Subtotal	14	12
Dead without metastasis	1	0
Alive without „recurrence“ (6–48 months after diagnosis, median 27 months)	28	8

Seven patients with interval carcinoma have already died from the disease, and another seven have generalized disease, as of May 1982 (Table 4). We do not yet have the exact figures for the control group, but, in spite of a relatively short follow-up, the case-fatality-recurrence rate among interval carcinomas, 28%, is much higher than among cases detected at screening. Of 14 patients who are dead or who have generalized disease, 12 had rapidly growing tumors, compared with only 8 of the 29 remaining cases of invasive carcinoma.

Conclusions

The incidence of interval carcinoma is related to:

1. The sensitivity of the screening mammography, which increases with age. This was reflected in a decreasing incidence with increasing age and also in a smaller proportion of advanced disease in older than in younger patients.
2. The experience of the radiologist. Most cases overlooked or misinterpreted at screening appeared in the first interval.
3. The availability of mammography between screenings. Of the interval carcinomas, 18% would probably not have been detected until at a subsequent screening had clinical mammography not been available.
4. The length of the interval between screenings. Most interval carcinomas were detected more than 12 months after the preceding screening. With increasing interval, the incidence would approach the natural incidence of carcinoma in the population.

Finally, there was a rather large proportion of aggressive tumors among the interval carcinomas. Most of these can probably not be picked up at screening, except with extremely short screening intervals, which seems unrealistic.

Detection Bias in Mammographic Screening for Breast Carcinoma

I. Andersson

Department of Diagnostic Radiology, Allmänna Sjukhuset, 214 01 Malmö, Sweden

The mammographic identification of carcinoma is based on the presence of a tumor or calcifications, or both. In the evaluation of a mass lesion, the border of the lesion and its relation to the surrounding tissues are of great importance. The appearance of the borderline zone varies considerably. At one end of the range is the spiculated tumor, which carries a very high probability of representing a carcinoma. At the other end is the circumscribed tumor with a smooth border, which bears a low probability of being a carcinoma. Furthermore, a small spiculated mass is comparatively easy to identify even in a glandular breast, but a small smoothly outlined tumor is often difficult or impossible to identify in a glandular breast and is not easily detectable even in a fatty breast.

Histologically, the majority of spiculated carcinomas are characterized by the presence of elastoid. They are designated "tubuloductal carcinomas" by Linell et al. (1980). There is increasing evidence that a pure tubular carcinoma, which usually also presents itself as a spiculated tumor, represents a precursor of this type of ductal carcinoma, a hypothesis put forward by Linell et al. (1980). The majority of circumscribed carcinomas are invasive comedocarcinomas. Medullary carcinomas with lymphoid infiltration and mucoid carcinomas are also usually smoothly outlined. It is generally believed that intraductal carcinoma precedes the invasive comedo carcinoma. It is possible that this also applies to medullary and mucinous carcinomas.

It is reasonable to assume that the varying sensitivity of mammography to reveal spiculated and circumscribed small tumors should be reflected in the distribution of histologic types in a sample obtained by mammographic screening compared with a clinical series. The data on the distribution of histologic types presented in Table 1 emanate from the ongoing screening project in Malmö. It appears that the proportion of the circumscribed type of carcinoma, i.e., ductal carcinoma of comedo type including medullary carcinoma with lymphoid infiltration and mucinous carcinoma, was lower among screening-detected cases than in the clinical series considered representative of breast cancer in Malmö in the age-group in question, i.e., females born 1908–1932. On the other hand, there was an overrepresentation of this type of carcinoma among patients appearing with carcinoma after a screening examination that was considered normal (interval carcinomas). Tubular carcinoma, which usually appears as a spiculated lesion, shows a different pattern, with an overrepresentation among screening-detected cases and an underrepresentation among interval cases. These distributions might, at least in part, be an expression of the different sensitivity of mammography to detect circumscribed and spiculated lesions. This could be considered a detection bias. Clearly, other explanations of the distributions, such as different growth rates of the tumors, are possible.

Many comedo carcinomas contain calcifications, which are often the clue to the diagnosis. Undoubtedly, most of the comedo carcinomas appearing as interval cases in this series

Recent Results in Cancer Research. Vol. 90

Table 1. Distribution of carcinomas by microscopic type. Classification according to Linell et al. (1980)

Type of carcinoma	Clinical series ($n = 238$) (%)	Screenings I–III ($n = 220$) (%)	Interval cases ($n = 50$) (%)
Tubular	15	30	8
Tubuloductal	34	24	30
Ductal of comedo type + medullary + mucinous	33	19	42
Lobular	11	10	6
Noninvasive			
Intraductal	5	14	10
Lobular	3	3	4

would have been detected at screening if they had produced calcifications. It is not clear why some comedo carcinomas do not give rise to calcifications.

The relative inability of mammography to detect circumscribed carcinomas early is of importance from a prognostic point of view. Although medullary carcinomas with lymphoid infiltration and mucinous carcinomas are considered to have a better than average prognosis it is our impression that the same does not apply to comedo carcinomas appearing as interval carcinomas.

Long-term follow-up of our screening series should provide opportunity to correlate histologic type of carcinoma with prognosis and, thus, to assess the importance of the detection bias.

Reference

Linell F, Ljungberg O, Andersson I (1980) Breast carcinoma. Aspects of early stages, progression and related problems. Acta Pathol Microbiol Scand [A] [Suppl] 272

Prognosis of Breast Cancer Related to Intramammary Lymph Nodes

M. B. McSweeney and R. L. Egan

Breast Imaging Center, Section of Radiology, Emory University School of Medicine, 1364 Clifton Road, Atlanta, GA 30322, USA

Introduction

While correlating radiographic findings with histopathologic changes in the breasts during the 1950s certain benign-appearing lesions were found to be intramammary lymph nodes (Egan 1960). These nodes have been disregarded by surgeons and anatomists and are often overlooked today. Since these nodes were rather common, we examined our material to see if these lymph nodes were of any prognostic significance.

Materials and Methods

Complete correlated clinical, radiographic, and pathologic studies on 173 intact breasts done from May 1965 to September 1969 were reviewed. This report is confined to the material from this whole-organ study. Primary operable breast carcinomas were present in 158 breasts, 153 female and one male. Of these carcinomas, four were simultaneous bilateral primaries (eight breasts), three were initial primaries, 13 were secondary primaries, and the remainder were unilateral primaries. There were also similar studies on 15 noncancerous breasts (13 women): seven followed previous mastectomy for carcinoma of the opposite breast; two were bilateral mastectomies (four breasts) for fibrocystic disease; two were unilateral mastectomies for fibrocystic disease; one had undergone previous biopsy for an ipsilateral positive axillary lymph node; and one contained cystosarcoma phylloides (by biopsy), and was borderline malignant. The follow-up period ranged from 13 to 17 years for all cases.

The method of preparing the breast specimens has been fully described (Egan 1970). The breast was neatly sliced into 5-mm thicknesses corresponding to the mediolateral mammogram with the first slice being most medial. Each slice was X-rayed with a low-kilovoltage high-detail technique, reviewed by the radiologist and pathologist, and each area of identifiable glandular tissue prepared for light-microscopic examination. By including as little adipose tissue as possible, readily recognized radiographically, 7-μm-thick histologic preparations of excellent quality were easily prepared. Hundreds of slides were prepared for each breast. All cases were reviewed on at least three occasions by the radiologist, surgeon, and pathologist.

Results

Intramammary lymph nodes were demonstrated in 45 breasts with carcinoma (29%) and in seven of the breasts with benign disease (47%). Fifteen breasts with carcinoma (10%)

Recent Results in Cancer Research. Vol. 90

Table 1. Distribution of intramammary lymph nodes in 173 whole-breast studies

Occurence	No. nodes	
	Benign	Malignant
No nodes	8	113
One positive node	0	13
One negative node	3	23
Negative and positive	0	2
Many negative	4	7

Table 2. Distribution of intramammary lymph nodes in 173 breasts

	No. breasts	No. nodes	UOQ	UIQ	LOQ	LIQ	Central
Malignant							
Single node positive	13	13	5	1	4	1	2
Single node negative	23	23	8	3	7	2	3
> 1 node positive	2	7	3	1	2	1	0
> 1 node negative	7	18	7	3	6	1	1
No nodes	113	0	0	0	0	0	0
Benign							
Single node	3	3	2	0	0	1	0
> 1 node	4	8	1	3	2	0	2
No nodes	8	0	0	0	0	0	0

UOQ, upper outer quadrant; *UIQ*, upper inner quadrant; *LOQ*, lower outer quadrant; *LIQ*, lower inner quadrant

contained at least one positive intramammary lymph node (Table 1). The nodes ranged in size from 3 mm to 15 mm with the positive nodes being 3 mm to 10 mm.

Intramammary lymph nodes occurred in all quadrants of the breast (Table 2). In breasts containing carcinoma, at least one node occurred in the same quadrant as the carcinoma in seven cases and in different quadrants in eight cases. One breast contained nine nodes with at least one node located in each of three quadrants; of these, two were positive and in the same quadrant as the carcinoma.

Positive intramammary lymph nodes were associated with stage I carcinoma in six cases and with stage II in nine cases. Of the stage I carcinomas with positive lymph nodes, only two had a 10-year survival. Of the nine cases of stage II carcinoma with positive intramammary lymph nodes, four survived 10 years (Table 3). The presence of positive intramammary lymph nodes per se had no demonstrable effect on prognosis in stage II but tended to indicate worsened prognosis in stage I.

Intramammary lymph node metastasis was associated with primary carcinoma of varied cell types – five invasive duct, four duct with scirrhous element, two duct with comedo component, one duct, tubular and mucoid, one duct with Paget's disease, one Paget's disease and duct with scirrhous element, and one mucoid.

Table 3. Ten-year survival with positive, negative, and absent intramammary (IM) lymph nodes in 158 cancerous whole-breast studies. Positive nodes considered precedent over negative nodes

	Positive IM nodes	Percent	Negative IM nodes	Percent	Absent IM nodes	Percent
Stage I						
Survival	2	33	15[a]	79	62[b]	83
Death	4	67	4	21	13	17
Stage II						
Survival	4	44	2	18	16	42
Death	5	56	9	82	22	58
Total	15	9.5	30	19	113	72

[a] Includes three cases of intraductal carcinoma
[b] Includes 13 cases of intraductal carcinoma

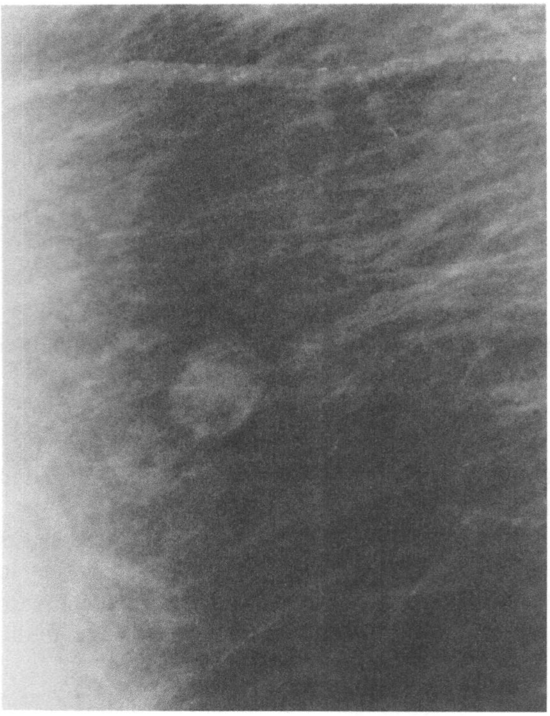

Fig. 1. Mammogram of a 63-year-old female with pendulous and painful breasts. No disease demonstrable. Incidental intramammary lymph node with fatty infiltration indicating a benign node. × 25

Discussion

There has been considerable confusion as to the existence, location, and classification of lymph nodes within the breast (Haagensen 1971). Nodes that actually represent low-lying axillary nodes or deep pectoral nodes have been mistaken for intramammary lymph nodes. Unless on histologic examination the node is completely surrounded by breast tissue, it cannot be considered a true intramammary lymph node.

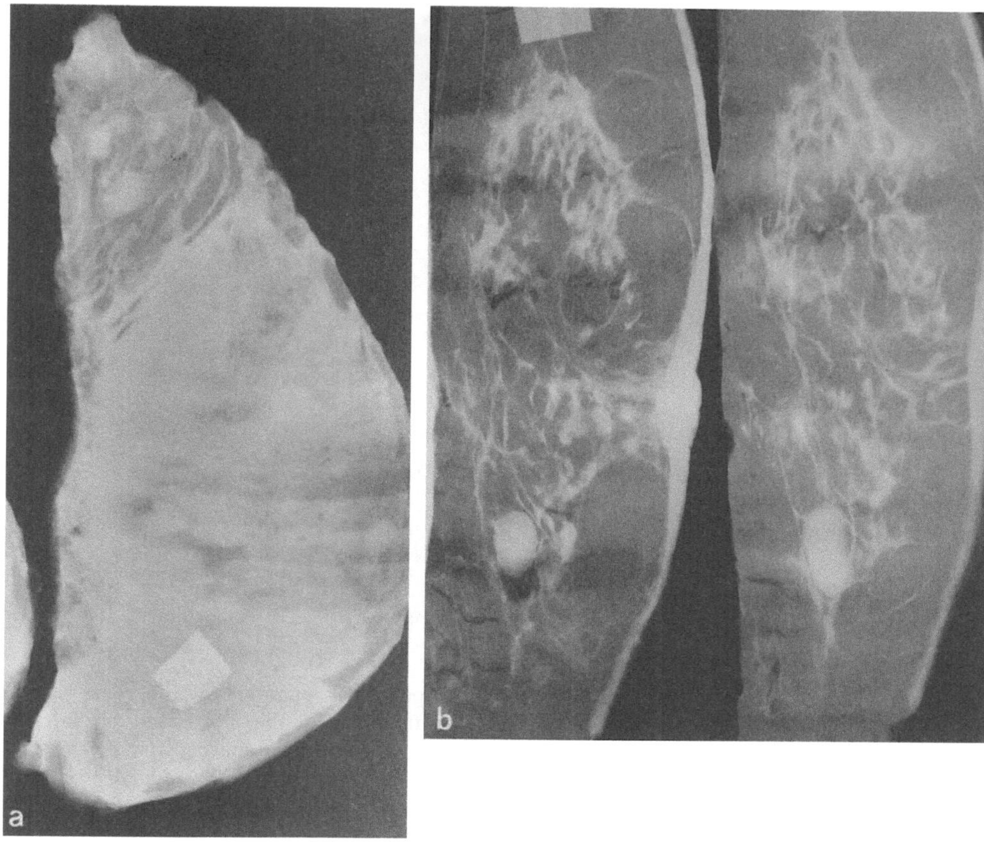

Fig. 2. a Longitudinal whole-breast 5-mm section of subcutaneous mastectomy radiograph showing dense glandular tissue and the axillary content. The three benign axillary lymph nodes are well beyond the breast tissues. **b** Whole breast slicer section radiograph demonstrating an intramammary lymph node within the fibroglandular tissues

There is some difficulty in making a precise diagnosis of intramammary lymph nodes on mammograms. A rounded, benign-appearing nodule that contains a hilar notch or central fatty replacement has the features of a node (Fig. 1). However, the intramammary lymph node must be surrounded with breast tissue (Fig. 2). In the upper outer quadrant of the breast it may be impossible to differentiate a low-lying axillary node from an intramammary node radiographically. The fibroglandular tissues may be superimposed over a low-lying axillary node, making it appear to be surrounded with breast tissue (Fig. 3). Most of the intramammary lymph nodes in this study were 5 mm or less in diameter and difficult to see on mammography if surrounded by dense fibroglandular tissue.

A potential source of histopathologic confusion would be metastasis to an intramammary lymph node completely replacing the node with malignant cells (Fig. 4). Without lymphoid tissue, this lesion could not be differentiated from another tumor nodule. A greater source of error, however, is failure to search for and examine intramammary lymph nodes in mastectomy specimens. It frequently requires the mammographer to alert the pathologist to the presence of these nodules before they are discovered for histopathologic examination. Otherwise, as in the past, these nodes may not be studied.

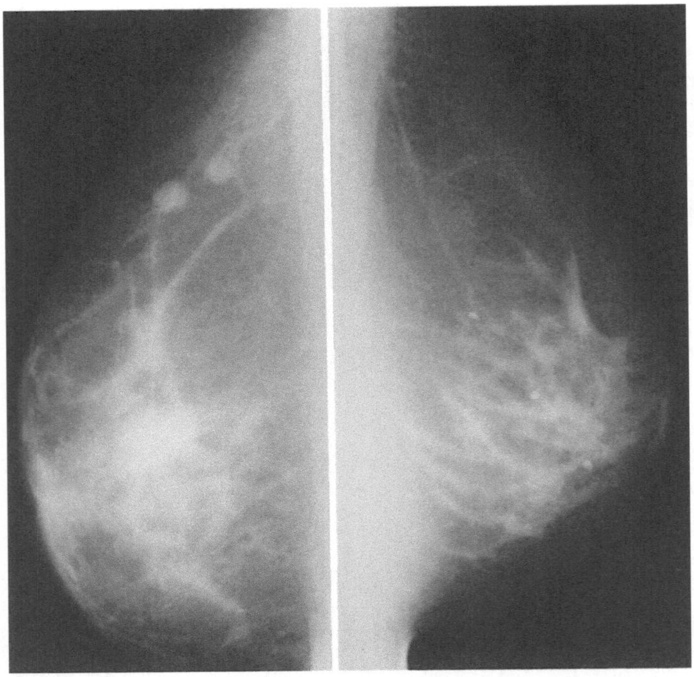

Fig. 3. A 56-year-old woman with a mass in the upper outer quadrant of the right breast. Mammography revealed an ill-defined carcinoma with flattening of the nipple and areola, two intramammary rounded nodules in the breast superiorly and one near the chest wall, and two low-lying axillary lymph nodes. Pathologically: infiltrating duct carcinoma with productive fibrosis; metastasis to the two superior intramammary lymph nodes but normal ones near the chest wall; all 15 axillary lymph nodes free of tumor

Histologic staging of breast cancer is imprecise. According to Fisher et al. (1978), 25% of carcinomas classified as stage I will actually be stage II on reexamination; a portion of stage II cancers will have decreased mortality and behave as stage I lesions. Prognostic factors such as tumor size, axillary lymph node status, and histologic type of carcinoma are of value but have failed to select that group of females with localized disease yet high mortality or those with regional disease and low mortality. Intramammary lymph node status as a prognostic indicator has received little attention but could indicate an intermediary phase between stage I and stage II breast carcinoma.

In this study, some of the numbers are small and not statistically significant. There was a trend toward a poorer prognosis in stage I carcinoma with positive intramammary lymph nodes although this may represent some of the histologically stage I carcinomas that are clinically stage II. In stage II lesions, positive intramammary lymph nodes seemed to have no direct effect on prognosis. Intramammary lymph nodes were more frequently associated with stage II disease and perhaps merely represented more advanced disease; their presence would indicate a greater likelihood of axillary metastatic disease. If these findings could be verified, intramammary lymph nodes could be of clinical importance.

Our observations have provided no connection of these intramammary lymph nodes with the usually accepted concept of lymphatic drainage of the breast toward the axillary or internal mammary lymph-node-bearing areas. For example, in Fig. 4, drainage apparently

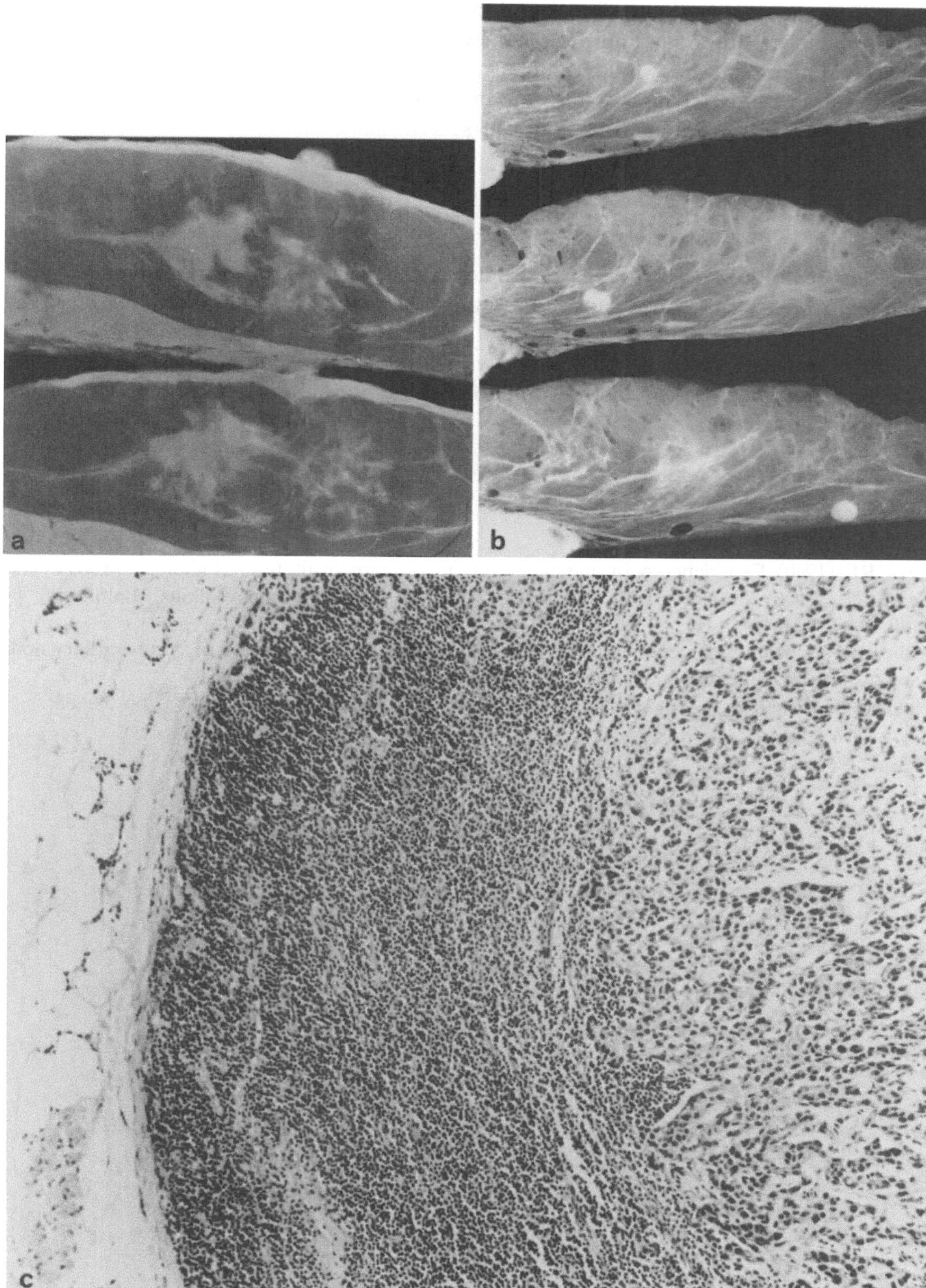

Fig. 4a–c. A 62-year-old woman with a large breast mass, clinically carcinoma. **a** Radiograph of the slicer section through the carcinoma at nipple level. **b** Radiographs of slicer sections at a distance from the carcinoma showing three separate intramammary lymph nodes. **c** Photomicrograph of the one positive node, central slicer

was in the contrary direction with a central carcinoma and a positive intramammary lymph node in the lower outer quadrant. In one medial lesion, metastasis occurred medially and inferiorly. Other metastases followed the usual pattern of drainage. About one-half of the positive intramammary lymph nodes were in the same quadrant as the main tumor mass, even when there were numerous nodes in several quadrants.

Conclusion

More investigation needs to be carried out regarding the role of intramammary lymph nodes and breast cancer prognosis. It is the role of the mammographer to alert the pathologist to their presence so that histopathologic studies can be performed. No specific pattern of lymphatic drainage is associated with intramammary lymph nodes. Conceivably, a stage Ia, positive intramammary lymph node(s) but normal axillary lymph nodes, could be defined and used.

References

Egan RL (1960) Experience with mammography in a tumor institution. Radiology 75:894–900

Egan RL (1970) Mammography and breast diseases. Williams and Wilkins, Baltimore, pp 70.19–70.131

Fisher ER, Swamidoss S, Lee CH et al. (1978) Detection and significance of occult axillary node metastases in patients with invasive breast cancer. Cancer 42:2025–2031

Haagensen CD (1971) Diseases of the breast, 2nd edn. Saunders, Philadelphia, pp 34–38

The Value of Mammography in Estimating the Prognosis for Patients with Breast Cancer

N. Bjurstam

Department of Diagnostic Radiology, University of Göteborg, Sahlgren's Hospital, 413 45 Göteborg, Sweden

Recent technical advances in the treatment of breast cancer have not had the impact on prognosis hoped for, and for the immediate future the diagnosis of breast cancer at an early stage in its development must remain the measure most likely to reduce the mortality of the disease. In patients with an established diagnosis of early breast cancer, it is important to define those at high risk in order to select the most rational treatment for each individual. Stoll stated in 1976: "Even the avoidance of deleterious treatment alone would undoubtedly lead to very marked improvement in the survival rates of breast cancer patients."

The chief aim of this paper is to assess the contribution of mammography in evaluating the prognosis in patients with breast carcinoma. The importance of a more reliable system for classifying patients with breast carcinoma is twofold. Firstly, it provides a more accurate guide to prognosis; and secondly, it ensures the proper selection of treatment for each patient. In earlier chapters of this book, the contribution of mammography in diagnosing multicentric carcinoma, bilateral cancer, and lymph node metastases are discussed. All these factors are of great importance in the identification of the high-risk patient. This report will be limited to patients with a single carcinoma in one breast. I will relate the radiographic appearance of the tumor to the outcome of the disease after treatment.

Material and Methods

The material consists of a consecutive series of 140 patients with unilateral invasive carcinoma examined clinically and by mammography in Göteborg, 1969 (Bjurstam 1978). All patients were treated with mastectomy or high-voltage radiotherapy or both. The majority (79%) were treated with radical mastectomy. The breast specimens were sliced, radiographed, and thoroughly examined by the pathologist. However, whole-organ sectioning was not performed. All 140 patients have been followed up for 10 years.

Survival rates for carcinoma can be expressed in three ways – crude survival rate, "corrected" or relative survival rate, and cancer survival rate corrected for intercurrent diseases. This latter method has been used in the present study (Johnsén et al. 1975).

Results

The survival rates are presented in Table 1. The 5-year survival rate is 71% and the 10-year survival rate is 63%. The results are in correspondance with those reported from the

Recent Results in Cancer Research. Vol. 90

Table 1. Relative survival rates in present material

	Survival rates (%)	
	5 years	10 years
All patients (140 cases)	71	63
Tumors ⩽ 5 cm (118 cases)	78	70

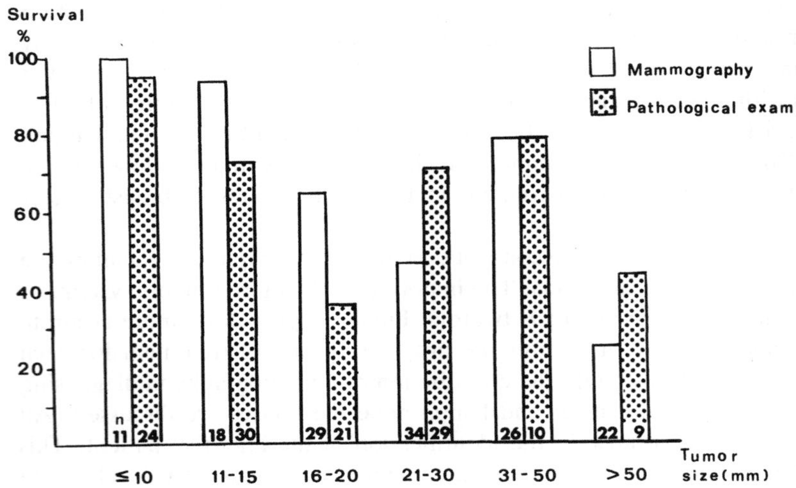

Fig. 1. Ten-year relative survival rate in relation to tumor size at mammography and pathologic examination

Stockholm region (Wallgren et al. 1976). If tumors 50 mm or larger are excluded, the 10-year survival rate is 70%. This subgroup in which large carcinomas are excluded will be used in the following analysis of certain mammographic findings.

In Fig. 1, the material is divided according to the largest tumor measured on the mammogram and the pathologic specimen, respectively. For patients with tumors smaller than 15 mm in the pathologic specimen and tumors measuring 30–49 mm in the mammogram, the survival rate is very high; on the other hand, for patients with tumors measuring, respectively, 15–30 mm and 50 mm or more the survival rate is significantly lower.

According to the rules of the Union International Contra le Cancrum (UICC) Commission for clinical staging of breast cancer with the TNM-system, the size of the tumor holds a dominating position. It is a well-known fact that there is good agreement between measurements made on the mammogram and the specimen. Conversely, the tumor diameter as determined by palpation is in most cases significantly greater. According to the UICC Commission, it is possible to use measurements made on the mammogram for TNM staging. The following example shows the value of using radiographic measurements and not measurements made by palpation.

Table 2. Gross contour of the tumor in relation to relative survival rates

Gross contour	Survival rates (%)	
	5 years	10 years
Well-delimited	87	77
Irregular	72	65

Table 3. Distribution of radiographic types of unilateral invasive carcinoma ≂ 5 cm

Radiographic type		Percent
Cluster of calcifications	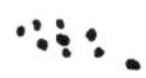	4
Circumscribed	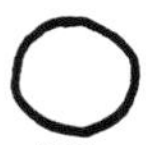	8
Lobulated	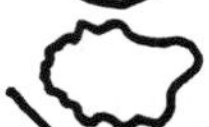	20
Spiculated	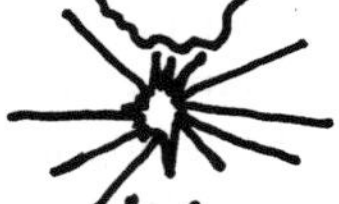	30
Intermediate	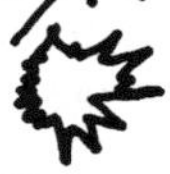	34
Diffuse		5

Table 4. Relative survival rates in relation to radiographic types of carcinoma

Radiographic type	Survival rates (%)	
	5 years	10 years
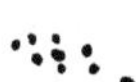	100	100
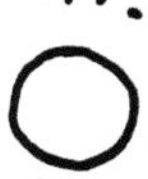	100	100
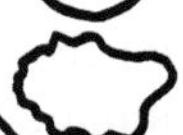	83	69
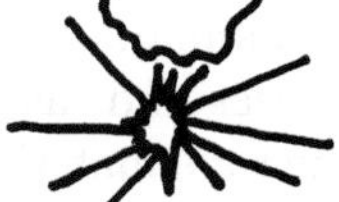	79	73
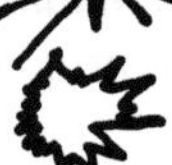	70	61
	50	50

Table 5. Ten-year cancer mortality rates and nodal involvement by radiographic type (cancer ≲ 50 mm)

Radiographic type	Positive nodes (%)	Mortality rate (%)
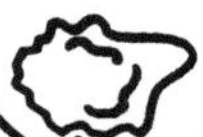	13	31
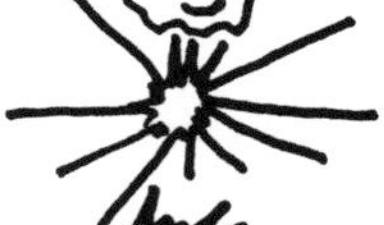	31	27
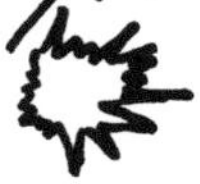	55	39
	83	50

A tumor whose greatest diameter is more than 5 cm is assigned to stage III in the TNM system even if there is no involvement of the skin and underlying tissue by axillary metastases. Consequently, such a tumor ($T_3\,N_0\,M_0$) comes into the same stage as a tumor with skin infiltration and lymph node metastases in the supraclavicular cavity or edema of the arm ($T_4\,N_3\,M_0$). By using tumor size measured on the radiographs instead of the tumor diameter determined by palpation, it is possible to reclassify a significant proportion of cases into stage III. As many as 43% (29 of 67) of cases of stage III can be correctly grouped into stage I or II.

The effect of the gross contour of the tumor on the survival rates is shown in Table 2. Patients with well-delimited tumors have a slightly higher survival rate than patients with irregular tumors. If the material is divided into the five radiographic types described by Bjurstam (1978) (Tables 3, 4), it is evident that the well-delimited tumors are composed of two different types with different survival rates. Circumscribed carcinomas have a very good prognosis while lobulated tumors do not differ significantly from the two irregular types of carcinoma. Clusters of calcifications also have a very favourable prognosis.

In Table 5, the nodal involvement and mortality for patients with different radiographic types of carcinoma are presented. Only 13% of the patients with lobulated-type tumors had lymph node metastases. On the other hand, the mortality was 31%. An interesting finding is that only one female with this type of tumor who died of cancer had lymph node metastases at the time of diagnosis and treatment. The results are quite different for diffuse carcinomas. Of patients with this type of tumor, 80% had lymph node metastases but the cancer mortality was 50%. The results indicate that different radiographic types of carcinoma differ biologically. The presence of axillary metastases has a much graver significance in tumors of the irregular variety than in tumors of the well-delimited type. Irregular tumors constitute two-thirds of all carcinomas in the present series and, as a consequence, lymph node metastases play a significant role in survival in the total material (Table 6). It is evident that the status of axillary lymph nodes is a very strong prognostic parameter in breast carcinoma.

In Table 7, the mean size for different types of carcinoma in relation to nodal involvement and cancer death is presented. There is remarkably little difference in the mean size for patients in the different groups. The results suggest that factors other than the size play a

Table 6. Effect of axillary node involvement on survival rates in tumors $\lesssim$ 5 cm

Nodal status	Number of patients	Survival rates (%)	
		5 years	10 years
No nodal involvement	68	91	86
Metastases			
Without perinodal growth	11	73	53
With perinodal growth	26	49	41
1–3 metastases	13	69	61
> 3 metastases	24	49	35

Table 7. Radiographic types and mean size of tumor at the time of diagnosis and treatment in relation to nodal involvement and cancer deaths in cancers $\lesssim$ 50 mm

Radiographic type	Mean size (mm)			
	Negative nodes	Positive nodes	No cancer deaths	Cancer deaths
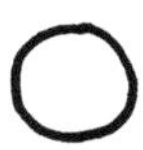	30	–	30	–
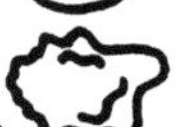	26	39	27	31
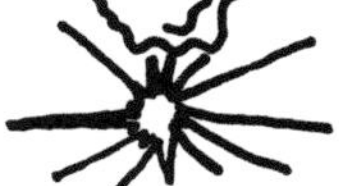	15	18	15	24
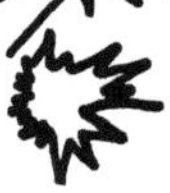	25	24	25	26

Table 8. Calcifications in carcinoma and relative survival rates

	Survival rates (%)	
	5 years	10 years
No calcifications	77	69
Calcifications typical of carcinoma	75	71
Less typical calcifications	81	70

decisive role in the outcome of disease in symptomatic patients with carcinomas smaller than 50 mm.

In Table 8, the material is divided according to the presence and type of calcification in the carcinoma. It is evident that the presence of calcifications has no effect on the survival rate. The effect of secondary skin involvement on the survival rates is shown in Table 9. There is only a slight difference in survival rates between patients with and without secondary skin lesions.

Table 9. Effect of secondary skin abnormalities on survival rates in tumors ≂ 5 cm

	Survival rates (%)	
	5 years	10 years
69 patients with skin abnormalities	72	63
49 patients without skin abnormalities	86	79

Conclusions

1. Tumor size measured on the radiograph instead of the tumor diameter determined by palpation should be used in the preoperative clinical classification of carcinomas.
2. Very few patients with carcinomas less than 1.5 cm in diameter will die of the disease over a 10-year period. On the other hand, only half of the symptomatic patients with carcinomas measuring 2–3 cm will survive 10 years, indicating the importance of diagnosing the tumor at an early stage before it becomes clinically manifest.
3. Patients with carcinomas in the form of calcification only and circumscribed tumors have a very high 10-year survival rate.
4. The presence of axillary lymph node metastases is a very strong prognostic marker in carcinomas of the irregular-tumor type. This emphasizes the importance of histopathologic examination of these nodes in the staging of breast carcinoma.

References

Bjurstam N (1978) Radiography of the female breast and axilla. Acta Radiol (Stockh) [Suppl] 357

Johnsén C, Bjurstam N, Hedberg K, Hultborn A, Johansson NT, Peterson L-E (1975) Breast disease. A clinical study with special reference to diagnostic procedures. Acta Chir Scand [Suppl] 454

Stoll BA (1976) Risk factors in breast cancer. In: New aspects of breast cancer, vol 2. Heineman, London

Union International Contra Cancrum (UICC) (1978) TNM classifications of malignant tumors, 3rd edn. Geneva

Wallgren A, Silfverswärd C, Eklund G (1976) Prognostic factors in mammary carcinoma. Acta Radiol Ther Phys Biol 15:1

*Screening for Breast Cancer in Europe: Achievements, Problems, and Future**

A. Gad, B. A. Thomas, and M. Moskowitz

Department of Clinical Pathology and Cytology, Falun Central Hospital, 791 82 Falun, Sweden

Summary

Several breast cancer screening programmes are being carried out in Europe. Clinical examination in combination with mammography is the screening method used in Guildford and Edinburgh (United Kingdom) as well as in Utrecht (Netherlands). Mammography is the only screening modality in the Swedish programmes of Falun (Kopparberg County), Linköping (Östergötland county), and Malmö and in Nijmegen (Netherlands). Clinical examination is the initial screening method in Turku (Finland).

The Swedish programmes are population-based, controlled, and randomised. They are designed to assess the impact of screening on the mortality of breast carcinoma. Comparing the results of all the European screening programmes is expected to give some answers to the hitherto unanswered questions concerning the screening method and ideal interval in different age groups.

The results achieved so far indicate that although mammography is a sensitive method for the detection of early breast cancer, clinical examination and an aggressive biopsy policy may be neccessary to reduce mortality from breast cancer in certain age groups. It is also evident that there is no universally applicable ideal screening method or rescreening interval for all age groups.

Introduction

The Health Insurance Plan of Greater New York (HIP) screening study is so far the only one of its kind, which by annual screening using mammography and clinical examination has provided evidence that screening affects survival and mortality from breast cancer (Shapiro et al. 1971; Shapiro 1977). Fourteen years after the beginning of the study, there are still fewer deaths in the study group than in controls in females 50–64 years old (Miller and Bulbrook 1982).

Tremendous advances have been achieved in the technique and quality of mammography and the radiation dose has been remarkably reduced during the last decade. However, the cost-effectiveness of clinical examination is still questionable. The Breast Cancer Detection and Demonstration Project (BCDDP) in the USA confirmed that modern mammography in combination with clinical examination can in self-selected females discover a large number of in situ and small breast cancers (Beahrs et al. 1979).

---

* This work was partly supported by a grant from Dalarna's Research Council

Recent Results in Cancer Research. Vol. 90

These two major developments in the continued efforts to reduce mortality from breast cancer focus interest on some important issues, namely, to confirm and if possible improve the HIP results in a mass-screening population-based trial, to assess the efficiency of mammography and clinical examination, separately or in combination, in reducing mortality in a cost-effective manner, to determine the ideal interval between two consecutive screens, and to investigate the possibility of extending the benefit of screening to females in the 40–49-year age group. Several screening programmes have started in Europe since 1970 designed in different ways to investigate these issues. These programmes are taking place in Florence in Italy (Cappellini et al. 1978), Utrecht and Nijmengen in the Netherlands (De Waard et al. 1978; Rombach 1980; Hendriks 1982), Falun (Kopparberg county), Linköping (Östergötland county), and Malmö in Sweden (Tabar et al. 1979; Tabar and Gad 1981; Andersson 1980), Turku in Finland (Räsänen et al. 1981), and Guildford and Edinburgh in the United Kingdom (UK Trial of Early Detection of Breast Cancer Group 1981; Thomas et al. 1981).

In Sweden, the single 45° oblique view was developed and tested in a nonrandomised study in Gävle (Lundgren and Helleberg 1982). This was followed by randomised and controlled screening programmes in the city of Malmö and in Kopparberg and Östergötland counties. One further study was started in Stockholm in 1981 and another is being planned in Gothenberg.

In 1976 the British department store chain Marks and Spencer started a nationwide nonrandomised noncontrolled screening programme for their employees using thermography, mammography, and clinical examination (A. K. Tucker, personal communication 1982). In 1979 a large-scale trial was started in the United Kingdom with the aim of evaluating the effectiveness of different methods for the early detection of breast cancer. Two populations, in Guildford and Edinburgh, are invited for annual screening by mammography and/or clinical examination. Two further populations in Huddersfield and one in the same age group in Nottingham are invited for education sessions in breast self-examination, and four control populations are offered no additional services beyond conventional diagnostic facilities (UK Trial of Early Detection of Breast Cancer Group 1981).

The aim of this paper is to familiarise the reader with the European screening programmes and to examine the possible outcome in the light of their achievements and shortcomings.

Screening Programmes and Methods

The information to be presented here is based on published data and personal communication with members of the different teams taking part in the various European screening programmes. Table 1 summarise the basic information about these programmes. Reference will be made to the results of the Cincinnati BCDDP when appropriate for the sake of comparison and to exemplify the aggressive approach in screening.

Population and Age Range

The total number of females throughout Europe invited to participate in breast screening programmes now exceeds 225,000 with a further 400,000 females in the control groups. Nijmegen and Turku are the only programmes to which women are admitted from the age of 35 years while Utrecht confines screening to women over 50 years of age. All other programmes commence screening at the age of 40–45 years. Females are not admitted for a first screening visit over the age of 64 years except in Malmö where the upper age limit is 69 years and in Florence where it is 70 years while Falun, Linköping and Nijmegen have no upper age limit.

The Control Group

The Dutch programmes have no individually identified females as controls. In Utrecht mortality figures will be compared with national figures, while in Nijmegen comparison will be made with the neighbouring town of Arnhem historically having similar incidence and mortality rates.

The Swedish programmes have defined control populations of about the same size as the active populations in Malmö and Linköping and half the size in Falun. Randomisation is carried out on the basis of parishes and municipalities in Falun and Linköping but on an individual basis in Malmö. The programmes in Kopparberg and Östergötland counties are the basis on which Swedish National screening policies will be decided.

The controls in the British trials consist of four populations of individually defined females quite separate from the study populations but having comparable incidence and mortality rates with the similarly defined study populations. In addition Edinburgh has a separate internal control group randomised on the basis of physician's practices.

Since 1970 women aged over 40 years living near Florence have been offered two-view mammography biennially, 20% being recalled for further investigation by mammography, clinical examination, thermography, and aspiration cytology. Unfortunately no contemporary incidence data are available for comparison. A full controlled population study is being planned in Italy.

In Finland clinical examination of the breasts by trained nurses is being undertaken in association with cervical cancer screening. Almost a quarter of the females were referred for single oblique-view mammography.

Primary Screening Method

Mammography. All major programmes include mammographic examination of the breasts. Mammographic techniques are varied: a single 45° oblique view being the sole procedure in Kopparberg and Linköping, a second cephalocaudal view is added in Malmö and Edinburgh, and may also be requested in the presence of a suspected clinical abnormality in Guildford. A true lateral view is the sole screening procedure in Nijmegen with a cephalocaudal view added if the radiographic technician suspects an abnormality on the lateral view. In Utrecht both these views are routinely used. With the exception of Utrecht, in which xeroradiography is used, all programmes use low-radiation-dosage film-screen systems allowing the screening procedure to be carried out with less than a 0.5-rad skin dose. In some programmes the dose is substantially less.

Interpretation of the films is undertaken by radiographic technicians in Utrecht and all xerograms are read by two observers. In Nijmegen, Falun, Linköping, and Malmö films are interpreted by a radiologist who specialises in mammography and does not undertake other radiological work. In Guildford and Edinburgh the films are interpreted by specially trained but nonradiologist physicians who refer films demonstrating a possible abnormality to a radiologist for a second opinion.

Table 1. Basic information about the European breast cancer screening programmes

Programme	No. screened, first cohort	Age and screening interval	Primary screening method: Mammography	Primary screening method: Film interpretation
Florence (Italy) 1970 No controls	24,907, 57% of population	40–70 years, 24–30 m since 1975, longer before	Mediolateral and craniocaudal	Radiologist
Utrecht (Netherlands) 1974 Control: national data	13,943, 71.5% of population	50–64 years, 12, 18, and 24 m	Mediolateral and craniocaudal xeroradiography	Two trained radiographic technicians
Nijmegen (Netherlands) 1974 Control: local town Arnhem	ca. 24,370, 69% of population	35–65 years, 35+ years after 1977, 3 × 24 m	Mediolateral and craniocaudal only if technician suspects abnormality	Radiologist
Falun (Kopparberg county, Sweden) 1977 Control: randomised communities in the county	34,187, 84% of population, 93% aged 40–70 years	40+ years, 18–30 m	Oblique	Radiologist
Malmö (Sweden) 1977 Control: randomised individual females in same population	15,748, 74% of population	45–69 years, 20–22 m	Oblique and craniocaudal	Radiologist
Turku (Finland) 1977 No controls	30,000, 84% of population	35–60 years, 60 m		Radiologist
Guildford (Surrey, UK) 1979 Control: four defined similar districts	16,586, 69% of registrations, ca. 75% of population	45–64 years, 3 × 24 m with clinical exam. in intermediate years	Oblique, craniocaudal may be requested if clinical abnormality found	Trained Dr. who examines subject, 2nd opinion by radiologist
Edinburgh (Scotland, UK) 1979 Control: as Guildford + a separate internal control group	> 12,000, ca. 60% of population	45–64 years, as Guildford	Oblique and craniocaudal	Trained Dr. with no access to clinical data, 2nd opinion by radiologist

Ca, cancer

Clinical examination	Second stage screening	Referral system	Cancer detected
Two Drs., a surgeon, and a radiologist	Clinical examination. Further mammographic views, thermography, galactography, and needle aspiration cytology	Report to family Dr.	3.1/1,000
Radiographic technician		Report to Dr. recommending referral for biopsy 18/1,000 or benign lesions found, additional biopsies 4.5/1,000 screened. Ca: benign 1: 1.4 or 1.9	7.6/1,000 6.5/1,000 invasive
		Radiological report to Dr. who decides referral policy. Referred 14.4/1,000, 10.5/1,000 biopsied. Ca: benign 1: 1	5.2/1,000 4.5/1,000 invasive
	Further mammographic views, magnification mammography, galactography, and needle aspiration cytology. 56/1,000 screened	Direct referral for specialist assessment, 18/1,000 screened, 12/1,000 biopsied. Ca: benign = 1: 0.5	6.9/1,000 6.3/1,000 invasive
	As Falun. 33/1,000 screened	Direct referral for specialist assessment, 17/1,000 screened, 12/1,000 biopsied. Ca: benign = 1: 0.7	7.5/1,000 6.3/1,000 invasive
Trained nurses	Oblique-view mammography in 23% of females (problematic females 35–55 and all over 60 years)		1.6/1,000
Trained Dr.	As Falun + specialist assessment, clinical examination. Ultrasound and further assessment. 88/1,000 screened	Direct referral to project surgeon, 20/1,000 screened, 15/1,000 biopsied. Ca: benign = 1: 1.8	5.5/1,000 4.7/1,000
Trained nurses	None but second clinical opinion available at screening visit if required	Referral via Dr. or direct to specialist, ca. 30/1,000 screened, 10/1,000 biopsied. Ca: benign = 1: 2	5.9/1,000 4.8/1,000 invasive

Clinical Examination. Only Utrecht, Guildford, and Edinburgh include clinical examination in the screening programme in association with mammography. In Utrecht this is carried out by the radiographic technician, in Guildford by the same physician who subsequently interprets the mammogram, and in Edinburgh by a trained nurse who may request a second opinion from a physician and whose findings are not available to the physician reading the mammograms. In the Swedish programmes the radiographic technician notes the presence of symptoms, scars, and moles but does not carry out clinical examination.

Second-Stage Screening

No second-stage investigations are available except in Falun, Linköping, Malmö, and Guildford. In the Swedish programmes subjects are recalled to the Mammography Department for further mammographic views and when appropriate specialised techniques such as magnification mammography, galactography, and pneumocystography may be used. Fine-needle aspiration of cysts and other lesions is also carried out in Falun.
In Guildford subjects are recalled to the screening centre for specialist assessment. They are re-examined clinically and the appropriate further investigations undertaken. These are similar to the methods used in the Swedish programmes except for the additional use of ultrasound examination. Galactography and pneumocystography are rarely used.

Referral Policy

The Swedish together with the Guildford studies refer investigated females directly to the surgeon. In Edinburgh subjects are referred from the screening clinic for further investigation by a specialist breast unit. The Dutch programmes report their findings to the subject's physician. In Nijmegen the physician decides upon the advisability of further investigation or treatment, whereas in Utrecht recommendation suggesting referral is made only for females having abnormalities considered to be suspicious for malignancy.

Rescreening Interval

In Utrecht alone the full screening procedure is repeated after 1 year, all other studies are based on the premise that improved mammographic techniques will allow the rescreening interval to be lengthened without impairing the improved mortality seen in the HIP study. The rescreening interval varies from 18 months for the second rescreening at Utrecht to almost 3 years for the rescreening of females 50 years and older in Falun and Linköping with most programmes having rescreening intervals of around 2 years. The British programmes differ in that Guildford and Edinburgh recall all females for clinical examination by a trained nurse 1 year after the full screening visit.

Results

At the first screening visit cancers were detected in all programmes at the rate of 5.5–7.6/1,000 subjects screened. Screening effected a detection rate of noninvasive cancer

Table 2. Distribution of screening-detected cancers according to size in five European programmes

<table>
<tr><th>Size</th><th>Utrecht</th><th>Falun</th><th>Guildford</th><th>Linköping</th><th>Malmö</th></tr>
<tr><td>In situ</td><td>26 (22%)</td><td>26 (8%)</td><td>16 (12%)</td><td>31 (11%)</td><td>29 (18%)</td></tr>
<tr><td>≤ 5 mm</td><td>7 (6%)</td><td>10 (3%)</td><td>11 (8%)</td><td rowspan="2">112 (38%)</td><td rowspan="2">71 (44%)</td></tr>
<tr><td>6–10 mm</td><td>18 (15%)</td><td>82 (23%)</td><td>27 (21%)</td></tr>
<tr><td>11–20 mm</td><td>43 (36%)</td><td>137 (39%)</td><td>36 (28%)</td><td>104 (35%)</td><td>47 (29%)</td></tr>
<tr><td>21–50 mm</td><td rowspan="2">19 (16%)</td><td>81 (23%)</td><td>17 (13%)</td><td>42 (14%)</td><td>12 (7%)</td></tr>
<tr><td>≥ 51 mm</td><td>14 (4%)</td><td>1 (1%)</td><td>5 (2%)</td><td>2 (1%)</td></tr>
<tr><td>Unknown</td><td>7 (6%)</td><td>–</td><td>22 (17%)[a]</td><td>–</td><td>–</td></tr>
<tr><td>Total</td><td>120</td><td>350</td><td>130</td><td>294</td><td>161</td></tr>
</table>

[a] Over 20 mm mammographically, not excised

of 0.6–1.3/1,000 subjects screened. In all programmes the detection rate represents an incidence of two to four times the expected annual incidence, being highest in the older age groups. In general the overall distribution of detected cancers according to size is similar in the controlled population studies. Two examples of screening by a single view alone, two by two-view mammography, one with the other without clinical examination, and one by single-view mammography combined with clinical examination are given in Table 2. The acceptance rate for females under 70 years of age was remarkably high (over 90%) and uniform in rural and urban areas in Falun and Linköping. In Malmö the rate was notably lower (73%). The remaining programmes follow the Malmö pattern. Following the initial screening further investigations were performed in around 50/1,000 subjects screened in Falun and Linköping with 12/1,000 eventually undergoing biopsy. In Malmö fewer are recalled though the biopsy rate remains the same. The biopsy rate in Guildford is only slightly higher – 15 of 1,000 females screened – though 88 of 1,000 screened had been recalled for specialist investigation. In the Dutch programmes no further investigation after the initial examination was undertaken, 14.4 of 1,000 screened were referred by their own doctors following the radiologist's report in Nijmegen and 10.5 of 1,000 underwent biopsy. In Utrecht 18 of 1,000 females screened had a biopsy recommended but a further 4.5 of 1,000 screened underwent biopsy at their practioners' instigation as a result of an abnormality detected by the screening process. Benign biopsy rates as a result of screening-detected abnormalities differed widely. Mammographic screening performed at Falun, Linköping, Malmö, and Nijmegen is associated with a low-cancer: benign-biopsy rate equal to or less than 1; while screening by two modalities is associated with ratios around 1 : 2.

Discussion

The major benefit from breast cancer screening must lie in a reduction in the mortality from the disease within the community as a whole in order to justify the financial and medical resources allocated to a national screening programme. Secondary benefits such as the possibility of decreased morbidity and longer survival are less easily quantifiable and thus less readily acceptable to the decision-makers.

The European programmes fall into two major categories, those designed to demonstrate a mortality change, including the Dutch, Swedish, and British, and those designed primarily to test the feasibility of using a specific screening programme or technique and assess its efficiency, as in Florence, Gävle, and Turku. Thus all programmes may be used as a basis for assessing the efficiency of a screening method to detect cancers at an early stage, but not all will yield information about the efficiency of screening programmes to influence mortality.

Trials designed to demonstrate a mortality change will yield such results valid only for the conditions of the trial. It must not be forgotten that the HIP study demonstrated such a change in a specific group of American females screened annually by clinical examination and mammography as compared with a control group of similar females. No other trial is repeating this work but all are using either a different screening method or a different rescreening interval. Should any trial fail to demonstrate a mortality change in all or certain age groups then it will be important to decide which variable was of most importance in producing such a result. It is in such circumstances that information gained from a comparison of the different programmes will be essential, and those trials that are concerned with screening methods alone will contribute.

The demonstration of a mortality change may be dependent upon the breast cancer status of the population on which the trial is carried out, the screening programme itself, and the control population with which the comparison is made.

The Trial Population

Possible benefit in terms of a cost-effective mortality reduction is governed by general principles relating to all screening programmes. Breast cancer must present an appreciable health hazard, both for the community and for the individual, this is not equally so in all communities. The incidence of the disease varies widely in different parts of the world, being relatively high in the European countries and North American where the majority of the screening trials are being carried out. Mortality rates in the different countries, however, do not always follow the same pattern, and countries with similar incidence rates may have widely different mortality rates. For example, annual incidence rates for Denmark, Sweden, the Netherlands, and Britain are around 50/100,000 females when standardised to the world population. Mortality rates on the same basis are almost 25/100,000 for all these countries except Sweden, where the figure is 25% lower at 18.7/100,000 women (Tulinius 1979). Since a 25% mortality reduction approaches the order of that obtained in the HIP study the discrepancy between Sweden and the other countries needs some consideration.

There are three main factors that could be operating here, the disease could be of a less malignant character in Sweden, treatment could be more effective, or the disease could be diagnosed at an earlier stage. Treatment methods do not appear to differ greatly in Sweden from those in use elsewhere and there seems to be no convincing reason to accept the first possibility. Preliminary data on the staging of breast cancer at diagnosis do, however, show marked differences assuming that Guildford and Falun are representative of the national situation prior to screening. Node-free tumours of 2 cm or less comprised under a quarter of the total cases in Guildford but over half in Falun. Conversely stage III and IV tumours accounted for about half the total in Guildford but only a fifth in Falun. Clearly the potential mortality reduction from screening programmes, even if equally efficient in detecting small cancers, will be different in these two communities since in Guildford a far higher proportion of females with cancer could benefit from earlier detection. A reduction in the incidence of stage III and IV disease is a necessary prerequisite for a mortality reduction in the short term, i.e., around 5 years, while a shift from stage II to I is more likely to be reflected over a longer period, possibly nearer 10 years. The control group in the HIP study resembled in British position, with screening producing a shift of stage III–IV disease to stage I and stage II disease relatively unchanged in incidence.

Screening programmes designed for a population with a relatively low mortality and the Swedish type of distribution of cancer staging to be cost-effective will need to be capable of detecting the majority of cancers at an earlier stage than that which they presented before screening. Programmes operating in countries resembling the British situation would be potentially able to produce a higher percentage mortality change and be more cost-effective even if they were somewhat less efficient. It is important in this connection to emphasize that any percentage mortality change cannot be assumed to be transferable to a different community by the implementation of the same screening system. In particular a screening programme that produced a small or delayed mortality change in the Swedish situation could, theoretically at least, be capable of producing a far larger mortality reduction at a much earlier time if carried out in a community with a higher incidence of stage III and IV disease resembling the British situation.

Questions need to be answered as to why there is this difference between countries having a similar incidence of the disease. The most likely explanation appears to lie in the awareness of the Swedish population of the value of early medical consultation in the event of breast symptoms and the general availability of specialist medical advice. The British trials, which include two populations where extensive health education programmes with open access to breast clinics are being carried out, should yield interesting information on this point.

The Screening Programme

Major factors affecting the efficiency of the screening programme include the following.

The population register on the basis of which screening invitations are despatched. The accuracy of this register in Sweden is probably one factor in the potential success of screening programmes in that country. In the British trials, inaccuracies in this register are one of the major problems with some 10% of females no longer living in the trial districts and, more important, some subjects forming part of the trial population being registered at old addresses and not easily accessible for early detection measures.

The acceptance rate for screening must contribute substantially to any possible mortality change, since clearly there is no screening benefit for nonattenders. A low acceptance rate must reduce the probable benefit of any screening method however efficient the method is in the detection of early cancer. Conversely a very high acceptance rate may enable a cheap and somewhat less efficient method to produce a worthwhile mortality change.

Such a screening method could not then be applied to a less compliant population and be expected to lead to a similar mortality change.

The Screening Age Group. Since breast cancer incidence rises rapidly with age, very high detection rates may be obtained from screening the elderly. When assessing screening methods for their ability to detect tiny cancers this factor must be considered, as a high

detection rate of small cancers in elderly females may be largely irrelevant in terms of mortality change.
This factor is of major importance when considering the high detection rates in some of the Swedish studies where, for example, in Falun 40% of the cancers detected at the first screening examination were in females aged 70 years or more. Such subjects were not screened in the other European studies and the Swedish data will be important in decisions concerning a possible upper age limit for participation in screening programmes.

The Screening Method. Clinical examination alone, even if backed by mammography when an abnormality is suspected, as in Turku, is clearly incapable of detecting the majority of cancers at a minimal stage. All other programmes are dependent on mammography, either alone or combined with clinical examination.
When all data are available it should be possible from a comparison of the staging of the cancers detected and the interval cancer rates in screened females to draw conclusions as to which mammographic technique is capable of producing the desired detection rate either in combination with clinical examination or alone. Even here caution must be used since decisions to recall subjects may differ between observers according to their selection criteria, which in turn may be dependent upon any secondary investigations accessible within the screening programme and the referrral arrangements. Technical considerations concering mammographic technique, films, processing, the number and type of projections, as well as the skill of those interpreting the films, whether radiologists or others, will be critical if any mammographic method of screening is envisaged on a national scale.
In younger females particularly, it is difficult to detect breast cancer while it is still minimal. Clinical examination is an important adjunct in these young subjects and must not be taken lightly (Moskowitz 1979a, to be published). Aggressive use of biopsy in younger females with a palpable abnormality and negative mammogram is justified if screening is to be carried out at all. We feel that lateral oblique-view mammography as a sole screening modality limits the process unduly (Moskowitz 1979a). Aggressive use of biopsy and/or aspiration increases the overall cost of screening by an inconsequential amount (Moskowitz and Fox 1979). An aggressive search for minimal breast cancer in a screening programme will contribute to the reduction of cancers occurring between screens, so called "interval cases".
While mammography is responsible for detecting most of the minimal breast cancers, we must not become so parochial and narrow as to believe that it is the only way to diagnose these lesions. In Cincinnati BCDDP screening practice, for example, 32 cancers, or 16% of all cancers detected, were discovered by clinical examination alone. Of these 32 cancers, 13 were minimal breast cancer. Thus approximately 17% of the minimal breast cancers were detected by physical examination *alone*. It is also interesting that there were 80 cancers detected by clinical examination, including those in which mammography was positive, and 22 were minimal. Similar, although not quite so striking, results have been observed in consultative practice as well. Biopsy for minimal lesions, based on clinical examination, was prompted by discovery of Paget's disease of the nipple, bleeding or discharge from the nipple, the presence of a small mass, or as the result of biopsy or aspiration of an apparently benign mass in which an incidental focus of nepolasm was found nearby.
Clinical examination detected almost 29% of the total minimal cancers diagnosed in the Cincinnati programme. However, the predictive value of positive clinical examination in detecting any cancer at any stage or size was 3% overall, and when clinical examination was the only positive finding there was only a 1.5% probability that breast cancer was present.

Table 3. Screening efficiency of European programmes after 1-year follow-up

	Age group (years)	First screening cancers/1,000 women screened	First year interval rate 1,000 women screened	First visit screening efficiency (%)
Utrecht	50–59	6.2	0.34	96
	60–65	9.5		
Gävle	40–49	1.0	0.46	68
	50–59	3.6	0.40	90
	60–69	5.9	0.40	94
Falun	40–49	2.3	0.67	78
	50–59	4.3	0.18	96
	60–69	8.9	0.55	94
Guildford	45–49	5.4	0.22	96
	50–59	4.6	0.46	93
	60–64	7.8	0.30	96

Therefore, while clinical examination has a sensitivity of about 17%–29% for minimal breast cancer, its specificity is very low. If one includes the mammographically positive cases found also by clinical examination, the true positive rate or sensitivity of clinical examination was 39% (Moskowitz, to be published). If one wishes to maximize the detection of small highly curable breast cancers, in our opinion, it is necessary to utilize clinical examination on a wider scale particularly in younger females.

Some tentative comparisons may even now be made from the European programmes by studying the data from Utrecht, Gävle, Falun, and Guildford, where 1-year follow-up figures are available (Table 3). For females aged 50-69 years, when the screening method is judged by its efficiency after 1 year, all programmes show an efficiency of 90%–95%. If screening were to be repeated at this time, as in Utrecht, then serious consideration would have to be given to the most cost-effective method in use, i.e. single-view mammography alone for primary screening. For females under the age of 50 years the picture is less clear. Only in Guildford where clinical examination is added to mammography does the efficiency remain at the same level; it falls below 80% in the Swedish studies. Whether this would be sufficient in view of the high acceptance rate of screening in the population remains to be answered. In Guildford it has already been noted that only in those under 50 years of age has clinical examination alone led to the suspicion of malignancy in a significant number of females.

It must also be remembered that in Guildford the mammograms are interpreted with knowledge of the clinical findings, and very minor mammographic abnormalities are more likely to influence a recall decision when it is known that a clinical abnormality is present. Perhaps a higher index of suspicion could improve the efficiency of single-view mammography in those under 50 years of age at the expense of a higher recall rate, or perhaps a second mammographic view would be helpful.

The Rescreening Interval. No trial has randomised varied rescreening intervals, and all are based on the premise that improved screening methods will make full annual screening, as in the HIP study, unnecessary. Such a premise may need revision for some or all age

Table 4. Screening efficiency of European programmes after 2-years follow-up

	Age group (years)[a]	Second year interval rate/ 1,000 females screened	First visit screening efficiency after 2 years
Gävle	40–49	0.55	50%
	50–59	0.48	80%
	60–69	0.32	89%
Falun	40–49	0.67	63%
	50–59	0.63	83%
	60–69	1.00	85%

[a] All ages relate to age at first screening visit

Table 5. Screening efficiency of Guildford programme

	Age group (years)[a]	Nurse clinical/ 1,000 females first screened	Second year interval	Screening efficiency	
				First screen only	First screen + nurse clinical exam.
Guildford	45–49	1.08	ca. 0.86	72%	86%
	50–59	0.58	ca. 0.34	77%	87%
	60–64	0.90	–	87%	96%

[a] All ages relate to age at first screening visit

groups. The rescreening interval must be linked to the efficiency of the screening method as judged at the end of the interval. Preliminary figures are available for Gävle, Falun, and Guildford, though in the latter they are based upon the 2-year follow-up of only two-thirds of the screened population as yet (Tables 4, 5). The position is complicated in Guildford by the clinical examination of screened females carried out 1 year after the first screening visit. This examination detected relatively few cancers, the staging of which was similar to that of the interval cancers, i.e. about half were stage I, the remainder more advanced. For the purposes fo this comparison this examination may be considered as the case finding of interval cancers, and the first full screening visit would be judged by its efficiency after 2 years as though all these cancers had developed during the 2nd year. It is, however, possible that all did not develop in this time, hence giving a falsely low 2-year efficiency level. Alternatively they may be considered as screening-detected cancers, which, as an indication of the efficiency of the programme as carried out, makes comparison of the initial screening method with the Swedish studies less straightforward.

All screening methods have a high efficiency of 85% or more after 2 years for females aged 60–69 years at the first screening visit. It seems likely that should screening lead to a reduction in mortality then single-view mammography alone at intervals of 2 years, or possibly longer, may be the most cost-effective method of attaining this for females over 60 years of age. For females aged 50–59 years the screening efficiency after 2 years is somewhat lower at around 80% for the initial screening examination and the screening interval probably cannot be extended further. However, it is not known as yet how low the efficiency at rescreening can be allowed to fall before the hoped-for change in mortality rate is lost. For females under the age of 50 years a different picture emerges with a screening method efficiency of only 50% at Gävle and 63% at Falun, the latter figure possibly being raised by some subjects having been rescreened after 20–24 months and so having a shorter follow-up period.

We may thus conclude that it is likely that single-view mammography alone at 2-yearly intervals for females under the age of 50 years does not constitute the ideal screening programme. The addition of clinical examination at the initial screening visit produces a 2-year efficiency of 72% at Guildford, again lower than is probably desirable for a biennial screening programme. The addition of the nurse clinical examination after 1 year raises the 2-year efficiency but whether in view of the staging of these cancers this examination itself is worthwhile remains to be determined.

On the present evidence the tentative conclusion must be that for females under the age of 50 years screening should be carried out on an annual basis and should include clinical examination in addition to mammography. Whether the addition of a second mammographic view will lead to an alteration of these tentative conclusions awaits the results from Malmö and Edinburgh.

It has been stated that no benefit from screening was demonstrated in the HIP study for females aged 40-49 years (Bailar 1976; Breslow et al. 1977; Shapiro 1977). In the early follow-up, in the analysis of either case fatality rates or mortality, this was indeed true. However, there are now new long-term follow-up data emerging from HIP that cast strong doubt on the earlier conclusions.

For females who were under the age of 50 years at the time of entry into screening, after 4 years of follow-up there were 11 deaths in the study group and 13 in the control group; after 5 years there were 19 versus 20 deaths, respectively. However, at the end of the 6th year after entry there were 27 deaths in the study group, while the control deaths rose to 31 (W. Venet, personal communication 1982). From that point forward there was a reduction in mortality due to breast cancer in the population of younger females offered screening. After 13 years there were a total of 45 deaths in the study group and 59 in the control group, a 24% reduction in mortality. The difference in mortality between study and control groups is not statistically significant for the younger or older females, taken separately. The lack of statistical significance is merely a reflection of the small numbers available when the groups are thus divided. Taken together, however, they are statistically significant at the $P = < 0.05$ level.

From an empirical point of view the exact mechanism leading to mortality reduction makes little difference. It is quite apparent that even an "inefficient" screen has the capacity to do so. The fact that the HIP mortality reduction for younger females was not observed until more than 5 years after entry should not be taken as unusual or require special explanation. On the contrary, in a disease of relative chronicity until death it would be unusual to expect a screening procedure to demonstrate a mortality reduction before 5–7 years. For breast cancer screening one would expect the maximum mortality reduction to appear after about 7 years, then as new cases occur in the postscreening period, this mortality benefit should be attenuated by the "noise" of postscreening mortality. In the younger females in the HIP study this is the course that is being followed.

Considering the high "miss" rate and interval cancer rate in younger females in the HIP study, any mortality benefit is remarkable. A more radical screening, detecting many tiny lesions, should result in a decreased interval cancer rate and earlier and greater mortality reduction. This would indicate that the course of some faster growing lesions can be interdicted by detecting them earlier. We have presented evidence that both of these events do occur (Moskowitz and Gartside 1982; Moskowitz 1979b). The data of Bloom and Field (1971) also suggest that for rapidly growing lesions favourable long-term case survival is more dependent on earlier detection than it is for indolent cancers.

The Referral and Treatment Policy. It is possible for a minimal cancer to be detected and no action to be taken as a result of the subject's refusal or the inaction of her medical advisers. This is essentially an educational problem that concerns some programmes more than others, but when present tends to negate a possible mortality change.

Pathologist Opinon. We start screening with the premise that the only way to diagnose breast cancer is tissue biopsy and/or aspiration cytology and that all other modalities are to be used as detecting rather than diagnostic tests. The pathologist in a screening programme is thus a central figure whose judgements do not affect only the way individual patients are to be treated but also radiologists and their selection criteria through the "feedback mechanism" initiated by pathology reports. More serious, especially in cases of significant rates of over – or under – diagnosis, is an overall muddling of statistics, which invalidates any serious attempt to analyse the screening programme in its entirety.

Analysis of the size of screening-detected cancers in five European programmes (Table 2) and comparing them with cancers detected in the BCDDP Cincinnati trial reveals very interesting information. The frequency of lobular and ductal carcinoma in situ (including Paget's disease of the nipple) is 8%–66% more in Cincinnati (24%) than in the European programmes, the difference being highest in programmes using one mammographic view without annual clinical examination. The difference is even more apparent when infiltrative cancers up to 5 mm in diameter are added to the in situ cancers (35% in Cincinnati). Of cancers detected in Malmö, 62% are in situ or infiltrative up to 10 mm in diameter compared with 34%, 41%, 43%, and 49% in Falun, Guildford, Utrecht, and Linköping, respectively. Cancers larger than 20 mm in diameter are more frequent in Guildford (31%) and in Falun (27%) than in other programmes, being lowest in Malmö (8%).

These differences can possibly be caused by the screening test or tests, the methodology of screening affecting pick-up (selection) and biopsy rates, periodicity of screening, and the diagnostic test, cytopathology. It is most unlikely that geographical factors contribute to these differences. This has stimulated us to undertake a blind prospective pathological study of a large number of minimal breast cancers examined by 12 pathologists, many of them engaged in European and American screening activities. The full results of this study are to be published in the near future but the preliminary data indicated that differences between pathologists cannot account for the variable rates of minimal cancers reported. Causes for these differences should be searched for in the screening test or tests, the pick-up and biopsy rates, and the periodicity of screening. We should not, however, fail to point out that there was an unacceptable divergence of opinion among a small group of pathologists taking part in this investigation. We found ourselves prompted to recommend that the pathologist responsible for any screening programme should be a breast specialist. A discussion of how to educate such specialists does not fall into the domain of this paper.

Controls

A mortality change can only be unequivocally demonstrated by reference to a control population, the type of which may well influence the apparent degree of any benefit. Controls may be, at the simplest level, merely the same population, prior to the introduction of the screening programme. Such *historical controls* are far from ideal and are not used in any of the present trials. It is however felt that they cannot be completely ignored since they form a second check on the validity of the trial data, in particular the control group should not have a higher mortality than the prescreening mortality. An indication of this may be obtained by comparing the pretrial staging of cancers in the trial population with those of the control population.

The "integrity" of the control group could be affected positively or negatively because of postscreening newly acquired attitudes by the physicians or the female population. More reliance on mammography as a diagnostic test and lower postscreening biopsy rates in the control group as well as increased awareness of the breast cancer problem are only a few examples of attitudes that could change the staging of the disease in either direction. *National mortality data* may be used as a basis for comparison as in Utrecht, but care must be taken that the screened population is truly representative of the national picture. It may be preferable to chose mortality data from a smaller population as at Nijmegen where a neighbouring town serves as the control population. In either case the controls are not named individually as are the screened population. More satisfactory is a control group composed of named individuals recruited to the trial by the same criteria as those used for the "screened" population, as in the British trials. Provided that the two populations are similar prior to the trials and that data collection is similarly organised in both populations, such controls can have positive advantages over those controls recruited from within the same community as the screening population.

One population may be randomly divided into screened and control groups. In Malmö individual females are randomised between the two groups, and in Kopparberg and Östergötland counties randomisation is on the basis of the parish or municipality in which the subject lives. Such randomised controlled population studies are usually considered to be highly desirable from the epidemiological viewpoint. In practice however it is likely that the control population will be influenced by a screening programme of the magnitude of the one in these studies and may not truly represent a basis for comparison with the situation if no screening had taken place.

Monitoring of the mortality in the control group in comparison with historical controls for the same population and present mortality rates in areas where there is no screening programme is essential if accurate conclusions are eventually to be drawn.

The Edinburgh screening project is of particular interest as not only does it have the same "named women" in separate population controls, as does Guildford, but it also has an additional control group taken from the Edinburgh population. This second control group consists of named women forming part of the same whole population, being randomised on the basis of physicians' practices. All females of whichever group are subject to a general health education campaign, thus overcoming one of the possible disadvantages of an internal control but complicating the assessment of the proportion of any mortality change attributable to the screening process or the health education measures.

No significant mortality differences should be expected from any of the European screening projects before 1985. In certain age-groups, particularly below 50 years, it is unlikely that convincing differences will emerge irrespective of the length of the follow-up period because of the small numbers involved.

References

Andersson I (1980) Mammographic screening for breast carcinoma. A cross-sectional randomised study of 45–69 year old women. M.D. Thesis, Lund University

Bailar JC (1976) Mammography; a contrary view. Ann Intern Med 84: 77–84

Beahrs OH, Shapiro S, Smart C (1979) Report of the working group to review the National Cancer Institute – American Cancer Society breast cancer detection demonstration projects. JNCI 62: 640–709

Bloom HJG, Field JR (1971) Impact of tumour grade and host resistance in survival of women with breast cancer. Cancer 28: 1580–1589

Breslow L, Henderson B, Massey F Jr, Pike M, Winkelstein W Jr (1977) Report of NCI ad hoc working group on the gross and net benefits of mammography in mass screening for the detection of breast cancer. In: Final reports of NCI ad hoc working groups. Department of Health, Education and Welfare, Publ no (NIH)-77-1400

Cappellini M, Ciatto S, Maltoni G (1978) Mass screening for early breast cancer detection. Tumori 64: 479–485

de Waard F, Rombach JJ, Colette HJA (1978) The DOM-project for early diagnosis of breast cancer in the city of Utrecht, Netherlands. UICC Tech Rep Ser 40: 183–200

Hendriks JHCL (1982) Population screening for breast cancer by means of mammography in Nijmegen 1975–1982. M.D. Thesis, Nijmegen University

Lundgren B, Helleberg A (1982) Single oblique-view mammography for periodic screening for breast cancer in women. JNCI 68: 351–355

Miller AB, Bulbrook RD (1982) Screening, detection, and diagnosis of breast cancer. Lancet 1: 1109–1111

Moskowitz M (1979a) Clinical examination of the breast by nonphysicians: A viable screening option? Cancer 44: 311–314

Moskowitz M (1979b) Screening is not diagnosis. Radiology 133: 265–268

Moskowitz M (to be published) The predictive value of certain mammographic signs in screening for breast cancer. Cancer

Moskowitz M, Fox SH (1979) Cost analysis of aggressive breast cancer screening. Radiology 130: 250–256

Moskowitz M, Gartside PS (1982) Evidence of breast cancer mortality reduction: aggressive screening in women under age 50. AJR 138: 911–916

Räsänen O, Auranen A, Grönroos M (1981) Breast cancer screening in Turku, Finland. Senologia 6: 155–158

Rombach JJ (1980) Breast cancer screening results and implications for diagnostic decision-making. Staflen's scientific publishing company. Alphen Aan den Rijn, Brussels

Shapiro S (1977) Evidence on screening for breast cancer from a randomised trial. Cancer 39: 2772–2782

Shapiro S, Strax P, Venet I (1971) Periodic breast cancer screening in reducing mortality from breast cancer. JAMA 215: 1777–1785

Tabar L, Gad A (1981) Screening for breast cancer: The Swedish trial. Radiology: 219–222

Tabar L, Gad A, Åkerlund E, Fors B, Fagerberg G, Baldetorp L, Gröntoft O, Lamke LO (1979) Screening for breast cancer in Sweden. A randomised controlled trial. In: Logan WW, Muntz EP (eds) Reduced dose mammography. Masson, Paris, pp 407–414

Thomas BA, Price JL, Boulter PS (1981) Breast cancer population screening by single view mammography with selective clinical examination. A pilot study. Clin Oncol 7: 201–204

Tulinius H (1979) Epidemiology of breast cancer, mortality and incidence. In: Early detection of breast cancer. Symposium arranged by the Swedish Society Against Cancer, Stockholm, pp 12–18

UK Trial of Early Detection of Breast Cancer Group (1981) Trial of early detection of breast cancer: Description of method. Br J Cancer 44: 618–627

The First Three Years of the Guildford Breast Screening Project

B. A. Thomas, J. L. Price, P. S. Boulter, and N. M. Gibbs

Guildford Breast Screening Project, Jarvis Screening Centre,
Stoughton Road, Guildford Surrey, England

Introduction

British trials for the early detection of breast cancer commenced in 1979. The death rates for breast cancer over 10–15 years are being studied in eight populations consisting of all females aged 45–64 years registerd with every general practitioner in the trial districts. Four districts act as controls, two are carrying out extensive educational programmes in breast self-examination, and two have instituted screening programmes of biennial clinical and mammographic screening with clinical examination alone in the intermediate years (UK Trial of Early Detection of Breast Cancer Group 1981).

This progress report gives some preliminary results of the first 3 years' activity of the Guildford Breast Screening Project.

Screening Method

Primary screening consists of a detailed clinical examination of the breasts by a female physician followed by mammography using a single 45° oblique projection, a supero-inferior view may be requested by the physician if a clinical abnormality has been found. Films are interpreted by the same physicians with a second opinion from the project radiologist as appropriate.

Any female who cannot be assured that no significant abnormality is present is recalled for specialist assessment at a review clinic where the subject undergoes a further clinical examination and whatever other investigations are relevant. These include further mammographic views, conventional or individual, macromammography, and ultrasound examination using a 5-MHz probe, which is of particular value in the assessment of impalpable solitary mammographic masses. Cysts are treated by aspiration. Cytological examinations are made of cyst aspirates, nipple discharges, and fine-needle biopsy specimens from palpable lesions. Intensive investigation at this stage is a major feature of this programme. Subjects thought to need further treatment are referred to the project surgeon (Thomas et al. to be published).

In the years between full screening examinations, all females screened in the previous year are invited to be clinically examined by a specially trained nurse. Should an abnormality be suspected the subject is recalled to the review clinic for single-view mammography followed by any specialist procedures deemed appropriate. Data concerning the incidence, staging, and follow-up of cancers are collected for females in the study population whether they attend the screening or not.

Recent Results in Cancer Research. Vol. 90

Table 1. Distribution of all cancers diagnosed[a] within 1 year in the study population, by age group and method of detection

Age group at time of invitation to screening (years)	No. of females in population	Attended for screening within 3 months	Benign biopsies	Screening-detected cancers				Interval cancers within 1 year	Cancers occurring within 1 year in subjects failing to attend	Total cancers in population	Screening efficiency (%)[b]	Programme efficiency (%)[c]
				Mam. only	Clin. only	Both	Total					
45–49	6,549	4,586 (70%)	46 10.1/1,000	5	5	15	25 5.4/1,000	1	1	27	96	93
50–54	6,048	4,326 (72%)	36 8.3/1,000	6	–	12	18 4.2/1,000	1	4	23	95	78
55–59	6,351	4,335 (68%)	50 11.5/1,000	7	–	15	22 5.1/1,000	3	4	29	88	76
60–64	5,121	3,339 (65%)	29 8.7/1,000	7	2	17	26 7.8/1,000	1	2	29	96	89
Total	24,069	16,586 (69%)	161 9.7/1,000	25	7	59	91 5.5/1,000	6	11	108	94	84

Mam., mammography; *Clin.*, clinical examination

[a] Excluding the less advanced cancers in the two instances of simultaneous bilateral disease

[b] Screening method efficiency: 91/97 = 94%

[c] Population programme efficiency: 91/108 = 84%

Results

The first population cohort consisted of 24,069 females, of whom 69% attended the initial screening examination. This represents nearer 75% of the true population since there is a 10%–15% inaccuracy rate in the Family Practitioner Committee's age/sex registers, which form the basis for comparisons in all trial districts. Details of all cancers occurring in the population within 1 year of the first screening visit are given in Table 1 and the staging of the screening-detected cancers is given in Table 2.

All females who attended the first screening visit, apart from those still under hospital care or known to have left the district, were invited for clinical examination, the results of which are shown in Tables 2 and 3. One case of cancer was diagnosed after a follow-up for over 1

Table 2. Staging of screening detected cancers by size

Pathology staging	First screening, cancers detected		Second screening, clinical, cancers detected		Third screening (half cohort), cancers detected	
	%	Number	%	Number	%	Number
Noninvasive	14	14	–	–	9	2
5 mm or under	10	9	–	–	4.5	1
6–10 mm	17	17 – (2)	31	4	36	8
11–15 mm	18	15 – (4)	8	1	23	5
16–20 mm	10	9 – (2)	15	2[a]	9	2
21–50 mm	15	15 – (6)	31	4 – (4)	4.5	1 – (1)
Over 50 mm	2	1	–	–	–	–
Not known (mam. over 20 mm)	13	11 – (9)	15	2 – (2)	14	3 – (1)
Total	100 (25)	91 – (23)	100 (46)	13 – (6)	100 (10)	22 – (2)

Figures in brackets denote node-positive cancers

[a] Includes one < 2 cm upon clinical and mammographic examination, treated by radiotherapy

Table 3. Details of attendance and recall for three screening visits

		First visit, clinical exam. + mammography	Second visit, clinical exam.	Third visit, clinical exam. + mammography
Subjects invited		24,069	16,416	10,296
Attended (% of invited)		16,586 (69%)	13,983 (85%)	7,236 (71%)
Reviewed	per 1,000 screened	88	97	58
Cysts aspirated	per 1,000 screened	8	5.5	7.5
Referred to surgeon	per 1,000 screened	20	6.4	8
Biopsy				
Benign	per 1,000 screened	9.7	2.8	3
Cancer	per 1,000 screened	5.5	0.9	3
Cancer: benign biopsies		1:1.77	1:3	1:1

year, of an abnormality detected at the first screening visit. Full follow-up data for the year following this second examination are not yet available for the whole cohort.

Two years after the first screening invitation, all females are invited to re-attend for full screening whether they accepted the first invitation or not, all addresses being checked on up-dated age/sex registers. Results are available for the first half of the cohort only; these are given in Tables 2 and 3. An assessment of the workload involved may be made from Table 3, which gives comparative figures for the three screening rounds.

Discussion

The combination of clinical examination and mammography, as would be expected, has resulted in a higher benign biopsy rate than purely mammographic screening methods (Lundgren 1980; Tabar and Gad 1981; Andersson 1980). However, a cancer: benign biopsy ratio of 1 : 1.77 at the prevalence screening round is considered to be acceptable.

Table 4. Staging based on pathological size

Noninvasive	Stage I	Stage II	Stage III/IV
Any size	≲2 cm node −ve or unknown but clinically −ve	≲2 cm node +ve >2 cm <5 cm node −ve or sample −ve including IM sample only for medial quadrant cancer	>5 cm >2 cm node +ve or unknown Any size − skin involved or chest wall involved or distant metastases

IM, internal mammary; −*ve*, negative; +*ve*, positive

Table 5. Incidence rates of cancers 1,000 females in total population − preliminary data

Screening round	Noninvasive	Stage I	Stage II	Stage III/IV	Total
First screening	0.58	1.74	0.71	0.75	3.77
Interval + FTA		0.33	0.04	0.33	0.71
Total 1st year	0.58	2.07	0.75	1.08	4.48
Second screening		0.32	0.17	0.09	0.57
Interval + FTA + Follow-up[a]	−	0.17	0.22	0.22	0.61
Total 2nd year		0.49	0.39	0.31	1.18
Third screening[a]	0.18	1.45	0.18	0.18	2.00
Control populations 1st year	0.02	0.38	0.40	0.70	1.50

FTA, cancers in females failing to attend for screening

[a] Rates based on first half of cohort only

Increasingly sophisticated investigatory techniques have helped reduce this to 1 : 1 in the third round. Clinical examination alone is much less satisfactory from this viewpoint with a 1 : 3 ratio; it is unfortunate that this policy did not reveal in situ disease in situations of clinical abnormality arising 1 year after a normal mammographic examination. It is interesting that clinical examination seems to be relatively more important in those under 50 years of age than in the older age groups.

The discovery of small or in situ cancers is not the primary justification for screening, and mortality data are awaited with interest. A significant mortality change must be preceded by a reduction in the rate of occurrence of those cancers that are known to be almost invariably fatal, that is stage III and IV disease. If population screening is to be justified on a national basis then this reduction of stage III and IV disease must be demonstrable in the population as a whole, not just in screened subjects. There is some evidence that this is starting to occur in the Guildford project population. Using a modified pathology staging (Table 4) the population incidence rates for the different stages may be considered and compared with those in the trial districts where the incidence resembles the prescreening situation in Guildord.

The population picture shows an apparent decrease in new stage III and IV disease as compared with the control population, which, if maintained, even allowing for the increased incidence detected in the first or prevalent disease screening round, should be reflected in a mortality change.

The incidence of stage I disease has shown a large increase, accounting for most of the overall increase in diagnosed disease. We look forward with confidence to the probability of an associated mortality change.

References

Andersson I (1980) Mammographic screening for breast carcinoma. Thesis, Malmo University

Lundgren B (1980) Single oblique view mammography, an efficient method for breast cancer screening. Thesis, Gavle University

Tabar L, Gad A (1981) Screening for breast cancer: The Swedish trial. Radiology 138: 219–22

Thomas BA, Price JL, Boulter PS, Gibbs NM (to be published) Cancers occurring in a total population one year after invitation to participate in a Breast Cancer Screening Programme. Clin Oncol

UK Trial of Early Detection of Breast Cancer Group (1981) Description of method. Br J Cancer: 44–618

Detection of Endocrine Responsiveness by Flow Cytometric DNA Analysis in Experimental Human Breast Cancer

N. Brünner, M. Spang-Thomsen, L. Vindeløv, A. Nielsen, and S. A. Engelholm

The University Institute of Pathological Anatomy, University of Copenhagen, Frederik V's Vej 11, 2100 Copenhagen, Denmark

Introduction

In human metastatic breast cancer, the response to endocrine therapy is approximately 30%, regardless of type of endocrine therapy applied (McGuire et al. 1975). Mainly based on this observation, it has been suggested that different kinds of endocrine treatment share the same ultimate mode of action (Rose 1982). However, in recent years it has been shown that different endocrine treatment modalities do not always show cross-resistance (Smith et al. 1982, Murray and Pitt 1982), suggesting different modes of action.

Two main types of in vitro tests have been conducted as predictive tests for endocrine sensitivity. One is based on the determination of treatment-induced cell kinetic changes of cells in culture (Israel and Saez 1978, Sanfilippo et al. 1979, Poulsen et al. 1982). The other test is based on steroid hormone receptor determinations (McGuire et al. 1975, Osborne et al. 1980). In this study, the effect of ablative (ovariectomy) and additive (estradiol) endocrine treatment on an estrogen- and progesterone-receptor-positive human breast carcinoma grown in nude mice was investigated. Flow cytometric DNA analysis (FCM) performed on tumor tissue obtained by fine-needle aspirations was used to estimate the effect on the cell cycle. The FCM data were compared with the effects on tumor growth.

The results demonstrate a correlation between FCM-monitored changes in the cell cycle distribution and changes in tumor growth, indicating a possible role for FCM in the assessment of endocrine sensitivity. Furthermore, the results suggest different modes of action of additive and ablative endocrine treatment.

Material and Methods

Tumor. The human breast carcinoma studied was kindly supplied by G. B. Bastert, Klinikum der Johann Wolfgang Goethe Universität, Frankfurt am Main. The tumor, a receptor-positive (ER+, PgR+) moderately differentiated ductogene carcinoma, was derived from the mastectomy specimen of a 54-year-old postmenopausal female. The tumor was serially grown in nude mice and was transferred to our laboratory in the 11th transplant generation. The present investigations were performed on tumors from the 17th and 18th passage in nude mice.

Animals. Specific pathogen-free (SPF) male and female NC/KH nude mice were kept under sterile conditions in a laminar flow clean bench. Room temperature was 25 ± 2° C; relative humidity was 55% ± 5%. Sterile food and water were given ad libitum.

Recent Results in Cancer Research. Vol. 90

Transplantation. Tumors were grown in intact female mice or in male mice, castrated at least 1 week before transplantation. A tissue block of approximately 2 mm was inoculated subcutaneously in each flank of the mice. The procedure was performed under general anesthesia with propanidid (Eponthol). Tumors were excluded in animals that died before the end of the experimental period, which was 28 days following the treatment. In addition, tumors in which growth was evident in less than six growth recordings prior to the day of treatment were excluded (Spang-Thomsen et al. 1981).

Endocrine Treatment. Castrated male mice were treated with 0.1 ml 17 β-estradiol (Progynon depot 10 mg/ml, Schering AG, Berlin) as a single intramuscular dose into the thigh. The treatment was given on day 44 after transplantation. Female nude mice were ovariectomized on day 45 after transplantation. There were in each group 11 treated and 12 untreated tumors in the estradiol experiment and 11 treated and 16 untreated tumors in the ovariectomy experiment.

Flow Cytometric DNA Analysis. The samples for FCM were obtained by sequential fine-needle aspirations. Tumors were aspirated three times a week for 3 weeks. At least one treated and one control tumor was aspirated each time. The aspiration procedure (Vindeløv 1977), storage of aspirates (Vindeløv et al. 1983a), and staining by propidium iodide (Vindeløv et al. 1983b) were performed as previously described. The flow cytometer used was a FACS III cell sorter (Becton Dickinson, Sunnyvale, CA, USA). The percentage of cells in the cell cycle phases was determined by statistical analysis of the DNA distribution (Christensen et al. 1978).

Growth Data. Tumors were measured three times a week and the growth data were used to construct rectilinear growth curves according to a transformed Gompertz function (Spang-Thomsen et al. 1980). On the basis of this function, two regression lines were constructed for all tumors, one before and one after the treatment. For the determination of each of these lines, six experimental points were used. The growth curves were normalized by correcting all growth data with the difference between the common mean tumor size at the time of treatment and the mean tumor size at the time of treatment in the individual treatment groups (Spang-Thomsen et al. 1981).

Results

The effect of estradiol and ovariectomy on the growth curves is shown in Figs. 1 and 2. Estradiol induced complete tumor regression of all treated tumors. The tumor shrinkage commenced approximately 12 days after treatment (Fig. 1). Regrowth was not observed. Ovariectomy had no effect on the growth curves (Fig. 2).
Representative sequences of the DNA distribution in the two treatment groups are shown in Fig. 3. Estradiol induced characteristic cell cycle perturbations in the tumors. The cell cycle changes, which could be detected from about day 5 after treatment (Fig. 3A–C), comprised an increase in the S phase fraction followed by an accumulation of polyploid cells after day 7 (Fig. 3B–C). Ovariectomy had no effect on the cell cycle distribution (Fig. 3D–F).

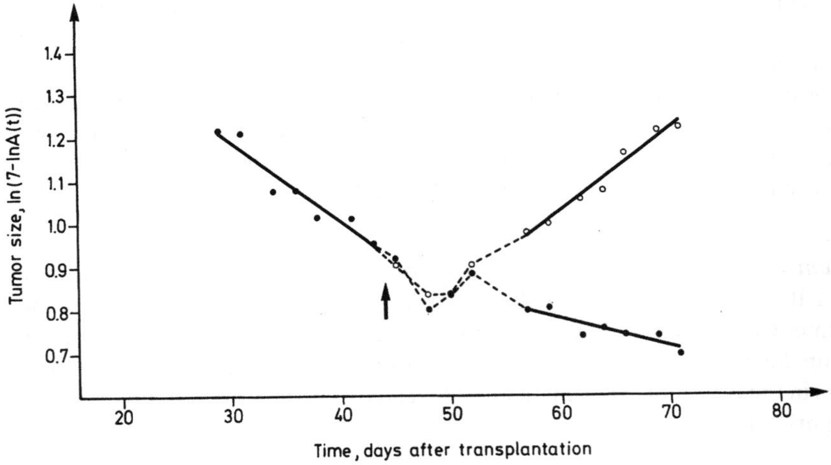

Fig. 1. Mean transformed Gompertz growth curves of a receptor-positive human breast carcinoma transplanted to nude mice on day 0 and treated with 0.1 mg 17 β-estradiol on day 44 *(arrow)*. The *points* represent mean values of experimental growth data of 11 treated (○) and 12 untreated (●) tumors

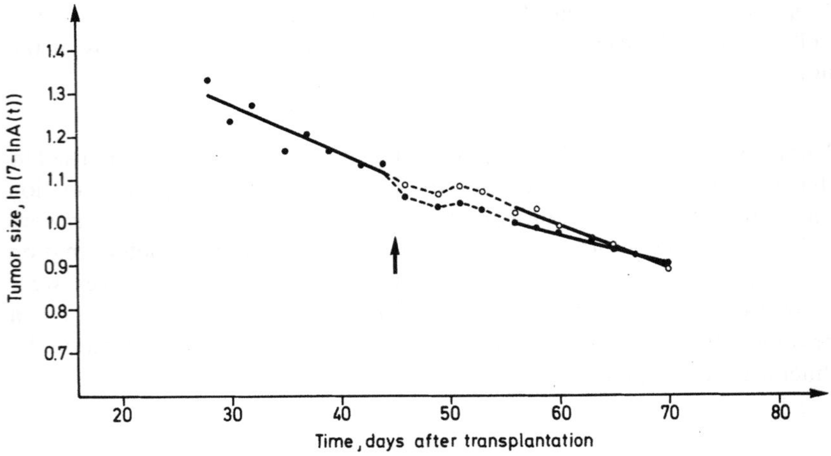

Fig. 2. Mean transformed Gompertz growth curves of a receptor-positive human breast carcinoma transplanted to nude mice on day 0 and treated with ovariectomy on day 45 *(arrow)*. The *points* represent mean values of experimental growth data of 11 treated (○) and 16 untreated (●) tumors

Discussion

The present study has demonstrated a correlation between the endocrine treatment-induced effect on growth curves and FCM-monitored cell cycle changes. The correlation was demonstrated in effective (estradiol) as well as in ineffective (ovariectomy) endocrine treatment. Thus, the results indicate that endocrine responsiveness, defined by tumor growth response, can be detected by FCM.

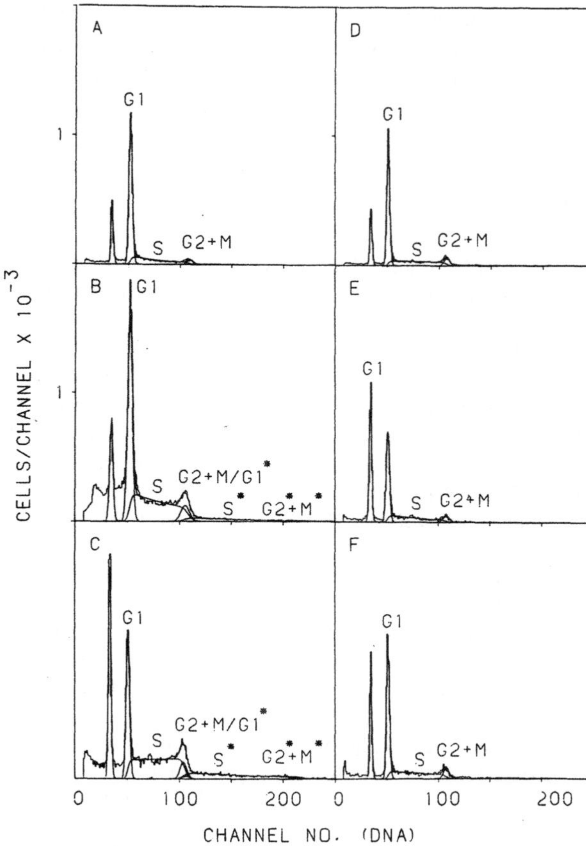

Fig. 3A–F. DNA distribution of a human mammary carcinoma grown in nude mice treated with estradiol **A–C** and with ovariectomy **D–F.** The histograms represent 0 **A** and **D,** 5 **B** and **E,** and 12 **C** and **F** days after the treatment. The parts of the DNA histograms produced by G_1, S, and G_2+M are indicated in the figure. *, polypolid cells

The effect of ablative and additive endocrine treatment has been suggested as being mediated by the same receptor (McGuire et al. 1975). The ablative treatment deprives the receptor of the stimulatory effect of endogenous estrogens and the additive treatment depletes cytoplasmic estrogen receptors, leaving the cells insensitive to endogenous estrogens. In this ER+, PgR+ mammary carcinoma, ablative and additive endocrine treatment resulted in different responses, which indicates either a more complex common mechanism of action or different mechanism of action.

Hypothetically, this tumor could have an aromatase system by which it sustains the hormone requirements for growth, despite the ablative procedure (Miller and Forrest 1974, Miller et al. 1982, Perel et al. 1982). This hypothesis is currently under investigation at our laboratory.

Evaluation of response to endocrine treatment in patients with breast cancer is usually based on treatment-induced changes in tumor size. In the present study, a correlation was demonstrated between the effect of endocrine treatment on tumor growth and on FCM-monitored cell cycle changes. Similar results were obtained in a recent study where an ER-, PgR- mammary carcinoma on nude mice was treated with estradiol (Brünner et al. 1983). Since the FCM method is simple to perform and results are available a few hours after the biopsy, the results indicate that FCM analysis may be used as an early and rapid method for the detection of endocrine responsiveness in human breast cancer.

References

1. Brünner N, Spang-Thomsen M, Vindeløv L, Nielsen A (1983) Effect of 17 β-oestradiol on growth curves and flow cytometric DNA distribution of two human breast carcinomas grown in nude mice. Br J Cancer 47: 641
2. Christensen IJ, Hartmann NR, Keiding N, Larsen JK, Noer H, Vindeløv L (1978) Statistical analysis of DNA distributions from cell populations with partial synchrony. In: Lutz D (ed) Pulse-Cytometry, vol 3. Euroean Press Medicon, Ghent, p 71
3. Israel N, Saez S (1978) Relation between steroid receptor content and the response to hormone addition in isolated human breast cancer cells in short-term culture. Cancer Res 38: 4314
4. McGuire WL, Carbone PP, Sears ME, Escher GC (1975) Estrogen receptors in human breast cancer: an overview. In: McGuire WL, Carbone PP, Volmer EP (eds) Estrogen receptors in human breast cancer. Raven New York, p 1
5. Miller WR, Forrest APM (1974) Oestradiol synthesis by a human breast carcinoma. Lancet 2: 866
6. Miller WR, Hawkins RA, Forrest APM (1982) Significance of Aromastase Activity in Human Breast Cancer. Cancer Res (Suppl) 42: 3365
7. Murray RML, Pitt P (1982) Aminoglutethimide in tamoxifen-resistant patients: The Melbourne experience. Cancer Res (Suppl) 42: 3437
8. Osborne CK, Yochmowitz MG, Knight WA, McGuire WL (1980) The value of estrogen and progesterone receptors in the treatment of breast cancer. Cancer 46: 2884
9. Perel E, Blackstein ME, Killinger DW (1982) Aromastase in human breast carcinoma. Cancer Res (Suppl) 42: 3369
10. Poulsen HS, Bichel P, Andersen J (1982) Short-term culture of human breast cancer: In vitro effects of hormones related to patient response. Br J Cancer 46: 67
11. Rose DP (1982) Postmenopausal oestrogen production and its inhibition. In: Stoll BA (ed) Endocrine relationships in breast cancer. Heinemann Medical, London, p 187
12. Sanfilippo O, Daidone MG, Di Fronzo G, Silvestrini R (1979) Short-term tissue culture of human breast cancer. Cancer 43: 2365
13. Smith IE, Harris AL, Morgan M, Gazet J-C, McKinna JA (1982) Tamoxifen versus aminoglutethimide versus combined tamoxifen and aminoglutethimide in the reatment of advanced breast carcinoma. Cancer Res (Suppl) 42: 3430
14. Spang-Thomsen M, Nielsen A, Visfeldt J (1980) Growth curves of three human malignant tumors transplanted to nude mice. Exp Cell Biol 48: 138
15. Spang-Thomsen M, Visfeldt J, Nielsen A (1981) Effect of single-dose x-irradiation on the growth curves of a human malignant melanoma transplanted into nude mice. Radiat Res 85: 184
16. Vindeløv L (1977) Flow microfluorometric analysis of nuclear DNA in cells from solid tumors and cell suspensions. Virchows Arch [Cell Pathol] 24: 227
17. Vindeløv L, Christensen IJ, Keiding N, Spang-Thomsen M, Nissen NI (1983a) Long-term storage of samples for flow cytometric DNA analysis. Cytometry 3: 31
18. Vindeløv L, Christensen IJ, Nissen NI (1983b) A detergent-trypsin method for the preparation of nuclei for flow cytometric DNA analysis. Cytometry 3: 323

The Reliability of Frozen-Section Diagnosis in Various Breast Lesions: A Study Based on 3451 Biopsies

N. J. Agnantis, N. Apostolikas, I. Christodoulou,
C. Petrakis, and J. Garas

Department of Pathology, Breast Division, Greek Anticancer Institute "Snt Savvas" Hospital, 7, D. Aginitou Street, Athens 611, Greece

Summary

In this study, we analyze breast biopsy material over a 5-year period and we compare the results of frozen-section diagnosis with the corresponding diagnosis of the permanent histologic sections. In this study, which represents the largest series in the available international literature, it is proven that frozen-section diagnosis of various breast lesions is a highly accurate procedure in spite of the difficulties facing the pathologist with the frequent borderline or premalignant lesions. The great responsibility of the pathologist is emphasized.

Introduction

The importance and the contribution of frozen-section diagnosis (FSD) during surgery is widely accepted. Until 1960, most pathology laboratories did not use the FSD procedure as a routine method because of the various technical disadvantages. After the introduction of the cryostat, the technique was greatly improved and during the last 20 years this procedure has become established as a routine method for all kinds of biopsy (Agnantis to be published; Azzopardi 1979; Rosai 1981; Rosen 1978; Sparkaman 1962).

With regard to the breast, the diagnosis at one time used to be very simple because physicians were faced with only the two extreme conditions, cancer or mastitis. More recently, with the introduction of mammography and other modern preoperative diagnostic methods, patients undergo surgery at earlier clinical stages of disease and, thus, FSD as become more difficult since the lesions detected show a more diverse character. So, the physician often finds himself obliged to make the final diagnosis by means of permanent paraffin sections. However, in our laboratory when a FSD is deferred, we always inform the surgeon of our reasons, our reservations about the accuracy of the final diagnosis, as well as our opinion as to what this diagnosis might be. We think that this is essential because the surgeon is then able, according to the gravity of the situation, to prepare the patient psychologically for any further treatment that may be necessary. Our final diagnosis is usually given within 24 h of receiving the surgical specimen for FSD. Before analyzing our material, it is useful to consider some principles and methods that every pathologist must consider at the time of a breast FSD:

1. Gross specimen examination.
2. Specimen X-ray examination.
3. Simultaneous frozen sections – additional technical procedures [imprint method – indications for this procedure and its advantages are reported in a previous publication (Agnantis et al. 1981b)].

Recent Results in Cancer Research. Vol. 90

4. Low power objective lens of microscope during FSD.
5. Discrepancies between histologic diagnosis and macroscopic evidence. Patient's case history should be considered.
6. Mistaken diagnosis can lead to needless amputation.
7. Pathologist should be experienced as personal responsibility is great.
8. Pathologist should avoid being influenced by other physicians during FSD.

Material and Methods, Results

Our material consists of 3451 breast frozen-section biopsies, which we obtained during a 5-year period (1976–1980). The number of biopsies is the number of specimens examined and not the number of patients operated upon, since sometimes we examined more than one specimen from the same patient. The technical procedures used in our department for breast biopsies are as follows: (a) specimen X-ray examination when appropriate [Indications for this procedure and its advantages are reported in previous publications (Agnantis 1982; Agnantis et al. 1980, 1981)] (b) metachromatic frozen-section stain (Azure A-Erie Garnet); (c) permanent frozen-section stain H & E; (d) normal H & E stain for permanent paraffin sections; and (e) special histochemical stains when needed.
Our reports on FSD are divided into three main groups: (a) negative for the benign cases; (b) deferred for the suspicious ones; and (c) positive for the obvious carcinomas. In the group (b) we recognize two subdivisions, those lesions with high reservation (hr) and those with low reservation (lr). The following list shows the indications for reservation according to the extent of the lesion, the degree of epithelial hyperplasia, and degree of cellular atypia, this reservation might be high or low:

1. Specimen size
   a) Large
   b) Small
2. Calcifications associated with fibrocystic disease (FCD)
3. Sclerosing adenosis
   a) Pseudoinfiltrating
   b) With apocrine metaplasia
   c) Microglandular
   d) In pregnancy
4. Cyst with thick walls
5. Duct or lobular hyperplasia
6. Papillary lesions – severe epitheliosis
7. Fat necrosis
8. Chronic granulomas
9. Plasma cell mastitis
10. Fibroadenoma with epithelial hyperplasia
11. Cystosarcoma phyllodes
12. Granular cell myoblastoma
13. Histiocytoma

In reviewing these 3451 breast frozen-section biopsies, we analyzed our results separately for each year and compared them with the corresponding permanent paraffin sections (see Table 1). Our findings are shown in Figs. 1–6.

Table 1. Comparative study of 3451 breast biopsies (1976–1980)

		1976			1977			1978			1979			1980			Total (years)		
		No. of cases		%	No. of cases		%	No. of cases		%	No. of cases		%	No. of cases		%	No. of cases		%
FSD	PSD	FSD	PSD		FSD	PSD		FSD	PSD		FSD	PSD		FSD	PSD		FSD	PSD	
–	–	318	317	99.7	365	362	99.2	510	507	99.4	357	357	100	208	207	99.5	1 758	1 750	99,6
	+		1	0.3		3	0.8		3	0.6		0	0		1	0.5		8	0.4
LR	–	12	12	100	47	42	89.4	99	96	97	181	177	97.8	232	210	90.5	571	537	94.1
(–)	+		0	0		5	10.6		3	3		4	2.2		22	9.5		34	5.9
																		HRG	
HR	–	7	1	14.3	6	1	16.7	16	7	43.8	41	29	70.7	67	48	71.7	137	86	62.8
(–)	+		6	85.7		5	83.3		9	56.2		12	29.3		19	28.3		51	37.2
–	–	133	0	0	126	0	0	213	0	0	262	0	0	251	1	0.4	985	1[a]	0.1
	+		133	100		126	100		213	100		262	100		250	99.6		984	99.9
Total			470			544			838			841			758			3451	

FSD, frozen-section diagnosis; *PSD*, permanent-section diagnosis; *HRG*, high-risk group; *LR*, low reservation; *HR*, high reservation

[a] Atypical juvenile papillomatosis

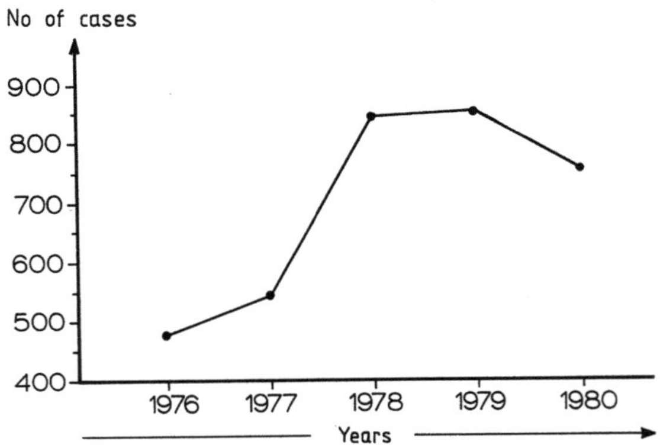

Fig. 1. Total number of FSD cases during the 5-year period

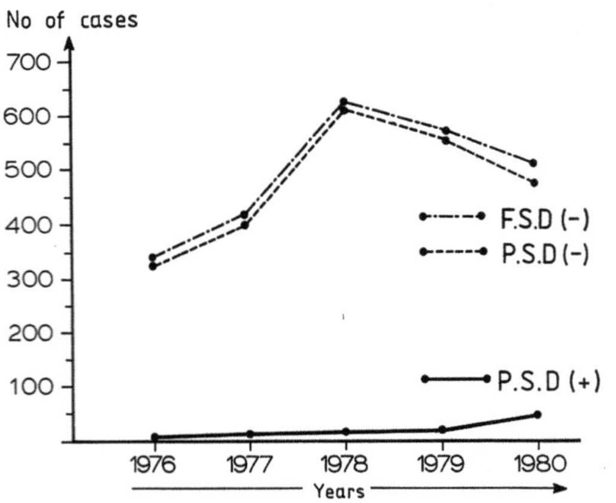

Fig. 2. The negative and differed cases. The curve of FSD is almost parallel to the curve of permanent-section diagnosis (PSD) except for the year 1980 when a small deviation is observed due to the increased number of false-negative diagnoses

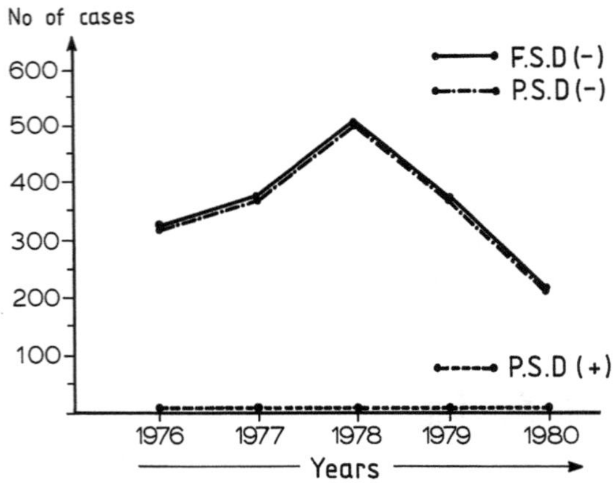

Fig. 3. The negative cases. Both curves (FSD and PSD) almost coincide. Here the percentage of false-negative diagnoses is extremely low

Discussion

The results of our study are basically in accordance with those in the available literature as far as the benign cases and the obvious carcinomas are concerned (Rosai 1981; Rosen 1978; Sparkaman 1962). However, for the deffered group our figures are higher, probably due to

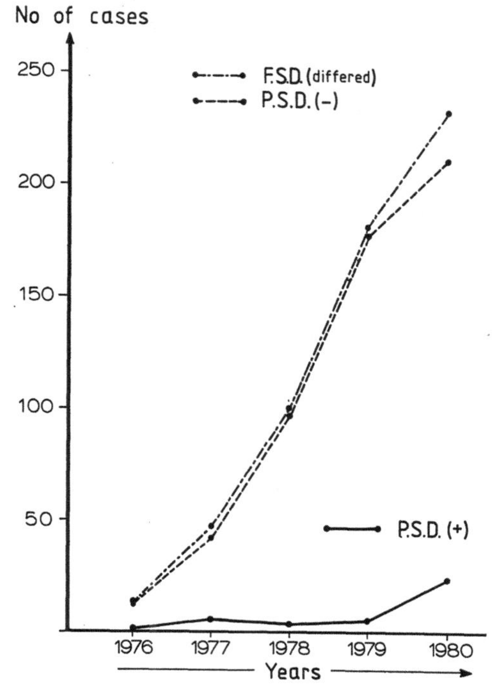

Fig. 4. The differed cases with low reservation. Here again a deviation for the year 1980 is observed with a corresponding increase in the number of false-negative diagnoses

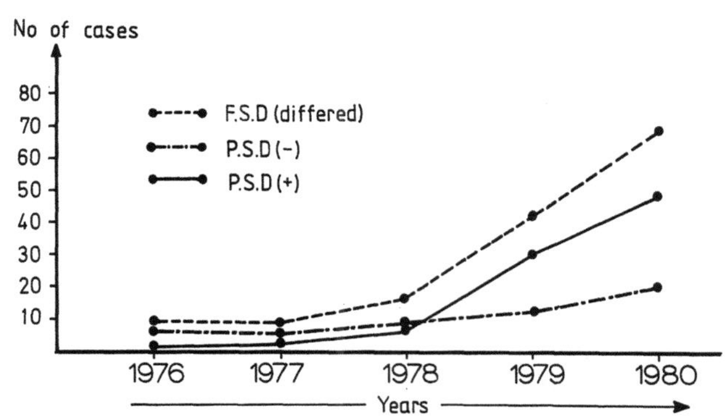

Fig. 5. The differed cases with high reservation. Here the deviation starts from the year 1978 increasing in the years 1979 and 1980. The curve of the false-negative diagnoses follows the same pattern

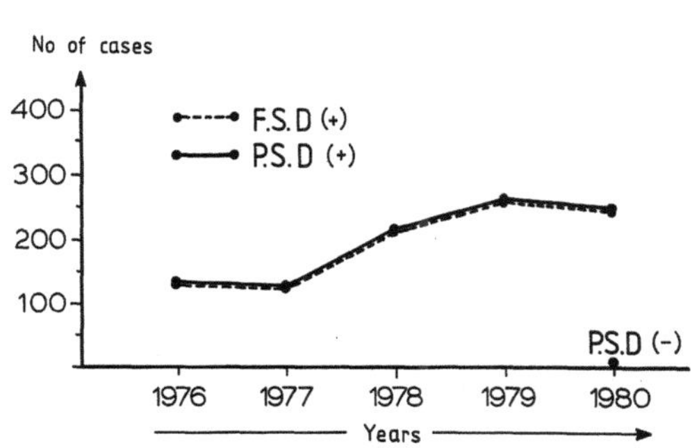

Fig. 6. The positive cases. Both curves (FSD and PSD) coincide entirely. There was only one false-positive case

the fact that we use a different system of classification and, more likely, because our study includes material examined more recently and for that reason is more difficult to interpret.

The latter part of Table 1 shows our results as a whole, on which we would like to make the following comments. There was no obvious tumor in the gross specimen in cases where a false-negative result was determined. Of 1758 negative cases of FSD, only eight were false-negative. In seven of these cases, carcinoma was detected in areas other than the one selected for frozen section. Only in one case was the cancer lesion in the selected section, and while it gave the impression of an inflammatory infiltration, in the paraffin sections it proved to be a small cell-infiltrating lobular carcinoma.

Of 708 deffered cases of FSD three-quarters of the false-negative results were cases of in situ carcinomas. The group of 137 deffered FSD with high reservation consisted of very difficult and complex lesions and thus the percentage of false-negative diagnoses was high.

Of 985 positive cases of FSD, there was only one false-positive case, which was initially interpreted as intraductal carcinoma and finally proved to be juvenile papillomatosis – Rosen's Swiss cheese disease (Rosen et al. 1980). This mistake could have been avoided if we had been better informed of the patient's clinical history and if the pathologist had been familiar with this particular lesion. Luckily, the surgeon did not proceed to undertake a mastetoctomy because the patient was only 30 years old and the FSD indicated in situ carcinoma.

From our study, which represents the largest series in the international literature, it is proven that FSD of various breast lesions is a highly reliable procedure in spite of the difficulties that the pathologist faces with the frequent borderline or premalignant lesions. Finally, we must again emphasize the great responsibility of the pathologist in FSD, and we totally agree with Azzopardi (1979) that as the life of the patient lies in the hands of one surgeon, so FSD belongs to the responsibility of one pathologist.

References

Agnantis N (1982) Frozen section diagnosis problems of breast lesions and the contribution of specimen mammography in their solution. (in Greek) Proceedings of the Medicosurgical Society of Athens, 1980, p 115

Agnantis N, Apostolikas N, Hondrou A, Claoudatou C, Karaiossifides C, Garas J (1980) Comparative study of specimen mammograms and histopathologic findings. A study based on 500 cases. (in Greek). Hell Oncol 16: 147

Agnantis N, Apostolikas N, Hondrou A, Claoudatou C, Kariossifides C, Garas J (1981) The contribution of specimen mammography in diagnosis difficult breast lesions (in Greek). Iatriki 40: 43

Agnantis N, Claoudatou C, Marnerou M, Nanopoulou V, Karaiossifides C (1983) Comparative study of breast biopsy imprints and corresponding histological findings. Hippocrates 8: 67

Azzopardi JG (1979) Problems in breast pathology. Saunders, Philadelphia

Rosai J (1981) Ackerman's surgical pathology, vol 1. Mosby, St Louis, p 1091

Rosen PP (1978) Frozen section diagnosis of breast lesions – recent experience with 556 consecutive biopsies. Ann Surg 187: 17

Rosen PP, Cantrell B, Mullen DL, DePalo A (1980) Juvenile papillomatosis (Swiss cheese disease) of the breast. Am J Surg Pathol 4: 3

Sparkaman RS (1962) Reliability of frozen section in the diagnosis of breast lesions. Ann Surgery 155: 924

Subject Index

Recent Results in Cancer Research

Sponsored by the Swiss League against Cancer. Editor in Chief: P. Rentchnick, Genève

For information about Vols. 1–9, please contact your bookseller of Springer-Verlag

10 Nelson, R. S.: Radioactive Phosphorus in the Diagnosis of Gastrointestinal Cancer.
11 Freeman, R. G. and J. M. Knox: Treatment of Skin Cancer.
12 Lynch, H. T.: Hereditary Factors in Carcinoma.
13 Tumours in Children, 2nd Edition. Edited by H. B. Marsden and J. K. Steward.
14 Odartchenko, N.: Production Cellulaire Erythropoïétique.
15 Sokoloff, B.: Carcinoid and Serotonin.
16 Jacobs, M. L.: Malignant Lymphomas and Their Management.
17 Normal and Malignant Cell Growth. Edited by R. J. M. Fry, M. L. Griem, and W. H. Kirsten (Symposium).
18 Anglesio, E.: The Treatment of Hodgkin's Disease.
19 Bannasch, P.: The Cytoplasm of Hepatocytes during Carcinogenesis. Electron- and Lightmicroscopical Investigations of the Nitrosomorpholineintoxicated Rat Liver.
20 Rubidomycin. A new Agent against Cancer. Edited by J. Bernard, R. Paul, M. Boiron, C. Jacquillat, and R. Maral.
21 Scientific Basis of Cancer Chemotherapy. Edited by G. Mathé (Symposium).
22 Koldovský, P.: Tumor Specific Transplantation Antigen.
23 Fuchs, W. A., J. W. Davidson, and H. W. Fischer: Lymphography in Cancer. With contributions by G. Jantet and H. Rösler.
24 Hayward, J.: Hormones und Human Breast Cancer. An Account of 15 Years Study.
25 Roy-Burman, P.: Analogues of Nucleic Acid Components. Mechanisms of Action.
26 Tumors of the Liver. Edited by G. T. Pack and A. H. Islami.
27 Szymendera, J.: Bone Mineral Metabolism in Cancer.
28 Meek, E. S.: Antitumour and Antiviral Substances of Natural Origin.
29 Aseptic Environments and Cancer Treatment. Edited by G. Mathé (Symposium).
30 Advances in the Treatment of Acute (Blastic) Leukemias. Edited by G. Mathé (Symposium).
31 Denoix, P.: Treatment of Malignant Breast Tumors. Indications and Results.
32 Nelson, R. S.: Endoscopy in Gastric Cancer.
33 Experimental and Clinical Effects of L-Asparaginase. Edited by E. Grundmann and H. F. Oettgen (Symposium).
34 Chemistry and Biological Actions of 4-Nitroquinolin 1-Oxide. Edited by H. Endo, T. Ono, and T. Sugimura.
35 Penn, I.: Malignant Tumors in Organ Transplant Recipients.
36 Current Concepts in the Management of Lymphoma and Leukemia. Edited by J. E. Ultmann, M. L. Griem, W. H. Kirsten, and R. W. Wissler (Symposium).
37 Chiappa, S., R. Musumeci, and C. Uslenghi: Endolymphatic Radiotherapy in Malignant Lymphomas. With contributions by G. Bonadonna, B. Damascelli, G. Fava, F. Pizzetti, U. Veronesi.
38 Koller, P. C.: The Role of Chromosomes in Cancer Biology.
39 Current Problems in the Epidemiology of Cancer and Lymphomas. Edited by E. Grundmann and H. Tulinius (Symposium).
40 Langley, F. A. and A. C. Crompton: Epithelial Abnormalities of the Cervix Uteri.
41 Tumours in a Tropical Country. A Survey of Uganda (1964–1968). Edited by A. C. Templeton.
42 Breast Cancer: A Challenging Problem. Edited by M. L. Griem, E. V. Jensen, J. E. Ultmann, and R. W. Wissler (Symposium).
43 Nomenclature, Methodology and Results of Clinical Trials in Acute Leukemias. Edited by G. Mathé, P. Pouillart, L.Schwarzenberg (Symposium).
44 Special Topics in Carcinogenesis. Edited by E. Grundmann (Symposium).
45 Koldovský, P.: Carcinoembryonic Antigens.
46 Diagnosis and Therapy of Malignant Lymphoma. Edited by K. Musshoff (Symposium).
47 Investigation and Stimulation of Immunity in Cancer Patients. Edited by G. Mathé and R. Weiner (Symposium).
48 Platinum Coordination Complexes in Cancer Chemotherapy. Edited by T. A. Connors and J. J. Roberts (Symposium).

49 Complications of Cancer Chemotherapy. Edited by G. MATHÉ and R. K. OLDHAM (Symposium).

50 Cancer Registry, Edited by E. GRUNDMANN and E. PEDERSEN (Symposium).

51 Gliomas. Current Concepts in Biology, Diagnosis and Therapy. Edited by J. HEKMATPANAH (Symposium).

52 The Ambivalence of Cytostatic Therapy. Edited by E. GRUNDMANN and R. GROSS (Symposium).

53 A. CLARYSSE, Y. KENIS, and G. MATHÉ: Cancer Chemotherapy.

54 Malignant Bone Tumors. Edited by E. GRUNDMANN.

55 MATHÉ G.: Cancer Active Immunotherapy, Immunoprophylaxis, and Immunorestoration.

56 Lymphocytes, Macrophages, and Cancer. Edited by G. MATHÉ, I. FLORENTIN, and M.-C. SIMMLER (Symposium).

57 Breast Cancer: A Multidisciplinary Approach. Edited by G. ST. ARNEAULT, P. BAND, and L. ISRAËL (Symposium).

58 B. S. SCHOENBERG: Multiple Primary Malignant Neoplasms.

59 Selective Heat Sensitivity of Cancer Cells. Edited by A. ROSSI-FANELLI, R. CAVALIERE, B. MONDOVI, and G. MORICCA.

60 Tumors of the Male Genital System. Edited by E. GRUNDMANN and W. VAHLENSIECK (Symposium).

61 D. METCALF: Hemopoietic Colonies.

62 Tactics and Strategy in Cancer Treatment. Edited by G. MATHÉ (Symposium).

63 Antitumor Antibiotics. Edited by S. K. CARTER, H. UMEZAWA, J. DOUROS, and Y. SAKURAI (Symposium).

64 Lymphoid Neoplasias I: Classification, Categorization, Natural History.

65 Lymphoid Neoplasias II: Clinical and Therapeutic Aspects.
Lymphoid Neoplasias I & II. Proceedings of the 1977 CNRS-EORTC International Colloquium. Editors: G. MATHÉ, M. SELIGMANN, M. TUBIANA. Devided into two volumes.

66 Carcinogenic Hormones. Edited by C. H. LINGEMAN.

67/68 Adjuvant Therapies and Markers of Post-Surgical Minimal Residual Disease I & II. Proceedings of the 1978 Annual Plenary Meeting of the EORTC. Editors: G. BONADONNA, G. MATHÉ, S. E. SALMON. Divided into two volumes.

67 Markers and General Problems of Cancer Adjuvant Therapies.

68 Adjuvant Therapies of the Various Primary Tumors.

69 Strategies in Clinical Hematology. Edited by R. GROSS and K.-P. HELLRIEGEL.

70 New Anticancer Drugs. Edited by S. K. CARTER

71 Endocrine Treatment of Breast Cancer. Edited by B. HENNINGSEN, F. LINDER, C. STREICHELE.

72 CAWLEY, J. C., BURNS, G. F., HAYHOE, F. G. J.: Hairy-Cell Leukaemia.

73 Thyroid Cancer. Edited by W. DUNCAN.

74 Cancer Chemo- and Immunopharmacology. 1. Chemopharmacology. Edited by G. MATHÉ and F. M. MUGGIA.

75 Cancer Chemo- and Immunopharmacology. 2. Immunopharmacology, Relations and General Problems. Edited by G. MATHÉ and F. M. MUGGIA.

76 New Drugs in Cancer Chemotherapy. Edited by S. K. CARTER, Y. SAKURAI, H. UMEZAWA.

77 K. STANLEY, J. STJERNSWÄRD, M. ISLEY: The Conduct of a Cooperative Clinical Trial.

78 Prostate Cancer. Edited by W. DUNCAN.

79 Chemotherapy and Radiotherapy of Gastrointestinal Tumors. Edited by H. O. KLEIN.

80 Adjuvant Therapies of Cancer. Edited by G. MATHÉ, G. BONADONNA, S. SALMON.

81 H. P. LOHRMANN and W. SCHREML: Cytotoxic Drugs and the Granulopoietic System.

82 Early Detection and Localization of Lung Tumors in High Risk Groups. Edited by P. R. BAND.

83 Colorectal Cancer. Edited by W. DUNCAN.

84 Modified Nucleosides and Cancer. Edited by G. NASS.

85 Urologic Cancer: Chemotherapeutic Principles and Management. Edited by F. M. TORTI.

86 Vascular Perfusion in Cancer Therapy. Edited by K. SCHWEMMLE, K. AIGNER.

87 F. HOLMES: Aging and Cancer.

88 Paediatric Oncology. Edited by W. DUNCAN.

89 Pain in the Cancer Patient. Edited by M. ZIMMERMANN, P. DRINGS, G. WAGNER.

90 Early Detection of Breast Cancer. Edited by S. BRÜNNER, B. LANGFELDT, P. E. ANDERSEN.

MIX
Papier aus verantwortungsvollen Quellen
Paper from responsible sources
FSC® C105338

If you have any concerns about our products,
you can contact us on
ProductSafety@springernature.com

In case Publisher is established outside the EU,
the EU authorized representative is:
Springer Nature Customer Service Center GmbH
Europaplatz 3, 69115 Heidelberg, Germany

Printed by Libri Plureos GmbH
in Hamburg, Germany